Diagnosis, Prevention and Treatment for Stroke

Diagnosis, Prevention and Treatment for Stroke

Editor

Aristeidis H. Katsanos

MDPI • Basel • Beijing • Wuhan • Barcelona • Belgrade • Manchester • Tokyo • Cluj • Tianjin

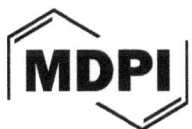

Editor
Aristeidis H. Katsanos
McMaster University and Population Health Research Institute
Canada

Editorial Office
MDPI
St. Alban-Anlage 66
4052 Basel, Switzerland

This is a reprint of articles from the Special Issue published online in the open access journal *Journal of Clinical Medicine* (ISSN 2077-0383) (available at: https://www.mdpi.com/journal/jcm/special_issues/research_stroke).

For citation purposes, cite each article independently as indicated on the article page online and as indicated below:

LastName, A.A.; LastName, B.B.; LastName, C.C. Article Title. *Journal Name* **Year**, *Article Number*, Page Range.

ISBN 978-3-03943-296-7 (Hbk)
ISBN 978-3-03943-297-4 (PDF)

© 2020 by the authors. Articles in this book are Open Access and distributed under the Creative Commons Attribution (CC BY) license, which allows users to download, copy and build upon published articles, as long as the author and publisher are properly credited, which ensures maximum dissemination and a wider impact of our publications.

The book as a whole is distributed by MDPI under the terms and conditions of the Creative Commons license CC BY-NC-ND.

Contents

About the Editor vii

Aristeidis H. Katsanos
Updates in Stroke Treatment, Diagnostic Methods and Predictors of Outcome
Reprinted from: *J. Clin. Med.* **2020**, *9*, 2789, doi:10.3390/jcm9092789 1

Jang-Hyun Baek, Byung Moon Kim, Jin Woo Kim, Dong Joon Kim, Ji Hoe Heo, Hyo Suk Nam and Young Dae Kim
Utility of Leptomeningeal Collaterals in Predicting Intracranial Atherosclerosis-Related Large Vessel Occlusion in Endovascular Treatment
Reprinted from: *J. Clin. Med.* **2020**, *9*, 2784, doi:10.3390/jcm9092784 9

Adam Wiśniewski, Joanna Boinska, Katarzyna Ziołkowska, Adam Lemanowicz, Karolina Filipska, Zbigniew Serafin, Robert Ślusarz, Danuta Rość and Grzegorz Kozera
Endothelial Progenitor Cells as a Marker of Vascular Damage But not a Predictor in Acute Microangiopathy-Associated Stroke
Reprinted from: *J. Clin. Med.* **2020**, *9*, 2248, doi:10.3390/jcm9072248 21

Chulho Kim, Sang-Hwa Lee, Jae-Sung Lim, Mi Sun Oh, Kyung-Ho Yu, Yerim Kim, Ju-Hun Lee, Min Uk Jang, San Jung and Byung-Chul Lee
Timing of Transfusion, not Hemoglobin Variability, Is Associated with 3-Month Outcomes in Acute Ischemic Stroke
Reprinted from: *J. Clin. Med.* **2020**, *9*, 1566, doi:10.3390/jcm9051566 37

Minho Han, Young Dae Kim, Jin Kyo Choi, Junghye Choi, Jimin Ha, Eunjeong Park, Jinkwon Kim, Tae-Jin Song, Ji Hoe Heo and Hyo Suk Nam
Predicting Stroke Outcomes Using Ankle-Brachial Index and Inter-Ankle Blood Pressure Difference
Reprinted from: *J. Clin. Med.* **2020**, *9*, 1125, doi:10.3390/jcm9041125 49

Yu-Sun Min, Jang Woo Park, Eunhee Park, Ae-Ryoung Kim, Hyunsil Cha, Dae-Won Gwak, Seung-Hwan Jung, Yongmin Chang and Tae-Du Jung
Interhemispheric Functional Connectivity in the Primary Motor Cortex Assessed by Resting-State Functional Magnetic Resonance Imaging Aids Long-Term Recovery Prediction among Subacute Stroke Patients with Severe Hand Weakness
Reprinted from: *J. Clin. Med.* **2020**, *9*, 975, doi:10.3390/jcm9040975 61

Adam Wiśniewski, Karolina Filipska, Joanna Sikora, Robert Ślusarz and Grzegorz Kozera
The Prognostic Value of High Platelet Reactivity in Ischemic Stroke Depends on the Etiology: A Pilot Study
Reprinted from: *J. Clin. Med.* **2020**, *9*, 859, doi:10.3390/jcm9030859 71

Giovanni Merlino, Carmelo Smeralda, Simone Lorenzut, Gian Luigi Gigli, Andrea Surcinelli and Mariarosaria Valente
To Treat or Not to Treat: Importance of Functional Dependence in Deciding Intravenous Thrombolysis of "Mild Stroke" Patients
Reprinted from: *J. Clin. Med.* **2020**, *9*, 768, doi:10.3390/jcm9030768 83

Young Dae Kim, Ji Hoe Heo, Joonsang Yoo, Hyungjong Park, Byung Moon Kim, Oh Young Bang, Hyeon Chang Kim, Euna Han, Dong Joon Kim, JoonNyung Heo, Minyoung Kim, Jin Kyo Choi, Kyung-Yul Lee, Hye Sun Lee, Dong Hoon Shin, Hye-Yeon Choi, Sung-Il Sohn, Jeong-Ho Hong, Jang-Hyun Baek, Gyu Sik Kim, Woo-Keun Seo, Jong-Won Chung, Seo Hyun Kim, Tae-Jin Song, Sang Won Han, Joong Hyun Park, Jinkwon Kim, Yo Han Jung, Han-Jin Cho, Seong Hwan Ahn, Sung Ik Lee, Kwon-Duk Seo and Hyo Suk Nam
Improving the Clinical Outcome in Stroke Patients Receiving Thrombolytic or Endovascular Treatment in Korea: from the SECRET Study
Reprinted from: *J. Clin. Med.* **2020**, *9*, 717, doi:10.3390/jcm9030717 . . . . **93**

Adam Wiśniewski, Joanna Sikora, Agata Sławińska, Karolina Filipska, Aleksandra Karczmarska-Wódzka, Zbigniew Serafin and Grzegorz Kozera
High On-Treatment Platelet Reactivity Affects the Extent of Ischemic Lesions in Stroke Patients Due to Large-Vessel Disease
Reprinted from: *J. Clin. Med.* **2020**, *9*, 251, doi:10.3390/jcm9010251 . . . . **109**

Marios-Nikos Psychogios, Ilko L. Maier, Ioannis Tsogkas, Amélie Carolina Hesse, Alex Brehm, Daniel Behme, Marlena Schnieder, Katharina Schregel, Ismini Papageorgiou, David S. Liebeskind, Mayank Goyal, Mathias Bähr, Michael Knauth and Jan Liman
One-Stop Management of 230 Consecutive Acute Stroke Patients: Report of Procedural Times and Clinical Outcome
Reprinted from: *J. Clin. Med.* **2019**, *8*, 2185, doi:10.3390/jcm8122185 . . . . **123**

Chrissoula Liantinioti, Lina Palaiodimou, Konstantinos Tympas, John Parissis, Aikaterini Theodorou, Ignatios Ikonomidis, Maria Chondrogianni, Christina Zompola, Sokratis Triantafyllou, Andromachi Roussopoulou, Odysseas Kargiotis, Aspasia Serdari, Anastasios Bonakis, Konstantinos Vadikolias, Konstantinos Voumvourakis, Leonidas Stefanis, Gerasimos Filippatos and Georgios Tsivgoulis
Potential Utility of Neurosonology in Paroxysmal Atrial Fibrillation Detection in Patients with Cryptogenic Stroke
Reprinted from: *J. Clin. Med.* **2019**, *8*, 2002, doi:10.3390/jcm8112002 . . . . **137**

Hyungjong Park, Minho Han, Young Dae Kim, Joonsang Yoo, Hye Sun Lee, Jin Kyo Choi, Ji Hoe Heo and Hyo Suk Nam
Impact of the Total Number of Carotid Plaques on the Outcome of Ischemic Stroke Patients with Atrial Fibrillation
Reprinted from: *J. Clin. Med.* **2019**, *8*, 1897, doi:10.3390/jcm8111897 . . . . **149**

Jens Eyding, Christian Fung, Wolf-Dirk Niesen and Christos Krogias
Twenty Years of Cerebral Ultrasound Perfusion Imaging—Is the Best yet to Come?
Reprinted from: *J. Clin. Med.* **2020**, *9*, 816, doi:10.3390/jcm9030816 . . . . **161**

About the Editor

Aristeidis H. Katsanos, MD, Ph.D., obtained his Medical Degree from the University of Ioannina, School of Medicine, Ioannina, Greece, in July 2011, and completed his training in Neurology (2014–2018) at the University of Ioannina School of Medicine, Ioannina, Greece, and at the National and Kapodistrian University of Athens, Athens, Greece. During the years 2011–2015 he also completed his Ph.D. thesis at the Department of Neurology, University of Ioannina, School of Medicine, Ioannina, Greece, investigating the contribution of transesophageal echocardiography in the diagnostic work-up of patients with stroke. After the completion of his Ph.D. thesis and training in Neurology, he was granted with a 6 month Research Fellowship by the European Academy of Neurology at the Ruhr University of Bochum, Bochum, Germany, for his research proposal to investigate the utility of transorbital sonography in patients with optic neuritis. Since July 1st 2019, he joined as a Clinical Fellow for Stroke Medicine at the Division of Neurology, McMaster University and Population Health Research Institute, Hamilton, Canada. Aristeidis has actively participated in numerous research projects and international collaborations on acute stroke treatment and secondary stroke prevention, and has published more than 160 papers in high-impact medical journals to date (2394 citations, H-index 29). He has served as an external consultant for research grants and as a peer-reviewer for over 50 medical journals. For the quality of his peer-reviewing in stroke literature, he received the Outstanding Reviewer Award in 2019 from Stroke Journal and an Award from Web of Science—Clarivate Analytics for being placed in the top 1% of reviewers for the year 2018–2019 in Neuroscience and Behavior on the Publons.

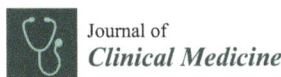

Editorial

Updates in Stroke Treatment, Diagnostic Methods and Predictors of Outcome

Aristeidis H. Katsanos

Division of Neurology, McMaster University/Population Health Research Institute, 237 Barton St E, Hamilton, ON L8L 2X2, Canada; ar.katsanos@gmail.com; Tel.: +1-365-888-1441

Received: 24 August 2020; Accepted: 26 August 2020; Published: 29 August 2020

1. Introduction

In recent years, there have been outstanding achievements in stroke diagnosis and care [1,2]. Our better understanding of the pathophysiological mechanisms and the advances in neuro-imaging have enabled us to diagnose stroke syndromes with remarkable precision and uncover underlying vessel pathologies that can be directly correlated with the stroke event [2]. Within a short period of time, endovascular thrombectomy (EVT) became the standard of care for patients with large vessel occlusions and symptom onset up to 24 h [3–5], while other recent trials introduced the use of perfusion imaging to guide intravenous thrombolysis in the extended time window [6].

This Special Issue of the Journal of Clinical Medicine features articles presenting considerations and improvements in acute stroke treatment, emerging neurosonology applications and novel predictors of stroke outcome.

1.1. Considerations and Improvements in Acute Stroke Reperfusion Therapies

Intravenous thrombolysis (IVT) in patients with a low National Institutes of Health Stroke Scale (NIHSS) score of 0–5 remains controversial. The Potential of rtPA for Ischemic Strokes with Mild Symptoms (PRISMS) trial was a phase 3, randomized, double-blind clinical trial that aimed to test the safety and efficacy of intravenous thrombolysis, with tissue plasminogen activator (tPA) administered within 3 h of symptom onset in acute ischemic stroke (AIS) patients with mild, non-disabling neurological deficits (baseline National Institutes of Health Stroke Scale (NIHSS) score equal to or less than 5) [7]. The study was prematurely terminated by the sponsor after the recruitment of 313 patients (one-third of the initially planned sample size) due to the low recruitment rates [7]. PRISMS investigators found comparable 3-month favorable functional outcomes between patients receiving IVT and aspirin, while highlighting an increased risk for symptomatic intracranial hemorrhage for patients randomized to intravenous tPA treatment [7].

Merlino et al. tested the hypothesis that the utility of intravenous tPA in patients with mild stroke symptoms may depend on their level of functional dependence at hospital admission [8]. Authors analyzed data form a prospectively collected database including 389 patients presenting with acute ischemic strokes and mild deficits [8]. Patients were stratified according to their baseline Barthel index (BI) score into those with functional dependence (BI score < 80) and those functionally independent (BI score ≥ 80) at baseline [8]. Merlino et al. found that intravenous thrombolysis with tPA was independently associated with more favorable functional outcomes at 3 months after stroke onset in patients that were judged to be dependent at hospital presentation [8]. The association between favorable 3-month outcomes and tPA administration was not evident for patients that were independent at their presentation, suggesting that the beneficial effect of tPA in patients with mild neurological syndromes on admission is influenced by their functional status at admission [8]. Despite the limitations of the present report, including the presence of unmeasured confounders due to the lack of randomization and bias by indication in the decision to deliver tPA, the authors address an important question that stroke physicians deal with in the everyday clinical practice. Until further studies provide compelling evidence for subgroups of patients with mild strokes for whom tPA treatment is futile or even harmful, eligible patients with disabling symptoms should not be excluded from prompt tPA administration.

Randomized controlled clinical trials have provided robust evidence on the benefit of both intravenous tissue tPA and EVT for improving the outcomes of acute ischemic stroke patients [9]. However, real world evidence is needed in order to unveil the real effectiveness of acute reperfusion stroke treatments in different countries and healthcare systems. Selection Criteria in Endovascular Thrombectomy and Thrombolytic Therapy (SECRET) is a prospective nationwide population multicenter registry that aims to explore the selection criteria and outcomes of patients who receive acute stroke reperfusion therapies in Korea [10]. SECRET investigators found significant increases in both the proportions of patients achieving successful recanalization (78.6% to 85.1%) and those discharged home (78.6% to 85.1%) from 2012 to 2017 [10]. A significant decrease in the time from hospital presentation to initiation of reperfusion therapy was also observed over the years 2012 to 2017 [10]. These data from Korea provide reassurance on the beneficial effect of reperfusion therapies in the real-world setting and the temporal improvements in treatment delivery. Population-based data are essential for the quality monitoring and optimal care delivery of acute reperfusion stroke therapies.

Rapid EVT delivery for acute ischemic stroke caused by large vessel occlusion leads to improved outcomes [11]. Optimizing intra-hospital management seems to be one of the most efficient ways to diminish treatment delays and decrease further the time from stroke onset to successful reperfusion. Direct transfer to the angiography suite, bypassing both the emergency department and the radiology room of the multidetector computed tomograph (CT), also known as one-stop management, has previously been suggested as an efficient method to reduce in-hospital delays [12]. In the angiography suite, patients with stroke symptoms receive a brain scan with the use of a flat-detector CT capable angiography-suite and, if eligible, they receive on the spot treatment with intravenous tPA and/or EVT [12]. Psychogios et al. examined if one-stop management can not only reduce intra-hospital treatment delays, but can also improve the functional outcomes of acute ischemic stroke patients with large vessel occlusion [13]. Large vessel occlusion was diagnosed in 72% and intravenous tPA was administered in 63% of the 230 total patients [13]. Compared to 43 case-matched patients triaged with multidetector CT, one-stop management was found to reduce the median door-to-reperfusion time by more than 40 min, and resulted in improved patient functional outcomes [13]. No safety concerns were noticed, as the incidence of intracranial bleeding and all-cause mortality was comparable between the two groups [13]. The authors correctly acknowledge in the limitations of their work that their findings might not be applicable to low volume stroke centers, as the number of patients with large vessel occlusions is expected to be much lower than the one described in the publication by Psychogios et al. [13]. The authors also state in their conclusion section that they have designed a prospective, randomized trial to evaluate the effectiveness and safety of their proposed one-stop protocol [13]. The results of this trial are expected to provide robust evidence on the optimal route selection for acute ischemic stroke patients with suspected large vessel occlusion and, if positive, change the flow of in-hospital stroke care delivery.

The underlying pathomechanism of a large vessel occlusion has been suggested to be associated with effectiveness of the EVT procedure and the outcomes of patients [14]. In a retrospective cohort study, Baek et al. investigated whether the status of leptomeningeal collaterals in the brain CT angiography can be a marker of the large vessel occlusion etiology [15]. Comparing leptomeningeal collateral patterns between patients with intracranial atherosclerotic disease and without, complete leptomeningeal collaterals were found to be more than two times more prevalent in patients with intracranial atherosclerotic disease [15]. Despite their fair negative predictive value, the presence of complete leptomeningeal collateral supply in baseline brain CT angiography was found to have an overall modest predictive value for the discrimination of the etiology of a large vessel occlusion [15]. The use of leptomeningeal collateral supply as a pre-procedural predictor for the stroke mechanism and outcomes of patients with large vessel occlusion treated with EVT deserves to be evaluated in multicenter prospective observational cohorts.

1.2. Emerging Applications of Neurosonology in Stroke

Although paroxysmal atrial fibrillation (AF) has been suggested to be present in at least a third of patients with cryptogenic stroke or transient ischemic attack (TIA) [16], current guidelines on secondary stroke prevention suggest that the clinical benefit of prolonged cardiac monitoring to uncover underlying paroxysmal AF after an acute ischemic stroke or TIA remains uncertain [17]. Identifying populations that might have a higher probability of underlying AF could lead to a more targeted use of prolonged cardiac monitoring for this patient population.

Liantinioti et al. sought to identify whether cardiac arrhythmia detection in spectral waveform analysis during neurosonology examinations with Carotid Duplex and Transcranial Doppler ultrasound may be associated with a higher likelihood of paroxysmal AF detection [18]. They evaluated 373 consecutive patients with recent cryptogenic strokes over a six-year period. The rate of AF detection on outpatient 24-h Holter ECG recording was 11% [18]. Arrhythmia detection during neurosonology evaluations was independently associated with a three-fold higher likelihood of PAF detection during follow-up [18]. The study by Liantinioti et al. highlights the importance of detecting and reporting cardiac arrhythmias during the neurosonology examination of patients with ischemic stroke, and further expands the utility of neurosonology in determining stroke etiology, by identifying those patients that have a higher probability of underlying paroxysmal AF and deserve more thorough cardiac rhythm monitoring. Given that antiplatelet treatment is known to confer inadequate protection, prompt anticoagulation in these patients can reduce the risk of future thromboembolic events [19].

Park et al. investigated the association between total carotid plaque number and long-term prognosis in ischemic stroke patients with AF [20]. Total plaque number was assessed with B-mode ultrasonography in 392 ischemic stroke patients with AF [20]. After a mean follow-up of 2.42 years, 28.8% of the patients suffered a major adverse cardiovascular event [20]. The presence of five plaques or more in the baseline carotid ultrasound was independently associated with an increased risk of both major adverse cardiovascular events and all-cause mortality [20]. Interestingly, the total plaque number along with the maximal plaque thickness and intima media thickness showed improved prognostic utility when added to the variables of the $CHAD_2DS_2$-VASc score [20]. Although Park et al. adjust their outcomes for baseline medications, it should be noted that there is a possibility for suboptimal medical management in their population, as 44% and 20% of patients were on antiplatelet and statin treatment, respectively, and despite the confirmed diagnosis of AF and history of stroke, only 22% patients were taking oral anticoagulant [20]. The findings by Park et al. suggest that patients with AF and high atherosclerotic burden are at increased risk for cardiovascular events. Carotid ultrasound could therefore serve as a valuable, non-invasive screening tool for identifying these high risk individuals.

CT perfusion imaging is used to guide systematic and endovascular stroke treatments for patients presenting in the extended time windows [4–6]. Ultrasound cerebral perfusion imaging techniques have been introduced and validated with different data acquisition and processing approaches [21]. In a very nice and comprehensive way, Eyding et al. summarize the evolution, different technical aspects and milestones in the use of cerebral ultrasound perfusion imaging over time [21]. The authors highlight future potential applications of cerebral ultrasound perfusion imaging as a bedside method of microcirculatory perfusion assessment [21]. Eyding et al. propose that in cases of the presence of sufficient temporal windows, a multi-modal approach for the detection of vessel occlusion, microvascular perfusion impairment or intracerebral hemorrhage is feasible with ultrasonographic techniques [21]. The evaluation of this method in the pre-hospital setting and the development of automated software algorithms are two directions that future research should focus on.

1.3. Novel Predictors of Stroke Outcome

Most physicians use their own clinical experience in predicting their patients' outcomes after a stroke, as accurate prognostic models and tests of functional recovery in stroke patients are lacking to date [22].

Min et al. performed a prospective cohort study to evaluate the usefulness of interhemispheric functional connectivity as a predictor of motor recovery in stroke patients with unilateral severe upper-limb paresis [23]. Functional connectivity was measured in resting-state functional magnetic resonance imaging (MRI) scans at 1 month from stroke onset [23]. Good recovery, assessed with the Brunnstrom stage of upper-limb function at 6 months, was associated with higher functional connectivity values [23]. The authors conclude that interhemispheric functional connectivity measurement using resting-state functional MRI scans may provide useful clinical information for predicting hand motor recovery during stroke rehabilitation [23]. The predictive value of functional connectivity assessment for long-term motor outcomes in subacute stroke patients has to be confirmed by independent large-scale studies. Future studies need also to evaluate the applicability of resting-state functional MRI for the prediction of the recovery of stroke patients with non-motor deficits (e.g., visual defects) and strokes of afferent vascular distributions.

Ankle-brachial blood pressure index (ABI) is calculated by the ratio of the systolic blood pressure of an ipsilateral ankle divided by the higher systolic blood pressure of the two arms [24]. Low ABI has previously been reported to identify patients with symptomatic and asymptomatic peripheral arterial disease, and has been associated with a higher risk of early recurrent stroke in patients with an acute ischemic stroke and no history of symptomatic peripheral arterial disease [24]. Han et al. investigated the association of high ABI difference between the two arms and systolic blood pressure difference between the two ankles with short- and long-term outcomes in acute ischemic stroke patients without peripheral artery diseases [25]. After analyzing data from 2901 patients with acute ischemic stroke, followed over a median of 3.1 years, the authors found that a high ABI difference either between arms or ankles is associated with poor functional outcomes, long-term cardiovascular events and all-cause mortality [25].

The impact of hemoglobin status and red blood cell transfusions (RBC) on acute ischemic stroke outcomes is controversial. Kim et al. aimed to investigate whether RBC transfusions and hemoglobin variability affects the outcome of patients after an acute ischemic stroke [26]. The authors analyzed data from 2698 patients with acute ischemic stroke admitted in three tertiary hospitals. In total, 32 patients (4.9%) were transfused with packed RBCs during their admission [26]. Patients transfused more than 48 h after hospitalization were found to have a higher probability of poor outcomes at 3 months [26]. Hemoglobin variability during hospitalization, however, was not found to be associated with patient outcomes [26]. Despite the inherent limitations of the study design of Kim et al., it being a retrospective cohort study with limited power and high risk of bias due to the presence of unmeasured confounders, it raises the need for further research in order to elucidate the potential impact of blood transfusions timing on the outcomes of patients with recent acute ischemic stroke.

Although platelet activation and aggregation has been suggested to play an important role in the pathogenesis of ischemic stroke, the association between platelet reactivity and ischemic lesions is still debatable. Ischemic stroke patients with high on-treatment platelet reactivity have previously been reported to be at increased risk of recurrent cerebrovascular ischemic events [27]. Wisniewski et al. aimed to assess the relationship between platelet reactivity and the extent of ischemic cerebral lesions according to stroke etiology [28]. The evaluation of platelet reactivity was performed within 24 h after stroke onset in 69 patients [28]. An ischemic brain volume measurement was performed in MRI sequences at day 2–5 after stroke onset [28]. In the subgroup of patients with large-vessel disease, a correlation between platelet reactivity and acute ischemic core volume was evident in aspirin-resistant subjects [28]. Based on their findings, authors propose that in patients with ischemic stroke due to large-vessel disease, high on-treatment platelet reactivity affects the extent of ischemic lesions [28].

Apririn resistance among patients with stroke in the study by Wisniewski et al. was estimated at 31.8% and at 7%, with the methods of impedance and optical aggregometry [28].

In a subsequent publication in the same issue of the Journal of Clinical Medicine, Wisniewski et al. assessed the relationship of platelet reactivity with early and late prognosis after an acute ischemic stroke, according to the stroke etiology [29]. Performing platelet function testing with two aggregometric methods in 69 individuals, they found higher platelet reactivity in patients with severe neurological deficits on day 90 after stroke onset, when compared to the group of patients experiencing mild neurological deficits [29]. In patients with acute ischemic stroke attributed to large vessel disease, a significant correlation between the platelet reactivity and functional status on the first day was also uncovered, with patients resistant to aspirin having a significantly greater possibility of severe neurological deficits on the first day of stroke compared to their aspirin-sensitive counterparts [29].

Endothelial progenitor cells are considered to be a marker of both endothelial damage and endothelium regeneration ability [30]. In a third publication, Wisniewski et al. assessed the number of endothelial progenitor cells in patients with acute ischemic or hemorrhagic stroke, and evaluated whether there exist relationships with clinical status, radiological findings, risk factors, selected biochemical parameters and prognosis [30]. The number of endothelial progenitor cells was determined in serum on the first and eighth day after stroke onset using flow cytometry in 66 patients with lacunar ischemic stroke, 38 patients with hemorrhagic stroke, and 22 control subjects without acute cerebrovascular incidents [30]. Although a significantly higher number of endothelial progenitor cells on the first day of stroke compared to the control group was identified, no relationships between the number of endothelial progenitor cells in the acute phase of stroke and biochemical parameters, vascular risk factors or clinical condition were uncovered [30]. The authors concluded that endothelial progenitor cells are an early marker in acute stroke regardless of etiology, with no prognostic value being identified [30].

2. Conclusions

Although real-world evidence confirms the beneficial effect of reperfusion therapies in the real-world setting, as well as the temporal improvements in stroke treatment delivery over the last few years, several research areas are still pending further investigation. The utility of intravenous tPA in patients with non-disabling stroke syndromes, the use of ultrasound cerebral perfusion imaging in the pre-hospital setting and the optimal in-hospital route for acute ischemic stroke patients with suspected large vessel occlusion are topics in acute stroke care that need to be further investigated. Ongoing research also needs to focus on the development of reliable radiologic, clinical and biomarkers predictors of stroke outcome.

Funding: This research received no external funding.

Conflicts of Interest: The author declares no conflict of interest.

Disclosures: A.H.K. serves as the invited editor for the Special Issue "Diagnosis, Prevention and Treatment for Stroke" in the Journal of Clinical Medicine.

References

1. Baek, J.-H.; Kim, B.M.; Kim, J.W.; Kim, D.J.; Heo, J.H.; Nam, H.S.; Kim, Y.D. Utility of Leptomeningeal Collaterals in Predicting Intracranial Atherosclerosis-Related Large Vessel Occlusion in Endovascular Treatment. *J. Clin. Med.* **2020**, *9*, 2784. [CrossRef]
2. Katsanos, A.H.; Hart, R.G. New horizons in pharmacologic therapy for secondary stroke prevention. *JAMA Neurol.* **2020**. [CrossRef]
3. Rabinstein, A.A. Update on treatment of acute ischemic stroke. *Continuum Minneap Minn* **2020**, *26*, 268–286. [CrossRef]

4. Tsivgoulis, G.; Safouris, A.; Katsanos, A.H.; Arthur, A.S.; Alexandrov, A.V. Mechanical thrombectomy for emergent large vessel occlusion: A critical appraisal of recent randomized controlled clinical trials. *Brain Behav.* **2016**, *6*, e00418. [CrossRef] [PubMed]
5. Nogueira, R.G.; Jadhav, A.P.; Haussen, D.C.; Bonafe, A.; Budzik, R.F.; Bhuva, P.; Yavagal, D.R.; Ribo, M.; Cognard, C.; Hanel, R.A.; et al. Thrombectomy 6 to 24 hours after stroke with a mismatch between deficit and infarct. *N. Engl. J. Med.* **2018**, *378*, 11–21. [CrossRef]
6. Albers, G.W.; Marks, M.P.; Kemp, S.; Christensen, S.; Tsai, J.P.; Ortega-Gutierrez, S.; McTaggart, R.A.; Torbey, M.T.; Kim-Tenser, M.; Leslie-Mazwi, T.; et al. Thrombectomy for stroke at 6 to 16 hours with selection by perfusion imaging. *N. Engl. J. Med.* **2018**, *378*, 708–718. [CrossRef] [PubMed]
7. Tsivgoulis, G.; Katsanos, A.H.; Malhotra, K.; Sarraj, A.; Barreto, A.D.; Köhrmann, M.; Krogias, C.; Ahmed, N.; Caso, V.; Schellinger, P.D.; et al. Thrombolysis for acute ischemic stroke in the unwitnessed or extended therapeutic time window. *Neurology* **2020**, *94*, e1241–e1248. [CrossRef]
8. Khatri, P.; Kleindorfer, D.O.; Devlin, T.; Sawyer, R.N., Jr.; Starr, M.; Mejilla, J.; Broderick, J.; Chatterjee, A.; Jauch, E.C.; Levine, S.R.; et al. Effect of alteplase vs aspirin on functional outcome for patients with acute ischemic stroke and minor nondisabling neurologic deficits: The PRISMS randomized clinical trial. *JAMA* **2018**, *320*, 156–166. [CrossRef] [PubMed]
9. Merlino, G.; Smeralda, C.; Lorenzut, S.; Gigli, G.L.; Surcinelli, A.; Valente, M. To treat or not to treat: Importance of functional dependence in deciding intravenous thrombolysis of "mild stroke" patients. *J. Clin. Med.* **2020**, *9*, 768. [CrossRef]
10. Tsivgoulis, G.; Katsanos, A.H.; Alexandrov, A.V. Reperfusion therapies of acute ischemic stroke: Potentials and failures. *Front. Neurol.* **2014**, *5*, 215. [CrossRef]
11. Kim, Y.D.; Heo, J.H.; Yoo, J.; Park, H.; Kim, B.M.; Bang, O.Y.; Kim, H.C.; Han, E.; Kim, D.J.; Heo, J.; et al. Improving the clinical outcome in stroke patients receiving thrombolytic or endovascular treatment in korea: From the SECRET study. *J. Clin. Med.* **2020**, *9*, 717. [CrossRef] [PubMed]
12. Bourcier, R.; Goyal, M.; Liebeskind, D.S.; Muir, K.W.; Desal, H.; Siddiqui, A.H.; Dippel, D.W.J.; Majoie, C.B.; van Zwam, W.H.; Jovin, T.G.; et al. Association of time from stroke onset to groin puncture with quality of reperfusion after mechanical thrombectomy: A meta-analysis of individual patient data from 7 randomized clinical trials. *JAMA Neurol.* **2019**, *76*, 405–411. [CrossRef] [PubMed]
13. Psychogios, M.N.; Behme, D.; Schregel, K.; Tsogkas, I.; Maier, I.L.; Leyhe, J.R.; Zapf, A.; Tran, J.; Bähr, M.; Liman, J.; et al. One-stop management of acute stroke patients: Minimizing door-to-reperfusion times. *Stroke* **2017**, *48*, 3152–3155. [CrossRef] [PubMed]
14. Wiśniewski, A.; Boinska, J.; Ziołkowska, K.; Lemanowicz, A.; Filipska, K.; Serafin, Z.; Ślusarz, R.; Rość, D.; Kozera, G. Endothelial progenitor cells as a marker of vascular damage but not a predictor in acute microangiopathy-associated stroke. *J. Clin. Med.* **2020**, *9*, 2248. [CrossRef]
15. Matias-Guiu, J.A.; Serna-Candel, C.; Matias-Guiu, J. Stroke etiology determines effectiveness of retrievable stents. *J. Neurointerv. Surg.* **2014**, *6*, e11. [CrossRef]
16. Psychogios, M.N.; Maier, I.L.; Tsogkas, I.; Hesse, A.C.; Brehm, A.; Behme, D.; Schnieder, M.; Schregel, K.; Papageorgiou, I.; Liebeskind, D.S.; et al. One-stop management of 230 consecutive acute stroke patients: report of procedural times and clinical outcome. *J. Clin. Med.* **2019**, *8*, 2185. [CrossRef]
17. Sposato, L.A.; Cipriano, L.E.; Saposnik, G.; Ruvz Vargas, E.; Riccio, P.M.; Hachinski, V. Diagnosis of atrial fibrillation after stroke and transient ischaemic attack: A systematic review and meta-analysis. *Lancet Neurol.* **2015**, *14*, 377–387. [CrossRef]
18. Kernan, W.N.; Ovbiagele, B.; Black, H.R.; Bravata, D.M.; Chimowitz, M.I.; Ezekowitz, M.D.; Fang, M.C.; Fisher, M.; Furie, K.L.; Heck, D.V.; et al. Guidelines for the prevention of stroke in patients with stroke and transient ischemic attack: A guideline for healthcare professionals from the american heart association/american stroke association. *Stroke* **2014**, *45*, 2160–2236. [CrossRef]
19. Liantinioti, C.; Palaiodimou, L.; Tympas, K.; Parissis, J.; Theodorou, A.; Ikonomidis, I.; Chondrogianni, M.; Zompola, C.; Triantafyllou, S.; Roussopoulou, A.; et al. Potential utility of neurosonology in paroxysmal atrial fibrillation detection in patients with cryptogenic stroke. *J. Clin. Med.* **2019**, *8*, 2002. [CrossRef]
20. Triantafyllou, S.; Katsanos, A.H.; Dilaveris, P.; Giannopoulos, G.; Kossyvakis, C.; Adreanides, E.; Liantinioti, C.; Tympas, K.; Zompola, C.; Theodorou, A.; et al. Implantable cardiac monitoring in the secondary prevention of cryptogenic stroke. *Ann. Neurol.* **2020**. [CrossRef]

21. Park, H.; Han, M.; Kim, Y.D.; Yoo, J.; Lee, H.S.; Choi, J.K.; Heo, J.H.; Nam, H.S. Impact of the total number of carotid plaques on the outcome of ischemic stroke patients with atrial fibrillation. *J. Clin. Med.* **2019**, *8*, 1897. [CrossRef] [PubMed]
22. Eyding, J.; Fung, C.; Niesen, W.D.; Krogias, C. Twenty years of cerebral ultrasound perfusion imaging—Is the best yet to come? *J. Clin. Med.* **2020**, *9*, 816. [CrossRef] [PubMed]
23. Jampathong, N.; Laopaiboon, M.; Rattanakanokchai, S.; Pattanittum, P. Prognostic models for complete recovery in ischemic stroke: A systematic review and meta-analysis. *BMC Neurol.* **2018**, *18*, 26. [CrossRef] [PubMed]
24. Min, Y.S.; Park, J.W.; Park, E.; Kim, A.-R.; Cha, H.; Gwak, D.-W.; Jung, S.-H.; Chang, Y.; Jung, T.-D. Interhemispheric functional connectivity in the primary motor cortex assessed by resting-state functional magnetic resonance imaging aids long-term recovery prediction among subacute stroke patients with severe hand weakness. *J. Clin. Med.* **2020**, *9*, 975. [CrossRef]
25. Tsivgoulis, G.; Bogiatzi, C.; Heliopoulos, I.; Vadikolias, K.; Boutati, E.; Tsakaldimi, S.; Al-Attas, O.S.; Charalampidis, P.; Piperidou, C.; Maltezos, E.; et al. Low ankle-brachial index predicts early risk of recurrent stroke in patients with acute cerebral ischemia. *Atherosclerosis* **2012**, *220*, 407–412. [CrossRef]
26. Han, M.; Kim, Y.D.; Choi, J.K.; Choi, J.; Ha, J.; Park, E.; Kim, J.; Song, T.-J.; Heo, J.H.; Nam, H.S. Predicting stroke outcomes using ankle-brachial index and inter-ankle blood pressure difference. *J. Clin. Med.* **2020**, *9*, 1125. [CrossRef]
27. Kim, C.; Lee, S.H.; Lim, J.S.; Oh, M.S.; Yu, K.-H.; Kim, Y.; Lee, J.-H.; Jang, M.U.; Jung, S.; Lee, B.-C. Timing of transfusion, not hemoglobin variability, is associated with 3-month outcomes in acute ischemic stroke. *J. Clin. Med.* **2020**, *9*, 1566. [CrossRef]
28. Fiolaki, A.; Katsanos, A.H.; Kyritsis, A.P.; Papadaki, S.; Kosmidou, M.; Moschonas, I.C.; Tselepis, A.D.; Giannopoulos, S. High on treatment platelet reactivity to aspirin and clopidogrel in ischemic stroke: A systematic review and meta-analysis. *J. Neurol. Sci.* **2017**, *376*, 112–116. [CrossRef]
29. Wiśniewski, A.; Sikora, J.; Sławińska, A.; Filipska, K.; Karczmarska-Wódzka, A.; Serafin, Z.; Kozera, G. High on-treatment platelet reactivity affects the extent of ischemic lesions in stroke patients due to large-vessel disease. *J. Clin. Med.* **2020**, *9*, 251. [CrossRef]
30. Wiśniewski, A.; Filipska, K.; Sikora, J.; Ślusarz, R.; Kozera, G. The Prognostic Value of High Platelet Reactivity in Ischemic Stroke Depends on the Etiology: A Pilot Study. *J. Clin. Med.* **2020**, *9*, 859. [CrossRef]

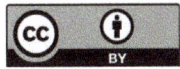

© 2020 by the author. Licensee MDPI, Basel, Switzerland. This article is an open access article distributed under the terms and conditions of the Creative Commons Attribution (CC BY) license (http://creativecommons.org/licenses/by/4.0/).

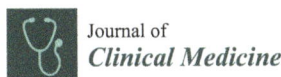

Article

Utility of Leptomeningeal Collaterals in Predicting Intracranial Atherosclerosis-Related Large Vessel Occlusion in Endovascular Treatment

Jang-Hyun Baek [1,2], Byung Moon Kim [3,*], Jin Woo Kim [4], Dong Joon Kim [3], Ji Hoe Heo [2], Hyo Suk Nam [2] and Young Dae Kim [2]

1. Department of Neurology, Kangbuk Samsung Hospital, Sungkyunkwan University School of Medicine, Seoul 03181, Korea; janghyun.baek@gmail.com
2. Department of Neurology, Severance Stroke Center, Severance Hospital, Yonsei University College of Medicine, Seoul 03722, Korea; jhheo@yuhs.ac (J.H.H.); hsnam@yuhs.ac (H.S.N.); neuro05@yuhs.ac (Y.D.K.)
3. Interventional Neuroradiology, Severance Stroke Center, Severance Hospital, Department of Radiology, Yonsei University College of Medicine, Seoul 03722, Korea; djkimmd@yuhs.ac
4. Department of Radiology, Gangnam Severance Hospital, Yonsei University College of Medicine, Seoul 06273, Korea; sunny-cocktail@hanmail.net
* Correspondence: bmoon21@hanmail.net; Tel.: +82-2-2228-7400

Received: 26 July 2020; Accepted: 27 August 2020; Published: 28 August 2020

Abstract: Earlier or preprocedural identification of occlusion pathomechanism is crucial for effective endovascular treatment. As leptomeningeal collaterals tend to develop well in chronic ischemic conditions such as intracranial atherosclerosis (ICAS), we investigated whether leptomeningeal collaterals can be a preprocedural marker of ICAS-related large vessel occlusion (ICAS-LVO) in endovascular treatment. A total of 226 patients who underwent endovascular treatment were retrospectively reviewed. We compared the pattern of leptomeningeal collaterals between patients with ICAS-LVO and without. Leptomeningeal collaterals were assessed by preprocedural computed tomography angiography (CTA) and basically categorized by three different collateral assessment methods. Better leptomeningeal collaterals were significantly associated with ICAS-LVO, although they were not independent for ICAS-LVO. When leptomeningeal collaterals were dichotomized to incomplete (<100%) and complete (100%), the latter was significantly more frequent in patients with ICAS-LVO (52.5% versus 20.4%) and remained an independent factor for ICAS-LVO (odds ratio, 3.32; 95% confidence interval, 1.52–7.26; $p = 0.003$). The area under the curve (AUC) value of complete leptomeningeal collateral supply was 0.660 for discrimination of ICAS-LVO. Incomplete leptomeningeal collateral supply was not likely ICAS-LVO, based on the high negative predictive value (88.6%). Considering its negative predictive value and the independent association between complete leptomeningeal collateral supply and ICAS-LVO, leptomeningeal collaterals could be helpful in the preprocedural determination of occlusion pathomechanism.

Keywords: atherosclerosis; computed tomography angiography; stroke; thrombectomy

1. Introduction

Mechanical thrombectomy has been primarily considered in most cases of endovascular treatment of acute intracranial large vessel occlusion [1]. However, mechanical thrombectomy might not be an optimal modality for a specific occlusion pathomechanism—that is, an in situ thrombo-occlusion of underlying intracranial atherosclerosis (intracranial atherosclerosis-related large vessel occlusion (ICAS-LVO)) [2,3]. ICAS-LVO is not a rare condition. In the Asian population, up to 30% of patients might have ICAS-LVO for their occlusion pathomechanism in endovascular treatment of anterior circulation [4]. More importantly, conventional mechanical thrombectomy modalities, such as stent retriever and thrombaspiration, are ineffective in ICAS-LVO. Mechanical thrombectomy was effective only in less than 20% of ICAS-LVO cases. Due to frequent reocclusion events, specific rescue endovascular modalities (i.e., intra-arterial glycoprotein IIb/IIIa inhibitor, balloon angioplasty, and intracranial stenting) were inevitable in most cases to achieve significant recanalization in ICAS-LVO [5–9].

On this point, earlier strategical consideration is crucial to shorten the time to recanalization [4]. For earlier strategical consideration, it could be more helpful if the occlusion pathomechanism is determined before endovascular treatment. However, the completion of such a preprocedural determination is challenging as the information available before endovascular treatment can be limited. In clinical practice, we are able to rely on only a few preprocedural clinical and imaging findings [7,10]. However, further reliable methods are sparse.

Leptomeningeal collaterals are one of the preprocedural factors which are potentially able to predict occlusion pathomechanism. Nevertheless, their association has not been clearly evaluated yet. Several experimental and clinical findings led us to focus on leptomeningeal collaterals. In these experimental findings, the vascular bed was more developed in chronic or long-term ischemic conditions [11–13]. Similarly, in patients with an intracranial stenosis due to ICAS, leptomeningeal collaterals were prominently developed to compensate for the diminished cerebral blood flow under chronic ischemia [11,12]. In one report, full and rapid leptomeningeal collateral filling was commented on as a finding, which suggests ICAS-LVO [7]. However, no specific evidence supported this comment. Instead, it was reported that initial infarct volume was smaller among patients with an ICAS-LVO. This merely indirectly suggested that leptomeningeal collaterals were better in ICAS-LVO [7,14].

If leptomeningeal collaterals are discriminatorily developed in patients with ICAS, we believe that they may be an indirect finding for ICAS-LVO. Thus, we hypothesized that (1) leptomeningeal collaterals would be different according to the occlusion pathomechanism—that is, robust or better leptomeningeal collaterals are associated with ICAS-LVO, and (2) based on this association, we could predict ICAS-LVO before endovascular treatment. Accordingly, this study aimed to evaluate (1) the association between leptomeningeal collaterals and ICAS-LVO, and (2) the predictability of preprocedural leptomeningeal collaterals for ICAS-LVO.

2. Methods

We retrospectively reviewed consecutive acute stroke patients between January 2010 and December 2018 who underwent endovascular treatment of intracranial vessel occlusion. Patients were selected from a prospective registry of a tertiary stroke center (Severance Stroke Center, Severance Hospital, Seoul, Korea). The registry consists of consecutive patients who underwent endovascular treatment, which was considered by the following criteria: (1) a computed tomography angiography (CTA)-determined, endovascularly accessible intracranial LVO associated with neurological symptoms; (2) within 8 h from stroke onset, though, in the later study period, patients falling within the window of 8 h to 12 h from stroke onset were also considered if they had an Alberta Stroke Program Early CT Score of seven points or more on initial non-contrast CT; and (3) a baseline National Institutes of Health Stroke Scale (NIHSS) score of four points or more. For patients eligible for intravenous tissue-type plasminogen activator treatment, the full dose of tissue-type plasminogen activator (0.9 mg/kg) was administered.

For this study, patients who had an M1 occlusion and CTA performed before endovascular treatment were selected from the registry. Conversely, those who presented with an internal carotid artery occlusion were excluded, as collateral flows through anterior or posterior communicating arteries can contribute to lesion-side cerebral flow. Additionally, patients with an occlusion of the distal artery or posterior circulation were also excluded because leptomeningeal collaterals could not be determined reliably in this population. We did not include patients with multiple intracranial artery occlusions because they could also affect leptomeningeal collaterals on middle cerebral artery territory.

The institutional review board approved this study and waived the requirement for obtaining informed consent prior to study inclusion based on the retrospective design.

2.1. Assessment of Leptomeningeal Collaterals (Collateral Assessment Methods)

Leptomeningeal collaterals were determined by CTA performed immediately before endovascular treatment. CTA collateral grade was assessed on 20-mm thickness maximum intensity projection images of single-phase CTA. In patients who underwent multiphase CTA imaging, we only used the first-phase images to evaluate leptomeningeal collaterals.

From among the various existing CTA-based collateral assessment methods, three different methods were adopted [15–17]. First, leptomeningeal collaterals were primarily assessed by a four-scale method previously reported as follows: (1) absent collateral supply to the occluded middle cerebral artery (MCA) territory of 0%, (2) collateral supply of greater than 0% but less than or equal to 50%, (3) collateral supply of greater than 50% but less than 100%, and (4) complete collateral supply of 100% (collateral assessment method 1; Tan's method; Figure 1) [15]. Second, the four grades were regrouped into a three-scale grade system as follows: (1) absent collateral supply to the occluded MCA territory of 0%, (2) collateral supply of greater than 0% but less than 100%, and (3) complete collateral supply of 100% (collateral assessment method 2; shortened from Mass' method) [16]. Third, the four grades were simply dichotomized into (1) collateral supply of 50% or less of the occluded MCA territory and (2) collateral supply of more than 50% (collateral assessment method 3; modified Tan's method) [17]. The four-scale grade of leptomeningeal collaterals was determined by two independent interventional neuroradiologists who were blinded to the clinical and procedural information. The kappa value for the interrater agreement was 0.85 (95% confidence interval, 0.79–0.91), which was similar to its original report [15]. Discrepant cases were resolved by consensus.

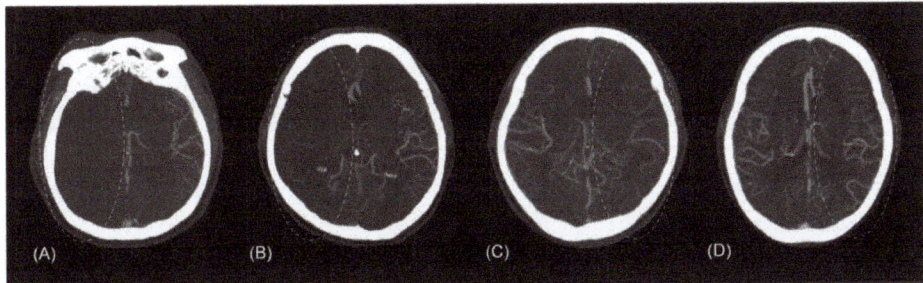

Figure 1. Assessment of leptomeningeal collaterals according to collateral assessment method 1 (Tan et al.'s method). Four computed tomography angiography maximum intensity projection axial images from different patients showing leptomeningeal collaterals. (**A**) Absent collateral supply to the occluded middle cerebral artery territory (circle), compared to the contralateral normal side. (**B**) Collateral supply of greater than 0% but less than or equal to 50%. (**C**) Collateral supply of greater than 50% but less than 100%. (**D**) Complete collateral supply of 100%.

2.2. Identification of ICAS-LVO

ICAS-LVO was determined angiographically. If the occlusion site was completely recanalized without any residual stenosis and reocclusion tendency, the occlusion pathomechanism was not considered as ICAS. In contrast, when significant fixed focal stenosis was noted on angiography, the case was considered as positive for ICAS-LVO [7]. For intractable cases whose occlusion was never recanalized, so that the focal stenosis could not be evaluated, occlusion at the arterial trunk was determined as indicative of ICAS-LVO [6]. ICAS-LVO was assessed independently by two other interventional neuroradiologists who were blinded to the CTA findings and clinical information. The kappa value for the interrater agreement was 0.92 (95% confidence interval, 0.86–0.98). Discrepant cases were also resolved by consensus.

2.3. Statistical Analysis

Based on the identification of ICAS-LVO, patients were assigned to the ICAS group or the non-ICAS group. First, we evaluated the association between leptomeningeal collaterals as determined by the three collateral assessment methods and ICAS-LVO. In this process, (1) basic demographics (age and sex), risk factors for atherosclerosis (hypertension diabetes, dyslipidemia, smoking, and coronary artery disease), typical clinical factors associated with occlusion pathomechanism (atrial fibrillation and initial NIHSS score), and leptomeningeal collaterals by each collateral assessment method were compared between the ICAS and non-ICAS groups. The Mann–Whitney U test, chi-squared test, and Fisher's exact test were used for comparison. Also, we summarized the study population by descriptive statistics. Continuous variables were expressed by a mean value with standard deviation or a median value with interquartile range, as appropriate. Categorical variables were expressed by a frequency with its percentage. Then, (2) to see whether better leptomeningeal collaterals were associated with ICAS-LVO, we performed binary logistic regression analyses for each collateral assessment method. To determine whether better leptomeningeal collaterals can be an independent variable for ICAS-LVO, variables with a p-value < 0.10 in the univariable analysis were entered into the multivariable model. Finally, (3) to evaluate the predictive power of leptomeningeal collaterals for ICAS-LVO, we calculated the sensitivity, specificity, positive predictive value (PPV), negative predictive value (NPV), and accuracy of each collateral assessment method. Receiver operating characteristic curve analyses were also performed to calculate the area under the curve (AUC) values and cutoff points, which were determined based on Youden's index.

Second, based on the results of logistic regression analyses and calculated cutoff points of each collateral assessment method, leptomeningeal collaterals were dichotomized into (1) incomplete collateral supply of less than 100% or (2) complete collateral supply of 100%. Then, the findings of complete and incomplete collateral supplies were compared between the ICAS and non-ICAS groups. To see whether complete leptomeningeal collateral supply was associated with ICAS-LVO, univariable and multivariable binary logistic regression analyses were performed in the same manner as the three collateral assessment methods. We also calculated sensitivity, PPV, NPV, accuracy, and AUC value for the dichotomization in predicting ICAS-LVO.

A p-value < 0.05 was considered statistically significant for the 95% confidence interval. All statistical analyses were performed using R software (version 3.5.0; R Foundation for Statistical Computing, Vienna, Austria).

3. Results

Among the 604 patients that underwent endovascular treatment for an intracranial vessel occlusion, 226 patients (mean age 69.0 ± 12.1 years; 54.4% male) were included (Figure 2). Patients with arterial dissection ($n = 5$), distal artery occlusion ($n = 132$), internal carotid artery occlusion ($n = 154$), and vertebrobasilar artery occlusion ($n = 79$) were excluded. In eight patients, leptomeningeal collaterals could not be determined by CTA because the arterial target was changed between CTA and endovascular treatment ($n = 2$; internal carotid artery occlusion on initial CTA was changed to M1 occlusion on cerebral angiography) or CTA was not performed before endovascular treatment ($n = 6$). Leptomeningeal collaterals were 0% in the occluded MCA territory in 15 patients (6.6%), greater than 0% but less than or equal to 50% in 57 (25.2%), greater than 50% but less than 100% in 95 (42.1%), and 100% in 59 (26.1%).

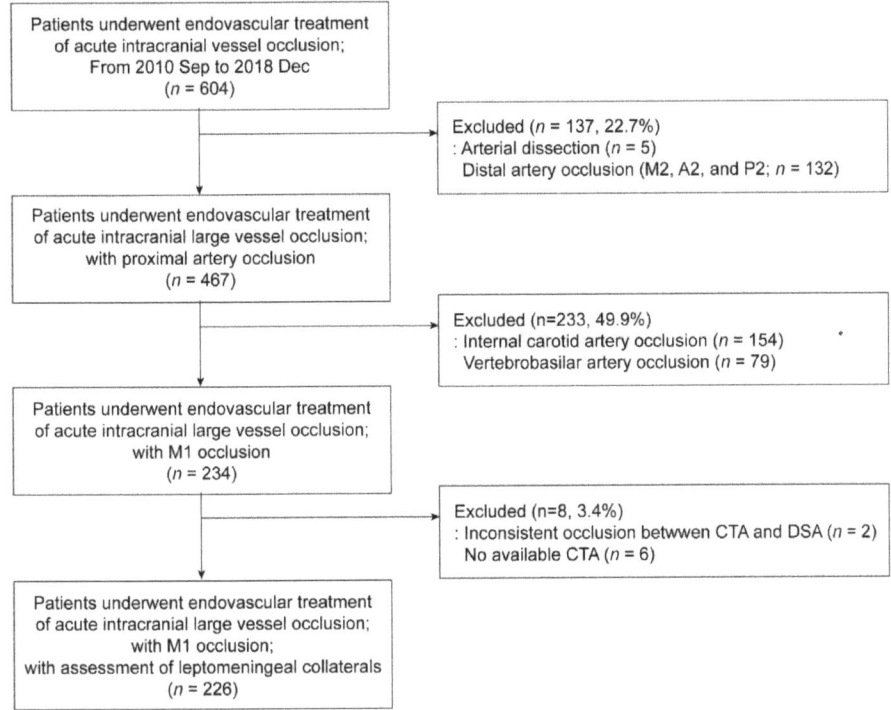

Figure 2. Patients selection flow chart. DSA, digital subtraction angiography.

3.1. Association Between Leptomeningeal Collaterals and ICAS-LVO

A total of 40 patients (17.7%) showed an ICAS-LVO as the occlusion pathomechanism. Based on the use of collateral assessment methods 1 and 2, patients with leptomeningeal collaterals of 0%, greater than 0% but less than or equal to 50%, and greater than 50% but less than 100% of occluded MCA territory were less common in the ICAS group, whereas cases of complete (100%) leptomeningeal collaterals were significantly more frequently found in the ICAS group (52.5% versus 20.4%; $p < 0.001$; Table 1). For collateral assessment method 3, more patients in the ICAS group had leptomeningeal collaterals of greater than 50% than the non-ICAS group (85.0% versus 64.5%; $p = 0.012$).

Table 1. Comparison of demographics, risk factors for stroke and atherosclerosis, and leptomeningeal collaterals between intracranial atherosclerosis (ICAS) and non-ICAS groups.

	All (n = 226)	ICAS (n = 40)	Non-ICAS (n = 186)	p-Value
Age, years	69.0 (±12.1)	66.2 (±16.4)	69.6 (±10.9)	0.222
Male sex	123 (54.4)	20 (50.0)	103 (55.4)	0.536
Hypertension	166 (73.5)	32 (80.0)	134 (72.0)	0.301
Diabetes	66 (29.2)	13 (32.5)	53 (28.5)	0.613
Dyslipidemia	48 (21.2)	12 (30.0)	36 (19.4)	0.135
Current smoking	42 (18.6)	16 (40.0)	26 (14.0)	<0.001
Coronary artery disease	52 (23.0)	11 (27.5)	41 (22.0)	0.457
Atrial fibrillation	119 (52.7)	11 (27.5)	108 (58.1)	<0.001
Initial NIHSS score	15.0 (11.0; 19.0)	12.0 (7.0; 17.0)	15.0 (12.0; 19.0)	0.001
Leptomeningeal collaterals				
Three assessment methods				
Method 1 (Tan)				
0%	15 (6.6)	1 (2.5)	14 (7.5)	<0.001
>0% but ≤50%	57 (25.2)	5 (12.5)	52 (28.0)	
>50% but <100%	95 (42.1)	13 (32.5)	82 (44.1)	
100%	59 (26.1)	21 (52.5)	38 (20.4)	
Method 2 (shortened Maas)				
0%	15 (6.6)	1 (2.5)	14 (7.5)	<0.001
>0% but <100%	152 (67.3)	18 (45.0)	134 (72.1)	
100%	59 (26.1)	21 (52.5)	38 (20.4)	
Method 3 (modified Tan)				
≤50%	72 (31.9)	6 (15.0)	66 (35.5)	0.012
>50%	154 (68.1)	34 (85.0)	120 (64.5)	
Dichotomization by cutoff				
Incomplete (<100%)	167 (73.9)	19 (47.5)	148 (79.6)	<0.001
Complete (100%)	59 (26.1)	21 (52.5)	38 (20.4)	

Age is represented by a mean value (±standard deviation); initial National Institutes of Health Stroke Scale (NIHSS) score by a median value (first and third quartile); all other variables by the number of patients (frequency, %).

On the logistic regression analyses for collateral assessment methods 1, 2, and 3, odds ratios for ICAS-LVO gradually increased as leptomeningeal collaterals improved (Figure 3). However, none were statistically significant in univariable and multivariable analyses (Table S1 and Figure 3). For multivariable analyses, each collateral assessment method was adjusted by current smoking, atrial fibrillation, and initial NIHSS score.

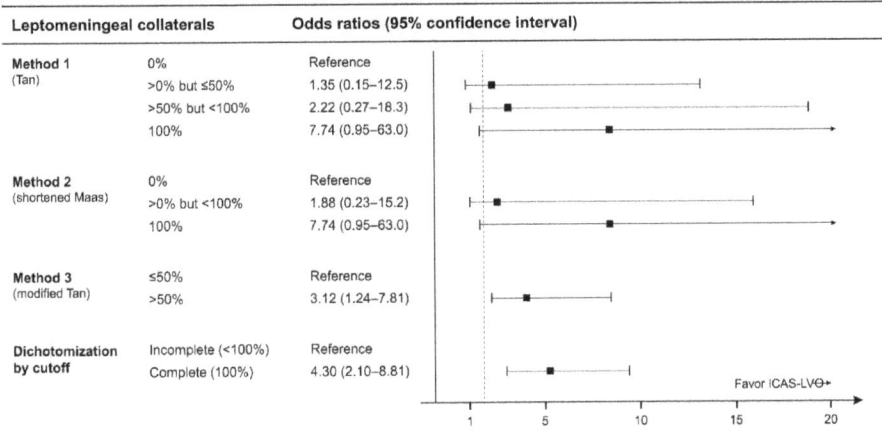

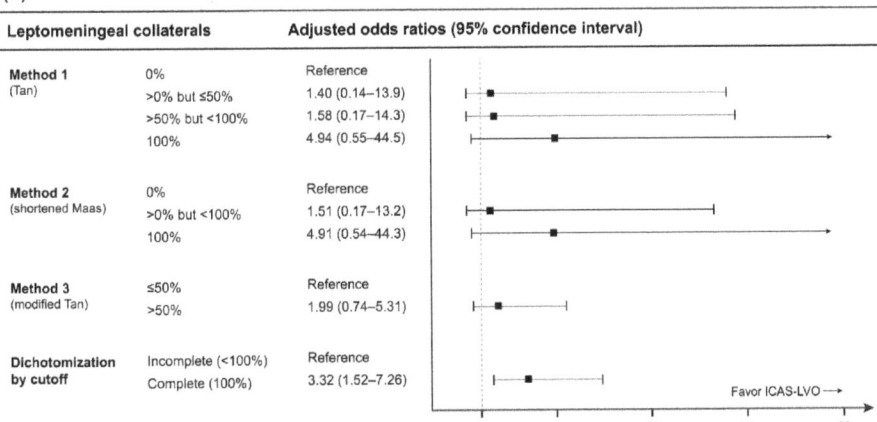

Figure 3. Univariable and multivariable logistic regression analyses of leptomeningeal collaterals for intracranial atherosclerosis-related large vessel occlusion (ICAS-LVO). Odds ratios with 95% confidence intervals from (**A**) univariable and (**B**) multivariable logistic regression analyses are plotted. In multivariable analyses, each leptomeningeal collateral assessment method was adjusted by current smoking, atrial fibrillation, and initial NIHSS score.

3.2. Predictive Power of Leptomeningeal Collaterals for ICAS-LVO

For collateral assessment methods 1 and 2, the calculated sensitivity, specificity, PPV, and NPV of leptomeningeal collaterals to predict ICAS-LVO were 52.5%, 79.6%, 35.6%, and 88.6%, respectively (Table 2). Collateral assessment method 3 showed higher sensitivity and lower specificity for ICAS-LVO than collateral assessment methods 1 and 2. AUC values of leptomeningeal collaterals were below 0.7 for all collateral assessment methods (each $p < 0.001$).

Table 2. Diagnostic performance of leptomeningeal collaterals for intracranial atherosclerosis-related large vessel occlusion.

Collateral Assessment Methods	Sensitivity (%)	Specificity (%)	PPV (%)	NPV (%)	Accuracy (%)	AUC
Method 1 (Tan) [1]	52.5	79.6	35.6	88.6	74.8	0.686
Method 2 (shortened Maas) [1]	52.5	79.6	35.6	88.6	74.8	0.668
Method 3 (modified Tan) [2]	85.0	35.5	22.1	91.7	44.2	0.602
Dichotomization by cutoff [1]	52.5	79.6	35.6	88.6	74.8	0.660

[1] For leptomeningeal collaterals of 100%; [2] for leptomeningeal collaterals of > 50%; PPV, positive predictive value; NPV, negative predictive value; AUC, area under curve.

3.3. Significance of Complete Leptomeningeal Collaterals in Predicting ICAS-LVO

Based on the results from the analyses of collateral assessment methods 1, 2, and 3, study participants' leptomeningeal collaterals were dichotomized to incomplete (less than 100%) and complete (100%). Patients in the ICAS group showed more complete leptomeningeal collateral supply ($p < 0.001$; Table 1). During multivariable analysis, complete leptomeningeal collateral supply remained an independent factor for ICAS-LVO (odds ratio, 3.32; 95% confidence interval, 1.52–7.26; $p = 0.003$; Table S1 and Figure 3). An AUC value for complete leptomeningeal collaterals was 0.660 (95% CI, 0.595–0.722; $p < 0.001$), with an NPV of 88.6% (Table 2).

4. Discussion

In this study, we found that leptomeningeal collaterals were associated with occlusion pathomechanism. Better leptomeningeal collaterals were significantly associated with ICAS-LVO in common collateral assessment methods. Nevertheless, during logistic regression analyses, only the use of a dichotomization method (incomplete versus complete) was independently associated with ICAS-LVO. Despite the independence, it achieved only a modest degree of predictability of ICAS-LVO. To the best of our knowledge, this study is the first study to evaluate the association of leptomeningeal collaterals with ICAS-LVO and its preprocedural possibility to predict ICAS-LVO.

This study was originally contrived from the necessity to enhance the preprocedural determination of occlusion pathomechanism in endovascular treatment of LVO. Because the optimal endovascular strategy—which includes selection of the most effective endovascular modality and when to switch from one modality to another—depends on the type of occlusion pathomechanism, the earlier determination of occlusion pathomechanism can be crucial in attaining significant recanalization [18,19]. However, unfortunately, there have been only a few practical factors identified that we can rely on to identify occlusion pathomechanism before an endovascular procedure. Common cardioembolic sources such as atrial fibrillation or valvular heart diseases are typically considered as evidence of an embolic occlusion of an intracranial artery [7]. Specific imaging findings—for example, a hyperdense artery sign on CT or a blooming artifact on magnetic resonance imaging—have also been regarded as markers of embolic occlusion [14,20]. Uniquely, the occlusion type observed on preprocedural CTA was significantly associated with occlusion pathomechanism. The occlusion type was superior to the atrial fibrillation and hyperdense artery sign in predicting the occlusion pathomechanism [10]. Patient demographics or a few risk factors for atherosclerosis can be referred to in order to assume the occlusion pathomechanism; however, they are quite indirect means [7]. Particular infarct patterns could also be helpful in determining the occlusion pathomechanism. However, the infarct pattern is less evident and may be limited in the preprocedural condition [14].

As we expected, leptomeningeal collaterals were significantly associated with occlusion pathomechanism in this study. In particular, complete leptomeningeal collaterals were consistently associated with ICAS-LVO with a modest level of predictability. In comparison with other preprocedural findings used to predict ICAS-LVO, the discriminative power of complete leptomeningeal collaterals seemed not so inferior. In this study population, the AUC value of complete leptomeningeal collaterals for ICAS-LVO was not lower than that of atrial fibrillation (0.653; 95% confidence interval, 0.587–0.715).

Furthermore, the AUC value of CTA-determined occlusion type for stent retriever success, one of the preprocedural findings presumed to be highly associated with ICAS-LVO, was less than 0.7 [5].

To the best of our knowledge, only one other study has commented on the association between leptomeningeal collaterals and ICAS-LVO in endovascular treatment [7]. In the literature, full and rapid leptomeningeal collaterals were significantly more frequent in patients with ICAS-LVO, which was consistent with our study. However, the result was unofficial from a small number of patients, so it was merely a piece of unpublished data in a review article. Additionally, leptomeningeal collaterals were not considered as a predictor of ICAS-LVO in the literature. Leptomeningeal collaterals were assessed by initial cerebral angiogram during endovascular treatment, not preprocedurally.

Complete leptomeningeal collaterals showed low sensitivity and PPV with a relatively higher NPV in discriminating ICAS-LVO. For practical use, the statistical parameters can be interpreted as follows: (1) in patients with ICAS-LVO, the probability of showing complete leptomeningeal collaterals was about 50% (low sensitivity); (2) even among cases showing complete leptomeningeal collaterals, ICAS-LVO was only present in about 40% of them (low PPV); and (3) if a patient showed incomplete leptomeningeal collaterals, occlusion pathomechanism was not likely to be ICAS-LVO up to 90% (high NPV).

The study results might be substantially affected by the chosen collateral assessment method. However, there has been no consensual grading system established to evaluate leptomeningeal collaterals on CTA. To avoid arbitrary grading, we tried to choose collateral assessment methods that have all been widely used in previous studies [21,22]. Based on the consistent findings from those collateral assessment methods, we regrouped the leptomeningeal collaterals by its cutoff value into incomplete or complete. Cerebral angiography can be a good modality with which to assess leptomeningeal collaterals. However, in most endovascular procedures, initial leptomeningeal collateral flow is not assessed on cerebral angiography because the arterial target is directly approached without taking the angiography of other cerebral vessels. We think that CTA might be the most rational modality to use to assess leptomeningeal collaterals in daily clinical practice. Multiphase CTA could be another collateral assessment method. However, multiphase CTA cannot be deployed in all centers; indeed, multiphase CTA was not performed in the early period of this study.

This study had a few limitations. First, it was performed retrospectively in a single tertiary stroke center. However, all patients were prospectively registered with a detailed description of their endovascular procedure. Furthermore, this study focused on objective findings, including imaging markers and angiographic findings rather than on clinical outcomes, thereby minimizing this limitation. Nevertheless, based on the retrospective nature of this study, there might be a possibility that the patients with better leptomeningeal collaterals were preferentially chosen for endovascular treatment. Although the predetermined protocol in our center did not regulate the leptomeningeal collateral status for endovascular treatment eligibility, the physician's clinical decision might be partly affected by the leptomeningeal collateral status.

Second, this study included patients only with M1 occlusion. Thus, the generalization of our study results to all anterior circulation strokes might be inappropriate. However, as described earlier, such use of this strict inclusion criterion was to ensure the improved evaluation of uncontaminated leptomeningeal collaterals. Study findings should be understood as providing verification of a general hypothesis that better leptomeningeal collaterals are associated with ICAS-LVO. In addition, generalization of the study results could also be limited because this study was performed in an Asian country where ICAS is more prevalent. As statistical power might be affected by the number of patients with ICAS-LVO, no one could precisely figure out the association of leptomeningeal collaterals with ICAS-LVO in other countries where ICAS is much less prevalent.

Third, this study also included patients with a tandem occlusion (M1 occlusion with cervical ICA occlusion/stenosis). Chronic ischemia, even due to severe cervical ICA stenosis, might be associated with robust leptomeningeal collaterals. Thus, theoretically, for the tandem occlusion, leptomeningeal collaterals could be abundant or complete, although its M1 occlusion is embolic from a cervical ICA lesion. In fact, about 5% patients of this study had an atherosclerotic cervical ICA occlusion. Fortunately, even after excluding the patients with tandem occlusions, the significance of the study results was not changed.

5. Conclusions

Leptomeningeal collaterals determined by preprocedural CTA were significantly associated with occlusion pathomechanism. Specifically, complete leptomeningeal collateral supply was independently associated with ICAS-LVO. Despite the association, however, leptomeningeal collaterals were simply predictive of ICAS-LVO in a modest degree. In clinical practice, one could assume that incomplete leptomeningeal collateral supply is not likely ICAS-LVO based on high NPV. In this way, leptomeningeal collaterals could be helpful in the preprocedural determination of occlusion pathomechanism.

Supplementary Materials: The following are available online at http://www.mdpi.com/2077-0383/9/9/2784/s1, Table S1: Multivariable analyses for the association with intracranial atherosclerosis-related large vessel occlusion.

Author Contributions: Conceptualization, J.-H.B. and B.M.K.; data curation, J.-H.B., B.M.K., J.W.K., D.J.K., J.H.H., H.S.N., and Y.D.K.; formal analysis, J.-H.B. and J.W.K.; funding acquisition, B.M.K.; methodology, J.-H.B. and B.M.K.; writing—original draft, J.-H.B.; writing—review and editing, J.-H.B. and B.M.K. All authors have read and agreed to the published version of the manuscript.

Funding: This research was supported by a grant of the Korea Health Technology R&D Project through the Korea Health Industry Development Institute (KHIDI), funded by the Ministry of Health and Welfare, Republic of Korea (HC15C1056).

Conflicts of Interest: The authors declare no conflict of interest.

References

1. Powers, W.J.; Rabinstein, A.A.; Ackerson, T.; Adeoye, O.M.; Bambakidis, N.C.; Becker, K.; Biller, J.; Brown, M.; Demaerschalk, B.M.; Hoh, B. Guidelines for the early management of patients with acute Ischemic stroke: 2019 Update to the 2018 guidelines for the early management of acute ischemic stroke: A auideline for healthcare professionals from the American Heart Association/American Stroke Association. *Stroke* **2019**, *50*, e344–e418. [PubMed]
2. Kang, D.-H.; Yoon, W.; Baek, B.H.; Kim, S.K.; Lee, Y.Y.; Kim, J.-T.; Park, M.-S.; Kim, Y.-W.; Hwang, Y.-H.; Kim, Y.-S. Front-line thrombectomy for acute large-vessel occlusion with underlying severe intracranial stenosis: Stent retriever versus contact aspiration. *J. Neurosurg.* **2020**, *132*, 1202–1208. [CrossRef] [PubMed]
3. Lee, J.S.; Lee, S.-J.; Hong, J.M.; Choi, J.W.; Yoo, J.; Hong, J.-H.; Kim, C.-H.; Kim, Y.-W.; Kang, D.-H.; Hwang, Y.-H.; et al. Solitaire thrombectomy for acute stroke due to intracranial atherosclerosis-related occlusion: ROSE ASSIST study. *Front. Neurol.* **2018**, *9*, e9. [CrossRef]
4. Tsang, A.C.O.; Orru, E.; Klostranec, J.M.; Yang, I.-H.; Lau, K.K.; Tsang, F.C.P.; Lui, W.M.; Pereira, V.M.; Krings, T. Thrombectomy outcomes of intracranial atherosclerosis-related occlusions. *Stroke* **2019**, *50*, 1460–1466. [CrossRef] [PubMed]
5. Baek, J.-H.; Kim, B.; Heo, J.H.; Nam, H.S.; Song, D.; Bang, O.Y.; Kim, D.J. Importance of truncal-type occlusion in stentriever-based thrombectomy for acute stroke. *Neurology* **2016**, *87*, 1542–1550. [CrossRef]
6. Baek, J.-H.; Kim, B.; Heo, J.H.; Kim, D.J.; Nam, H.S.; Kim, Y.D. Outcomes of endovascular treatment for acute intracranial atherosclerosis–related large vessel occlusion. *Stroke* **2018**, *49*, 2699–2705. [CrossRef]
7. Lee, J.S.; Hong, J.M.; Kim, J.S. Diagnostic and therapeutic strategies for acute intracranial atherosclerosis-related occlusions. *J. Stroke* **2017**, *19*, 143–151. [CrossRef]
8. Park, H.; Baek, J.-H.; Kim, B. Endovascular treatment of acute stroke due to intracranial atherosclerotic stenosis-related large vessel occlusion. *Front. Neurol.* **2019**, *10*, e308. [CrossRef]
9. Kang, D.-H.; Yoon, W. Current opinion on endovascular therapy for emergent large vessel occlusion due to underlying intracranial atherosclerotic stenosis. *Korean J. Radiol.* **2019**, *20*, 739–748. [CrossRef]
10. Baek, J.-H.; Kim, B.; Yoo, J.; Nam, H.S.; Kim, Y.D.; Kim, D.J.; Heo, J.H.; Bang, O.Y. Predictive value of computed tomography angiography-determined occlusion type in stent retriever thrombectomy. *Stroke* **2017**, *48*, 2746–2752. [CrossRef]

11. Brozici, M.; Van Der Zwan, A.; Hillen, B. Anatomy and functionality of leptomeningeal anastomoses: A review. *Stroke* **2003**, *34*, 2750–2762. [CrossRef] [PubMed]
12. Shuaib, A.; Butcher, K.; A Mohammad, A.; Saqqur, M.; Liebeskind, D.S. Collateral blood vessels in acute ischaemic stroke: A potential therapeutic target. *Lancet Neurol.* **2011**, *10*, 909–921. [CrossRef]
13. Liebeskind, D.S. Collateral circulation. *Stroke* **2003**, *34*, 2279–2284. [CrossRef] [PubMed]
14. Suh, H.I.; Hong, J.M.; Lee, K.S.; Han, M.; Choi, J.W.; Kim, J.S.; Demchuk, A.M.; Lee, J.S. Imaging predictors for atherosclerosis-related intracranial large artery occlusions in acute anterior circulation stroke. *J. Stroke* **2016**, *18*, 352–354. [CrossRef]
15. Tan, I.; Demchuk, A.; Hopyan, J.; Zhang, L.; Gladstone, D.J.; Wong, K.-K.; Martin, M.; Symons, S.; Fox, A.; Aviv, R. CT angiography clot burden score and collateral score: Correlation with clinical and radiologic outcomes in acute middle cerebral artery infarct. *AJNR Am. J. Neuroradiol.* **2009**, *30*, 525–531. [CrossRef]
16. Maas, M.B.; Lev, M.H.; Ay, H.; Singhal, A.B.; Greer, D.M.; Smith, W.S.; Harris, G.J.; Halpern, E.; Kemmling, A.; Koroshetz, W.J.; et al. Collateral vessels on CT angiography predict outcome in acute ischemic stroke. *Stroke* **2009**, *40*, 3001–3005. [CrossRef]
17. Kim, B.; Baek, J.-H.; Heo, J.H.; Nam, H.S.; Kim, Y.D.; Yoo, J.; Kim, D.J.; Jeon, P.; Baik, S.K.; Suh, S.; et al. Collateral status affects the onset-to-reperfusion time window for good outcome. *J. Neurol. Neurosurg. Psychiatry* **2018**, *89*, 903–909. [CrossRef]
18. Tian, C.; Cao, X.; Wang, J. Recanalisation therapy in patients with acute ischaemic stroke caused by large artery occlusion: Choice of therapeutic strategy according to underlying aetiological mechanism? *Stroke Vasc. Neurol.* **2017**, *2*, 244–250. [CrossRef]
19. Kim, B.M. Causes and solutions of endovascular treatment failure. *J. Stroke* **2017**, *19*, 131–142. [CrossRef]
20. Kim, S.K.; Baek, B.H.; Lee, Y.; Yoon, W. Clinical implications of CT hyperdense artery sign in patients with acute middle cerebral artery occlusion in the era of modern mechanical thrombectomy. *J. Neurol.* **2017**, *264*, 2450–2456. [CrossRef]
21. McVerry, F.; Liebeskind, D.; Muir, K.W. Systematic review of methods for assessing leptomeningeal collateral flow. *AJNR Am. J. Neuroradiol.* **2012**, *33*, 576–582. [CrossRef] [PubMed]
22. Kim, B.; Chung, J.; Park, H.-K.; Kim, J.Y.; Yang, M.-H.; Han, M.-K.; Jeong, C.; Hwang, G.; Kwon, O.-K.; Bae, H.-J. CT angiography of collateral vessels and outcomes in endovascular-treated acute ischemic stroke patients. *J. Clin. Neurol.* **2017**, *13*, 121–128. [CrossRef] [PubMed]

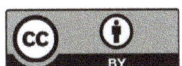

© 2020 by the authors. Licensee MDPI, Basel, Switzerland. This article is an open access article distributed under the terms and conditions of the Creative Commons Attribution (CC BY) license (http://creativecommons.org/licenses/by/4.0/).

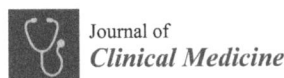

Article

Endothelial Progenitor Cells as a Marker of Vascular Damage But not a Predictor in Acute Microangiopathy-Associated Stroke

Adam Wiśniewski [1,*], Joanna Boinska [2], Katarzyna Ziołkowska [2], Adam Lemanowicz [3], Karolina Filipska [4], Zbigniew Serafin [3], Robert Ślusarz [4], Danuta Rość [2] and Grzegorz Kozera [5]

- [1] Department of Neurology, Collegium Medicum in Bydgoszcz, Nicolaus Copernicus University in Toruń, Skłodowskiej 9 Street, 85-094 Bydgoszcz, Poland
- [2] Department of Pathophysiology, Collegium Medicum in Bydgoszcz, Nicolaus Copernicus University in Toruń, Skłodowskiej 9 Street, 85-094 Bydgoszcz, Poland; joanna_boinska@cm.umk.pl (J.B.); katarzyna_stankowska@cm.umk.pl (K.Z.); drosc@cm.umk.pl (D.R.)
- [3] Department of Radiology, Collegium Medicum in Bydgoszcz, Nicolaus Copernicus University in Toruń, Skłodowskiej 9 Street, 85-094 Bydgoszcz, Poland; adam.lemanowicz@cm.umk.pl (A.L.); serafin@cm.umk.pl (Z.S.)
- [4] Department of Neurological and Neurosurgical Nursing, Collegium Medicum in Bydgoszcz, Nicolaus Copernicus University in Toruń, Łukasiewicza 1 Street, 85-821 Bydgoszcz, Poland; karolinafilipskakf@gmail.com (K.F.); robert_slu_cmumk@wp.pl (R.Ś.)
- [5] Medical Simulation Centre, Medical University of Gdańsk, Faculty of Medicine, Dębowa 17 Street, 80-208 Gdańsk, Poland; gkozera1@wp.pl
- * Correspondence: adam.lek@wp.pl; Tel.: +48-790-813-513

Received: 3 June 2020; Accepted: 14 July 2020; Published: 15 July 2020

Abstract: Background: The aim of the study was to assess the number of endothelial progenitor cells (EPCs) in patients with acute stroke due to cerebral microangiopathy and evaluate whether there is a relationship between their number and clinical status, radiological findings, risk factors, selected biochemical parameters, and prognosis, both in ischemic and hemorrhagic stroke. Methods: In total, 66 patients with lacunar ischemic stroke, 38 patients with typical location hemorrhagic stroke, and 22 subjects from the control group without acute cerebrovascular incidents were included in the prospective observational study. The number of EPCs was determined in serum on the first and eighth day after stroke onset using flow cytometry and identified with the immune-phenotype classification determinant (CD)45−, CD34+, CD133+. Results: We demonstrated a significantly higher number of EPCs on the first day of stroke compared to the control group (med. 17.75 cells/µL (0–488 cells/µL) vs. 5.24 cells/µL (0–95 cells/µL); $p = 0.0006$). We did not find a relationship between the number of EPCs in the acute phase of stroke and the biochemical parameters, vascular risk factors, or clinical condition. In females, the higher number of EPCs on the first day of stroke is related to a favorable functional outcome on the eighth day after the stroke onset compared to males ($p = 0.0355$). We found that a higher volume of the hemorrhagic focus on the first day was correlated with a lower number of EPCs on the first day (correlation coefficient (R) = −0.3378, $p = 0.0471$), and a higher number of EPCs on the first day of the hemorrhagic stroke was correlated with a lower degree of regression of the hemorrhagic focus (R = −0.3896, $p = 0.0367$). Conclusion: The study showed that endothelial progenitor cells are an early marker in acute microangiopathy-associated stroke regardless of etiology and may affect the radiological findings in hemorrhagic stroke. Nevertheless, their prognostic value remains doubtful in stroke patients.

Keywords: endothelial progenitor cells; ischemic stroke; hemorrhage; prognosis; clinical outcome

1. Introduction

Stroke is an important social and medical problem in the 21st century, as it is one of the main causes of morbidity and long-term disability and the second most frequent cause of death in the world [1]. Ischemic stroke associated with disturbances of the blood flow to the brain tissue, leading to necrosis of the part of the brain covered by ischemia (80–85%), is the most common. Hemorrhagic stroke (15–20%) associated with extravasation of blood to the brain is less common but has greater mortality [2]. Stroke may be the result of endothelial dysfunction (in the course of cerebral microangiopathy), as well as the cause of vascular endothelial damage. Stroke due to small vessel disease, i.e., lacunar stroke, is associated with pathological changes (classical atherosclerosis, fibrosis, enamel, and calcification) of small cerebral vessels (diameter below 600 μm), and accounts for approximately 20–25% of all ischemic strokes [3]. Among hemorrhagic strokes, the most common, typical location (deep) intracerebral hemorrhage, seems to have been most related to microangiopathy. It results from blood extravasation from stabbing branches (most often lenticular-striatum arteries) supplying the basal ganglia and thalamus. It is related to pathological changes of the vessel's walls (including cells of the endothelium) in the course of improperly treated hypertension [4].

Endothelial progenitor cells (EPCs) are a recognized marker of both the degree of endothelial damage and the ability to regenerate the endothelium. Due to their multiplication potential, they can differentiate into many cells, but most often, they proliferate into mature circulating endothelial cells. Thanks to mediators, such as VEGF (vascular endothelial growth factor), SDF-1 (stromal-derived factor), and G-CSF (granulocyte colony-stimulating factor), they migrate to damaged areas of the brain affected by ischemia. They play an important role in the regeneration of the nervous tissue, glial cell nutrition, reduction of neuronal apoptosis, and blood–brain barrier stabilization. They are associated with postnatal angiogenesis, especially in neovascularization of blood vessels damaged by ischemia [5–7]. This is particularly important in patients with stroke. As a result, they are increasingly considered as a potential treatment method for stroke patients, especially with ischemic stroke, and the initial results of their use in studies on mice and rats seem encouraging [8–12]. However, the role and importance of these cells in stroke patients is still the subject of controversy, and reports on this subject are scarce and often ambiguous. It is believed that a large number of EPCs, due to their regenerative and repairing properties, may affect the size of the ischemic focus and even the clinical and functional status of the patients, and thus, the prognosis [13]. Therefore, the aim of this study was to assess the number of EPCs in the blood serum and their potential relationship with the clinical condition, radiological image, and prognosis in patients in the acute phase of stroke caused by cerebral microangiopathy.

2. Material and Methods

2.1. Study Design and Participants

The study was conducted in accordance with the Declaration of Helsinki and the protocol was approved by the Bioethics Committee of Nicolaus Copernicus University in Torun at Collegium Medicum of Ludwik Rydygier in Bydgoszcz (KB No. 769/2014). The study included subjects who, having read the study protocol, signed the informed consent to participate in the study. The researchers explained all stages of the study to the subjects and presented all potential risks associated with the research.

The definition of stroke, updated in 2013 by the American Heart Association/American Stroke Association (AHA/ASA), was used, which is an episode of a sudden neurological disorder caused by focal cerebral, spinal, or retinal ischemia lasting over 24 h or corresponding to the morphological features of ischemia of the central nervous system [14].

The study was conducted from February 2015 to December 2017 in the Department of Neurology at Collegium Medicum in Bydgoszcz of Nicolaus Copernicus University in Torun in the University Hospital No. 1 in Bydgoszcz. This prospective and observational study included stroke patients with cerebral microangiopathy: 66 patients with lacunar ischemic stroke, 38 patients with typical location intracerebral hemorrhage, and 22 people from the control group.

The group of patients with lacunar stroke included patients with no significant hemodynamic stenoses of large pre-skull vessels or cardiogenic-embolic background, and the performed neuroimaging confirmed the presence of a lacunar focus and/or revealed chronic vascular changes with a typical location and morphology (subcortical lesions, periventricular lesions, leukoaraiosis features) [15]. The typical location intracerebral hemorrhage was diagnosed based on the results of a computed tomography scan performed during the patient's admission. Patients with symptomatic cerebral hemorrhage in the course of taking oral anticoagulants and patients with extensive lobal hemorrhage during amyloid angiopathy were excluded. We included only stroke subjects admitted to the hospital with a duration of stroke symptoms no longer than 12 h. The control group consisted of people of similar age and vascular risk factors hospitalized in the Department of Neurology for reasons other than acute cerebrovascular disease and did not represent cerebrovascular incidents in the last 3 years.

Exclusion criteria included lack of the patient's consent to participate in the study or inability to express it consciously (stroke with aphasia or quantitative disturbances of consciousness); patients with documented oncological history; patients with chronic inflammatory processes, e.g., chronic venous thrombosis of the lower limbs or chronic ischemia of the lower limbs; patients with a stroke or TIA during the last 3 years; and patients with severe bleeding in the last 2 years, e.g., gastrointestinal bleeding, level of hemoglobin < 9 g/dL, hematocrit value < 35%; and duration of stroke symptoms more than 12 h before hospital admission.

Routine laboratory tests were performed at the Laboratory Diagnostics Department of the University Hospital No. 1 in Bydgoszcz in the morning within 24 h from the onset of stroke symptoms. About 6 mL of blood were collected from the veins of the forearm from patients to determine the following biochemical parameters in the blood serum: C reactive protein (CRP), fibrinogen, and homocysteine (Atellica Solution, Siemens Healthcare, Erlangen, Germany).

In all patients, computed tomography without contrast was performed at the time of admission to the hospital in the Hospital Emergency Department of A. Jurasz University Hospital No. 1 in Bydgoszcz using a 64-row Brilliance computer CT scanner (Phillips, Eindhoven, The Netherlands). In subjects with hemorrhagic stroke, the volume of hemorrhagic focus was assessed in mL on the 1st and 8th day of the stroke using the special Philips software. The degree of hemorrhagic focus regression was the volume difference between the 1st and 8th day.

2.2. Flow Cytometry

Determination of EPCs in blood in stroke subjects was performed on admission, within the first 24 h (1st day), and on the 8th day of the disease, using flow cytometry. In the control group, cell determinations were made on the 1st day of the hospital stay. The method for the determination of the level of circulating EPCs was based on previous reports [16,17]. Fresh blood (4.5 mL) with minimal stasis was collected into cooled tubes (Becton Dickinson Vacutainer® System, Plymouth, UK) containing potassium ethylenediaminetetraacetic acid (K2EDTA) and analyzed within 2 h. The samples were obtained in the morning between 8 and 10 a.m., after a 12-h period of overnight fasting. The approach of the current study was to use three concurrent markers of classification determinant (CD)45−, CD34+, CD133+, to increase the accuracy of endothelial progenitor detection. Cells were further confirmed by a fluorescent-activated cell sorting (FACS) Calibur flow cytometer (Becton Dickinson, San Diego, USA) using monoclonal antibodies directed against antigens specific for circulating endothelial progenitor cells (Figure 1). The data acquired was analyzed by using CellQuest software (Becton Dickinson). Circulating EPC counts were assessed by flow cytometry according to the procedure provided by Mancuso et al. [16]. Fresh peripheral blood (50 µL) was incubated with Peridinin-Chlorophyll-Protein–Cyanine (PerCP-Cy5.5)-conjugated anti-CD45 (concentration 25 µg/mL), as well as allophycocyanin (APC)-conjugated anti-CD34 antibodies (concentration 25 µg/mL) (all BD Biosciences, Pharmingen, San Diego, CA, USA), and phycoerythrin (PE)-conjugated anti-CD133 (concentration 50 µg/mL) (Miltenyi Biotec, Bergisch Gladbach, Germany). EPCs were defined as negative for hematopoietic marker CD45, positive for endothelial progenitor marker CD133, and positive for endothelial cell marker CD34, showing expression on early hematopoietic and vascular-associated tissue. At least 100,000 events were measured in each sample. The total cell count was calculated by TruCount tubes (BD Biosciences, San Jose, CA, USA) containing a calibrated number of fluorescent beads, and 'lyse-no-wash' procedures were used in the present study to improve the sensitivity [17]. Absolute EPCs numbers (cells/µL) were calculated based on the following pattern: Number of measured EPCs/number of fluorescent beads counted × number of beads/µL.

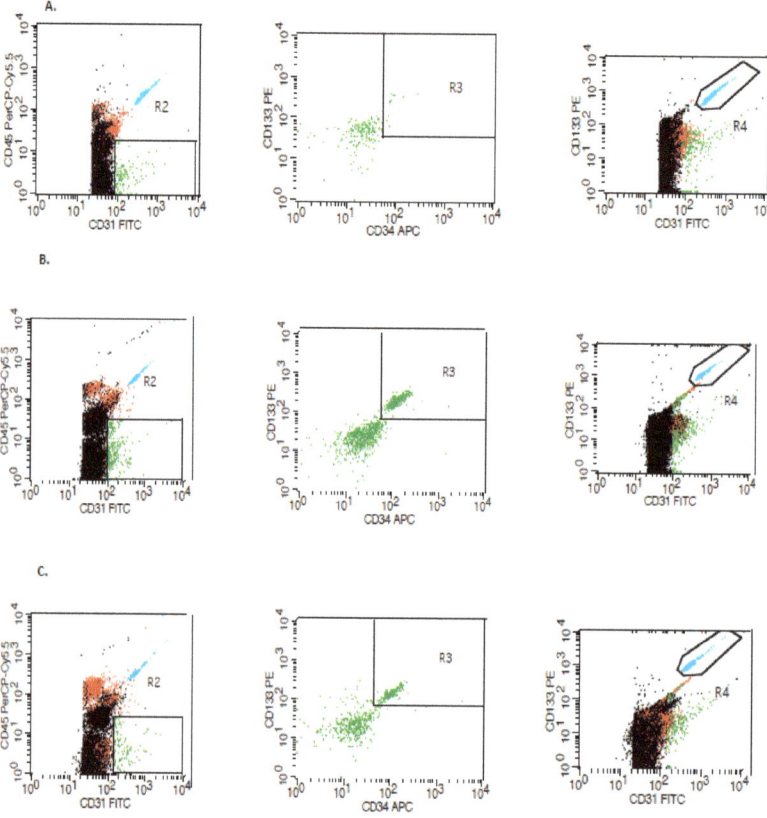

Figure 1. Sample of selected flow cytometric plots for the identification of circulating endothelial. progenitor cells in the control group (**A**), in patients with ischemic stroke (**B**), and hemorrhagic stroke (**C**). Peridinin-Chlorophyll-Protein–Cyanine-conjugated anti-CD45 (CD45 PerCP-Cy5.5), allophycocyanin-conjugated anti-CD34 antibodies (CD34 APC), phycoerythrin-conjugated anti-CD133 (CD133 PE), fluorescin isothiocyanate anti-CD31 (CD31 FITC). R2,R3,R4—regions defined in flow-cytometric dot plots for the detection of relevant surface markers of mononuclear cells, R2—gate for CD45 PerCP-Cy5.5/CD31 FITC; R3—gate for CD133 PE/CD34 APC; R4—gate for CD133 PE/CD31 FITC.

2.3. Clinical Outcome

Both the clinical and functional condition were assessed by means of standardized research tools: the National Institute of Health Stroke Scale (NIHSS) and the Modified Rankin Scale (mRS) [18,19], within the first 24 h after admission to the hospital (1st day) and on the 8th day of hospitalization. Two subgroups of stroke patients were identified based on the stroke severity: A subgroup with a mild and moderate neurological deficit (0–10 points on the NIHSS scale), and a subgroup with a severe neurological deficit (>10 points on the NIHSS scale). Due to the functional condition, two subgroups of patients with stroke were identified: Those with a favorable prognosis (0–2 points on the mRS scale) and those with an unfavorable prognosis (3–5 points on the mRS scale).

2.4. Statistical Analysis

The statistical analysis of collected data was performed with the help of the statistical program STATISTICA—version 13.1 (Dell Inc., Round Rock, TX, USA). Due to the unfulfilled assumptions related to the possibility of using parametric tests (Shapiro–Wilk for normality and Levene's for homogeneity of variance), non-parametric tests were used in the analysis, namely the Mann–Whitney U test, Wilcoxon test, Kruskal–Wallis test, Spearman's rank correlation test, and independence chi-square test. Variables not characterized by normal distribution were described using the median (median value), quartile distribution, and range. Multivariate regression analysis (MANOVA) was conducted to estimate relations between EPCs and clinical or functional condition. The significance level $p < 0.05$ was considered statistically significant.

3. Results

The general characteristics and comparison of the population of the studied patients are presented in Table 1. Patients with hemorrhagic stroke were in a significantly worse functional condition (mRS) on the first day compared to ischemic stroke subjects.

Table 1. Comparison of selected anthropometric, biochemical parameters, risk factors, and clinical status in patients with ischemic stroke, hemorrhagic stroke, and in the control group.

Parameter	Ischemic Stroke	Hemorrhage	Control Group	p-Values
Sex, male, (%) [1]	62.1	55.3	36.4	0.1088
Sex, female, (%) [1]	37.9	44.7	63.6	0.1267
Age (median, range) [3]	69 (45–88)	73.5 (45–91)	63.5 (50–82)	0.1034
Smoking, (%) [1]	32.6	28.9	24.5	0.3457
Hypertension, (%) [1]	90.9	94.7	81.8	0.2555
Hyperlipidemia, (%) [1]	60.6	50	54.5	0.566
Diabetes, (%) [1]	37.9	21.8	27.3	0.186
CRP (mg/L), (median, range) [2]	4.50 (0.39–58.12)	5.79 (0.38–70.1)	-	0.2117
Homocystein (µg/mL) (median, range) [2]	11.05 (3.52–30.92)	9.22 (2.65–42.8)	-	0.6341
Fibrinogen (g/L), (median, range) [2]	284 (59–590)	315.5 (157–463)	-	0.2985
NIHSS 1st day (points) (median, range) [2]	6 (2–21)	6 (1–21)	-	0.6103
NIHSS 8th day (points) (median, range) [2]	3 (0–15)	3 (0–14)	-	0.7086
mRS 1st day (points) (median, range) [2]	4 (2–5)	5 (3–5)	-	0.0001 *
mRS 8th day (points) (median, range) [2]	2 (0–5)	3 (0–4)	-	0.2377

[1] chi square test, [2] Mann–Whitney U test, [3] Kruskal–Wallis test, * statistical significance, CRP, C-reactive protein; NIHSS, National Institute of Health Stroke Scale; mRS, modified Rankin Scale.

There was a significantly higher number of EPCs in the blood on the first day of stroke (regardless of etiology) compared to the control group (respectively, med. 17.75 cells/µL (0–488 cells/µL) vs. 5.24 cells/µL (0–95 cells/µL); $p = 0.0006$). There was a significantly higher number of EPCs in the blood serum on the first day of ischemic stroke compared to the control group (med. 18.65 cells/µL (0–278 cells/µL) vs. 5.24 cells/µL (0–95 cells/µL); $p = 0.0011$) and on the first day of hemorrhagic stroke compared to the control group (med. 17.17 cells/µL (0–488 cells/µL) vs. 5.24 cells/µL (0–95 cells/µL); $p = 0.0034$) (Figure 2).

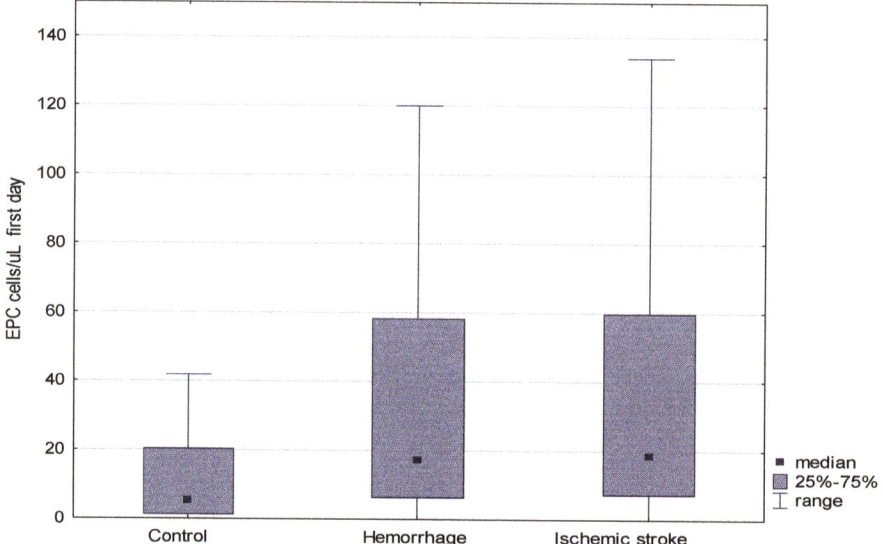

Figure 2. Comparison of the number of endothelial progenitor cells (EPCs) on the first day between the patients with ischemic stroke, hemorrhagic stroke, and the control group.

There were no significant differences in the number of EPCs between patients with ischemic and hemorrhagic stroke both on the first day and on the eighth day of the disease. Prospective analysis did not show significant changes in the number of EPCs in the blood of patients with stroke (regardless of etiology) between the first and eighth day of the disease.

The number of EPCs did not differ significantly in men and women, both in the whole population and in the group with stroke (regardless of etiology) on the first day or in the group with stroke on the eight day of the disease. There were no significant correlations between the age and the number of EPCs on the first day in the whole population ($R = 0.0370$, $p = 0.6809$), and in patients with hemorrhagic stroke on the first ($R = 0.0783$, $p = 0.6402$) and eighth day ($R = -0.0762$, $p = 0.6489$) and ischemic stroke on the first ($R = -0.0326$, $p = 0.7949$) and eighth day ($R = 0.0939$, $p = 0.4529$).

There were no significant relationships between the number of EPCs on the first and eighth day after a stroke event with hypertension, hyperlipidemia, smoking, and diabetes in ischemic stroke (Table 2), as well as in hemorrhagic stroke (Table 3).

Table 2. Comparison of the number of endothelial progenitor cells (EPCs) on the first and eighth day of ischemic stroke between patients with present and absent vascular risk factors.

Parameter	EPCs/µL 1st Day			EPCs/µL 8th Day		
	Present	Absent	p-Values *	Present	Absent	p-Values *
Hypertension	17.14 (0–278.11)	23.24 (2.77–112.21)	0.8847	24.45 (0.46–316.89)	62.47 (18–323.29)	0.0536
Hyperlipidemia	14.69 (0–178.86)	25.55 (4.12–278.11)	0.1785	25.02 (0.40–316.89)	25.72 (2.03–323.29)	0.4724
Diabetes	14.47 (0–178.86)	25.12 (1.01–278.11)	0.0701	31.16 (0.40–323.29)	24.51 (0.46–316.89)	0.7014
Smoking	16.32 (0–178.86)	22.13 (2.77–112.21)	0.1654	27.85 (0.40–323.29)	31.69 (2.03–323.29)	0.1324

* Mann–Whitney U test. Results are median (range) in cells/µL.

Table 3. Comparison of the number of endothelial progenitor cells (EPCs) on the first and eighth day of hemorrhagic stroke between patients with present and absent vascular risk factors.

Parameter	EPCs/µL 1st Day			EPCs/µL 8th Day		
	Present	Absent	p-Values *	Present	Absent	p-Values *
Hypertension	17.75 (0–488.41)	4.43 (3.75–5.11)	0.0722	17.93 (0–325.43)	22.44 (0.10–44.78)	0.4522
Hyperlipidemia	31.23 (0.62–338.00)	15.51 (0–488.41)	0,7042	37.62 (1.21–325.43)	11.64 (0–233.20)	0.1443
Diabetes	17.48 (6.36–58.38)	16.47 (0–488.41)	0.7608	17.15 (3.01–10020)	17.93 (0–325.43)	0.7608
Smoking	25.67 (0.62–338.00)	21.98 (0–488.41)	0.6983	23.68 (1.21–325.43)	17.44 (0.10–233.20)	0.6684

* Mann–Whitney U test Results are median (range) in cells/uL.

There were no significant correlations between EPCs on the first and eighth day after a stroke event with the selected biochemical parameters, both in ischemic and hemorrhagic stroke (Table 4).

Table 4. Correlations between the number of endothelial progenitor cells (EPCs) on the first and eighth day of ischemic and hemorrhagic stroke and the selected biochemical parameters.

	EPCs/µL 1st Day				EPCs/µL 8th Day			
	Ischemic Stroke		Hemorrhage		Ischemic Stroke		Hemorrhage	
	R	p	R	p	R	p	R	p
CRP	0.1630	0.1909	−0.0242	0.8854	0.0986	0.4308	−0.1526	0.3602
fibrinogen	−0.1731	0.1644	0.1135	0.4974	0.1095	0.3816	−0.0459	0.7840
homocystein	−0.0879	0.4827	0.0578	0.7309	−0.0376	0.7639	0.2465	0.1356

Spearman's rank correlation, CRP, C-reactive protein, R, correlation coefficient.

There were no significant correlations between the number of EPCs on the first day of stroke (regardless of etiology) and the clinical condition (NIHSS scale) on the first day (R = 0.0128; p = 0.8790) and on the eighth day (R = 0.1300; p = 0.1882), as well as between the number of EPCs on the eighth day of stroke and the clinical condition on the first day (R = 0.1846; p = 0.0607) and on the eighth day (R = 0.1243; p = 0.2085). There were no significant relationships between the number of EPCs on the first day of stroke (regardless of etiology) and the functional condition (mRS scale) on the first day (R = 0.0318; p = 0.7480), and on the eighth day (R = −0.1239; p = 0.2099), as well as between the number of EPCs on the eighth day of stroke and the functional condition on the first day (R = 0.0049; p = 0.9606) and on the eighth day (R = 0.0672; p = 0.4973). Considering the etiology of stroke, there were no significant correlations between the number of EPCs on the first and eighth day of the disease and the clinical or functional condition, both in ischemic and hemorrhagic stroke (Table 5).

Table 5. Correlations between the number of endothelial progenitor cells (EPCs) on the first and eighth day of ischemic and hemorrhagic stroke and the clinical and functional status on the first and eighth day of stroke.

	EPCs/µL 1st Day				EPCs/µL 8th Day			
	Ischemic Stroke		Hemorrhagic Stroke		Ischemic Stroke		Hemorrhagic Stroke	
	R	p	R	p	R	p	R	p
NIHSS 1st day	−0.0469	0.7084	0.0932	0.5778	0.1842	0.1387	0.2108	0.2038
NIHSS 8th day	−0.1469	0.2388	−0.0888	0.5959	0.1446	0.2465	0.0857	0.6085
mRS 1st day	0.1359	0.2765	−0.1228	0.4624	0.0230	0.8544	0.0837	0.6171
mRS 8th day	−0.1355	0.2766	0.1300	0.1882	0.0858	0.4933	0.0648	

Spearman's rank correlation, NIHSS, National Institute of Health Stroke Scale, mRS, modified Rankin Scale. R, correlation coefficient.

There were no significant differences between patients with severe and mild neurological deficit on the first day of stroke in relation to the number of EPCs on the first day (total $p = 0.4802$; ischemic stroke $p = 0.7837$; hemorrhagic stroke $p = 0.4166$) and on the eighth day (total $p = 0.1794$; ischemic stroke $p = 0.2969$; hemorrhagic stroke $p = 0.4457$). Similarly, there were no significant differences between patients with severe and mild neurological deficit on the eighth day of stroke in relation to the number of EPCs on the first day (total $p = 0.4545$; ischemic stroke $p = 0.3248$; hemorrhagic stroke $p = 0.9568$) and on the eighth day (total $p = 0.6479$; ischemic stroke $p = 0.2069$; hemorrhagic stroke $p = 0.5335$). There were no significant differences between patients with favorable and unfavorable prognosis on the first day of stroke in relation to the number of EPCs on the first day (total $p = 0.9383$; ischemic stroke $p = 0.8786$; hemorrhagic stroke $p = 0.8903$) and on the eighth day (total $p = 0.9072$; ischemic stroke $p = 0.9264$; hemorrhagic stroke $p = 0.9278$). Similarly, there were no significant differences between patients with a favorable and unfavorable prognosis on the eighth day of stroke in relation to the number of EPCs on the first day (total $p = 0.1470$; ischemic stroke $p = 0.2369$; hemorrhagic stroke $p = 0.4559$) and on the eighth day (total $p = 0.6969$; ischemic stroke $p = 0.9485$; hemorrhagic stroke $p = 0.4559$).

In the multivariate model of regression adjusted for sex, type of stroke, and clinical or functional condition, we demonstrated that in females, a higher number of EPCs on the first day of stroke is related to a favorable outcome on the eighth day after the stroke onset compared to males ($p = 0.0355$) (Figure 3). There were no significant correlations regarding the other analyzed dependencies.

There was a negative but significant correlation between the volume of hemorrhagic focus on the first day of hemorrhage and the number of EPCs on the first day of hemorrhagic stroke ($R = -0.3378$, $p = 0.0471$) (Figure 4).

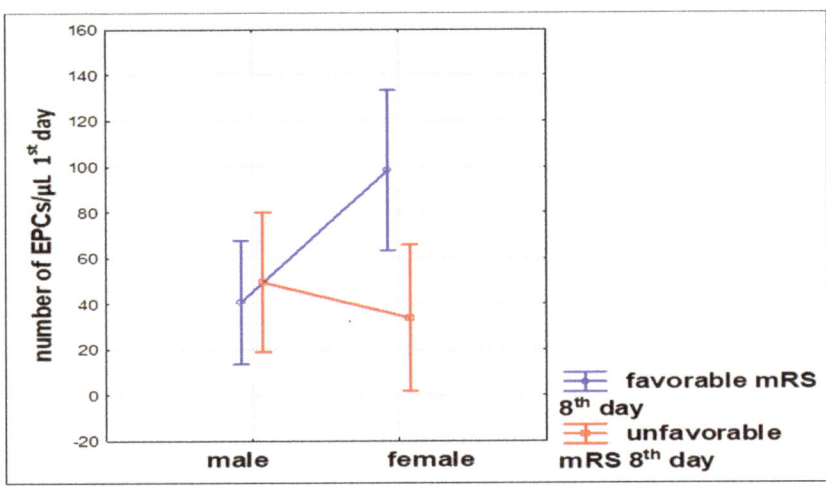

Figure 3. Multivariate analysis between the number of endothelial progenitor cells (EPCs) on the first day of stroke, sex, and functional outcome on the eighth day in the modified Rankin scale (mRS).

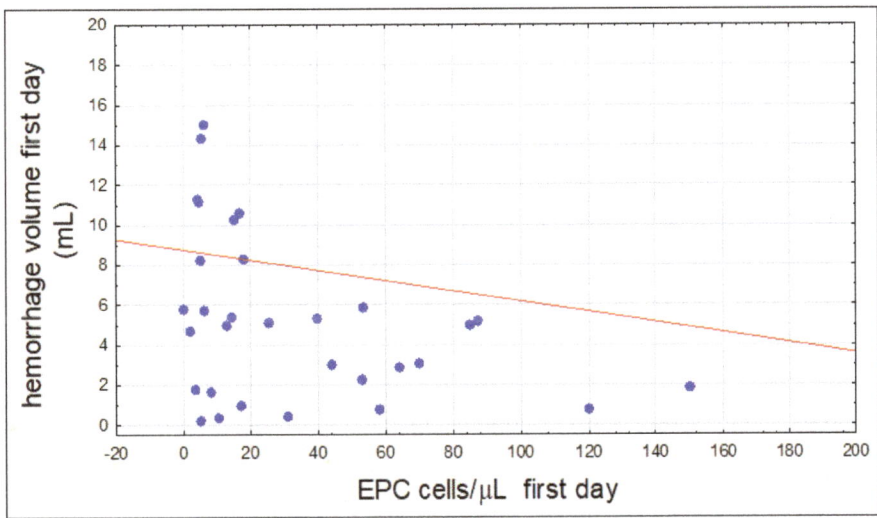

Figure 4. Correlation between the number of endothelial progenitor cells (EPCs) on the first day of hemorrhagic stroke and the volume of hemorrhagic focus on the first day of stroke.

There were no significant correlations between the number of EPCs on the eighth day of hemorrhagic stroke with the volume of hemorrhagic focus on the first day ($R = -0.0791, p = 0.6513$) and on the eighth day ($R = -0.0002, p = 0.9897$), as well as between the number of EPCs on the first day and the volume of hemorrhagic focus on the eighth day ($R = -0.1294, p = 0.4803$). A negative correlation between the number of EPCs on the first day of hemorrhagic stroke and the degree of regression of the hemorrhagic focus was demonstrated ($R = -0.3896, p = 0.0367$) (Figure 5).

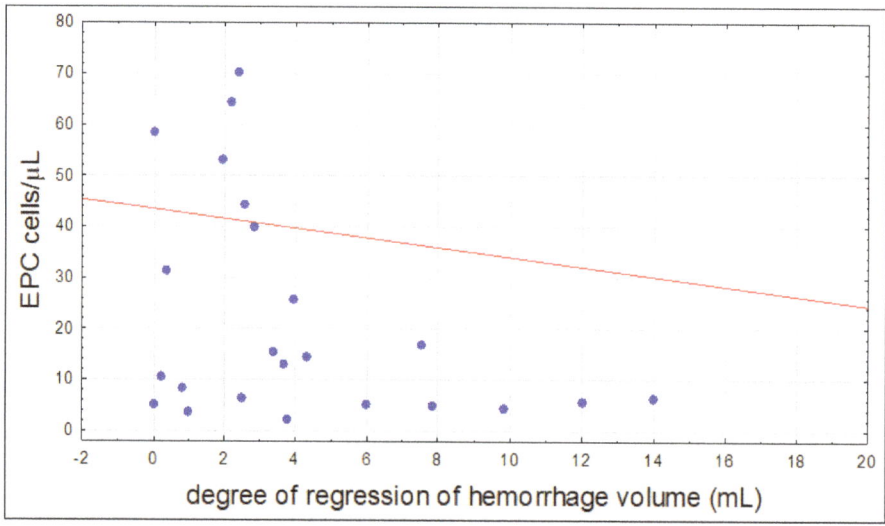

Figure 5. Correlation between the number of endothelial progenitor cells (EPCs) on the first day of hemorrhagic stroke and the degree of regression of the hemorrhagic focus.

4. Discussion

The results of this study showed that, in the acute phase of ischemic and hemorrhagic stroke, a significantly higher number of EPCs were observed than in the control group. This confirms that damage to the cerebral endothelium, whether in the course of acute ischemia or mechanical damage to the vascular wall, leads to significant mobilization and proliferation of EPCs. This is probably the mechanism of differentiation into mature endothelial cells, which, due to the production of numerous cytokines, are actively involved in the repair and neovascularization of damaged brain tissues [7]. Similar conclusions were drawn by Yip et al., Meamar et al., and Regueiro et al. [20–22], who, assessing patients in the acute phase of ischemic stroke, also found a significantly higher number of EPCs than in control. Similarly, Paczkowska et al. [23] obtained a higher number of EPCs in the acute stage of hemorrhagic stroke in comparison to the control group. The results of our research and the above show that regardless of the etiology, it is the state of sudden damage to vascular endothelium (similar to acute myocardial infarction and acute limb ischemia) that clearly activates EPCs' proliferation, where EPCs are the main repair and regenerative element of the damaged endothelial cells [24,25]. It is worth noting that Ghani et al. and Deng Y et al. [26,27] in their studies obtained different results and a lower number of EPCs in the acute phase of ischemic stroke than those in the control group, and Zhou et al. [28] noted a lower number of EPCs in patients with both acute ischemic and hemorrhagic stroke, compared to the control group. The differences in the results of the above studies could have resulted from a different population of patients and a different configuration of superficial antigens used in flow cytometry to detect EPCs.

The data in the literature show that, in acute cerebrovascular incidents, EPCs are activated within the first 24 h, reach their maximum blood level around the 7th day, and gradually decrease after 21–28 days. Most authors assessed only patients with ischemic stroke [27,29,30] and only a few assessed patients with either ischemic or hemorrhagic stroke [28]. Taguchi et al. and Marti-Fabregas et al. [29,30] showed statistically significantly more EPCs after 7 days of acute ischemic stroke than during the first 24 h. Zhou et al. [28] also obtained similar results but in both ischemic and hemorrhagic stroke. In this work, although in both types of stroke the number of cells was higher on the eighth day of the disease than on the first day, these differences did not reach statistical significance. Nevertheless, the results of this study confirmed that mobilization of EPCs occurs within a few hours after the onset of symptoms of stroke; within 24 h, the number of EPCs in the blood serum reaches a very high level, and the state of high activation persists for at least the first week of the disease. Due to the fact that the area of interest was the acute phase of cerebrovascular incidents, the number of EPCs on day 21–28 was not assessed. In addition, in this study, the number of EPCs did not differ significantly in patients with ischemic and hemorrhagic stroke (similar results were presented by Zhou et al.), both on the first and on the eighth day, which suggests that acute brain endothelial damage, and not its etiopathogenesis, plays a leading role in the activation of EPCs.

In this research, no significant correlations were found between the number of EPCs and the selected biochemical parameters of blood (CRP, homocysteine, fibrinogen), as well as risk factors of vascular diseases, which suggests their potential lack of influence on the number of activated EPCs. It is suggested that the above factors may affect the chronic number of EPCs in the blood, without affecting their mobilization and activation capacity in acute endothelial damage, such as in stroke.

In the present study, it was not shown that the number of EPCs in the acute phase of stroke significantly affected the clinical and functional status of the patients or was associated with early prognosis. There were no significant correlations between the number of EPCs on the first and eighth day of the stroke and the score on the mRS or NIHSS scale on the first and eighth day, both in ischemic and hemorrhagic stroke. In addition, the division of patients into groups with a favorable and unfavorable prognosis and with a mild and severe neurological deficit did not differentiate both types of strokes based on the number of EPCs. Zhou et al. also did not demonstrate the effect of the number of EPCs on the clinical state and prognosis of patients (both in ischemic and hemorrhagic stroke) and Marti-Fabregas et al. did not find a significant correlation in ischemic stroke [28,30]. In contrast, Sobrino et al. [31] noted that a large number of EPCs on the seventh day of ischemic stroke is associated with a better clinical condition, expressed by a lower score of the NIHSS scale. However, it should be noted that they were only evaluating patients with non-lacunar stroke, while the analysis of this work is related only to patients with lacunar stroke. On the other hand, Yip et al. [20] noted that a small number of EPCs on the second day of ischemic stroke is associated with a worse clinical deficit, expressed by a higher score on the NIHSS scale. However, they took into account all patients with ischemic stroke, regardless of the etiopathogenesis, i.e., both patients with lacunar and non-lacunar strokes. Pias-Peleteiro et al. [32] analyzed the relationships between the number of EPCs and the functional condition and prognosis in patients with hemorrhagic stroke and showed that a higher number of EPCs on the seventh day is associated with a better distant prognosis expressed by a small number of points on the mRS scale on the 12th month from the hemorrhage. Conversely, Sobrino et al. [33] noted that a large number of EPCs on the seventh day of hemorrhagic stroke is associated with a better prognosis and functional state of patients in the third month from the hemorrhage, also expressed by lower scores on the mRS scale. Nevertheless, ambiguous and often contradictory results of studies on the impact of EPCs on the prognosis of stroke patients suggest further research in this subject.

Multivariate analysis showed that the relation between the number of EPCs and functional condition may depend on the sex. In females, a higher number of EPCs is related with a favorable functional status. This preliminary finding reported in this study underlines the potential impact of sex hormones for a possible role of EPCs in stroke prognosis. More research is required to improve these initial findings.

The results of this study showed that a large number of EPCs on the first day of hemorrhagic stroke is associated with a smaller volume of the hemorrhagic focus. Zhou et al. [26] also analyzed similar relationships but found no significant association between the number of EPCs in the acute stage of hemorrhagic stroke and the volume of the hemorrhagic focus. In contrast, Pias-Peleteiro et al. and Sobrino et al. [32,33] showed a similar significant negative correlation between the number of EPCs on the seventh day of hemorrhagic stroke and the volume of the residual hemorrhagic focus, respectively, on the third and sixth month after the hemorrhage. Other authors analyzed the volume of the ischemic focus and showed that a large number of EPCs in the acute phase of ischemic stroke is associated with a relatively smaller volume of the ischemic focus in the diffusion sequence (DWI) [31,34]. In the present study, the relationship between the number of EPCs and the volume of the ischemic focus was not analyzed.

To our best knowledge, this is the first study analyzing the relationship between the number of EPCs and the degree of regression of the hemorrhagic focus. The significant negative correlation obtained in this research is a novelty in this field and is in contradiction to the well-known repair and regenerative function of EPCs suggested by most authors. Subjects with a higher number of EPCs on the first day presented with the lowest regression level of the hematoma volume. The results reported in this study may shed new light on the role of EPCs in hemorrhagic stroke and significantly undermine and raise doubt to their repair properties. Most of the recent pre-clinical studies in animal models demonstrated a protective and regenerative function of EPCs after cerebrovascular insult [12,35–38]. Several mechanisms of possible action were reported, especially by suppressing oxidative stress, apoptosis, mitochondrial impairment, and inflammation processes [35–37]. The essential role of EPCs in increasing brain angiogenesis has been highlighted in animal models of stroke [12,38]. However, the lack of references in the literature and the small number of patients with hemorrhagic stroke in this study suggest that verification of the obtained data and further research in this area in multi-center randomized trials is needed.

This study has its limitations. The effect of the number of EPCs on the distant prognosis in patients with stroke was not analyzed. The moderate number of patients and small control group is also a limitation. However, these numbers seemed sufficient to draw conclusions. Conversely, for formal reasons (conscious consent for the study for the bioethics committee), the analysis did not include patients with a severe neurological deficit, e.g., patients with consciousness disorders, so the study did not include the actual cross-section of patients with stroke but only patients with a milder clinical condition. Determination of EPCs by only one measurement at different times within the first 24 h of stroke is also a main limitation and could have a great impact on the results. The authors are aware that for the dynamic changes in the function and number of EPCs under ischemic or inflammatory conditions, the use of microbeads and Q-dot-based nanoparticles is superior to conventional flow cytometry. Most statistical analyses were univariate, which could have reduced the reliability of the results.

5. Conclusions

The study showed that endothelial progenitor cells are an early marker of cerebral vascular damage, both in ischemic and hemorrhagic stroke. The research highlights, for the first time, a negative correlation between the level of EPCs and the degree of regression of a hemorrhagic focus and that this relation between the number of EPCs and functional condition may depend on the sex. However, the prognostic value of EPCs for the clinical condition and early prognosis of stroke patients remains doubtful.

Author Contributions: Conceptualization, A.W.; methodology, A.W., G.K., J.B., K.Z.; software, J.B., K.Z. validation, G.K., D.R.; formal Analysis, A.W., K.F., and G.K.; investigation, A.W.; resources, D.R., Z.S.; data curation, J.B., A.L.; writing—original draft preparation, A.W. and K.F.; writing—review and editing, A.W.; visualization, A.W.; supervision, G.K., D.R., R.Ś.; project administration, A.W. and G.K. All authors have read and agreed to the published version of the manuscript.

Funding: This research received no external funding.

Conflicts of Interest: The authors declare no conflict of interest.

References

1. Naghavi, M.; Wang, H.; Lozano, R.; Davis, A.; Liang, X.; Zhou, M.; Vollset, S.E.; Ozgoren, A.A.; Abdalla, S.; Abd-Allah, F.; et al. Global, regional, and national age-sex specific all-cause and cause-specific mortality for 240 causes of death, 1990-2013: A systematic analysis for the Global Burden of Disease Study 2013. *Lancet* **2015**, *385*, 117–171.

2. Mozaffarian, D.; Benjamin, E.J.; Go, A.S.; Arnett, D.K.; Blaha, M.J.; Cushman, M.; de Ferranti, S.; Despres, J.P.; Fullerton, H.J.; Howard, W.J.; et al. Heart disease and stroke statistics—2015 update: A report from the American Heart Association. *Circulation* **2015**, *131*, 434–441. [CrossRef]
3. Giwa, M.O.; Williams, J.; Elderfield, K.; Jiwa, N.S.; Bridges, L.R.; Kalaria, R.N.; Markus, H.S.; Esiri, M.M.; Hainsworth, A.H. Neuropathologic evidence of endothelial changes in cerebral small vessel disease. *Neurology* **2011**, *78*, 167–174. [CrossRef] [PubMed]
4. Grysiewicz, R.A.; Thomas, K.; Pandey, D.K. Epidemiology of Ischemic and Hemorrhagic Stroke: Incidence, Prevalence, Mortality, and Risk Factors. *Neurol. Clin.* **2008**, *26*, 871–895. [CrossRef]
5. Li, Y.-F.; Ren, L.-N.; Guo, G.; Cannella, L.A.; Chernaya, V.; Samuel, S.; Liu, S.-X.; Wang, H.; Yang, X. Endothelial progenitor cells in ischemic stroke: An exploration from hypothesis to therapy. *J. Hematol. Oncol.* **2015**, *8*, 33. [CrossRef]
6. Du, F.; Zhou, J.; Gong, R.; Huang, X.; Pansuria, M.; Virtue, A.; Li, X.; Wang, H.; Yang, X.F. Endothelial progenitor cells in atherosclerosis. *Front. Biosci.* **2012**, *17*, 2327–2349. [CrossRef] [PubMed]
7. Chu, K.; Jung, K.-H.; Lee, S.-T.; Park, H.-K.; Sinn, D.-I.; Kim, J.-M.; Kim, N.-H.; Kim, J.-H.; Kim, S.-J.; Song, E.-C.; et al. Circulating endothelial progenitor cells as a new marker of endothelial dysfunction or repair in acute stroke. *Stroke* **2008**, *39*, 1441–1447. [CrossRef]
8. Gutiérrez-Fernández, M.; Otero-Ortega, L.; Ramos-Cejudo, J.; Rodríguez-Frutos, B.; Fuentes, B.; Tejedor, E.D. Adipose tissue-derived mesenchymal stem cells as a strategy to improve recovery after stroke. *Expert Opin. Boil. Ther.* **2015**, *15*, 873–881. [CrossRef]
9. Moubarik, C.; Guillet, B.; Youssef, B.; Codaccioni, J.L.; Pierchecci, M.D.; Sebatier, F.; Lionel, P.; Dou, L.; Foucault-Bertaud, A.; Velly, L.; et al. Transplanted late outgrowth endothelial progenitor cells as cel therapy product for stroke. *Stem Cell Rev.* **2011**, *7*, 208–220. [CrossRef]
10. Nakamura, K.; Tsurushima, H.; Marushima, A.; Nagano, M.; Yamashita, T.; Suzuki, K.; Ohneda, O.; Matsumura, A. A subpopulation of endothelial progenitor cells with low aldehyde dehydrogenase activity attenuates acute ischemic brain injury in rats. *Biochem. Biophys. Res. Commun.* **2012**, *418*, 87–92. [CrossRef]
11. Fan, Y.; Shen, F.; Frenzel, T.; Zhu, W.; Ye, J.; Liu, J.; Chen, Y.; Su, H.; Young, W.L.; Yang, G.-Y. Endothelial progenitor cell transplantation improves long-term stroke outcome in mice. *Ann. Neurol.* **2009**, *67*, 488–497. [CrossRef] [PubMed]
12. Rosell, A.; Morancho, A.; Navarro-Sobrino, M.; Martinez-Saez, E.; Guillamon, M.M.H.; Lope-Piedrafita, S.; Barceló, V.; Borrás, F.; Penalba, A.; Garcia-Bonilla, L.; et al. Factors Secreted by Endothelial Progenitor Cells Enhance Neurorepair Responses after Cerebral Ischemia in Mice. *PLoS ONE* **2013**, *8*, e73244. [CrossRef] [PubMed]
13. Liao, S.; Luo, C.; Cao, B.; Hu, H.; Wang, S.; Yue, H.; Chen, L.; Zhou, Z. Endothelial Progenitor Cells for Ischemic Stroke: Update on Basic Research and Application. *Stem Cells Int.* **2017**, *2017*. [CrossRef] [PubMed]
14. Sacco, R.L.; Kasner, S.E.; Broderick, J.P.; Caplan, L.R.; Connors, J.J.; Culebras, A.; Elkind, M.S.; George, M.G.; Hamdan, A.D.; Higashida, R.T.; et al. An updated definition of stroke for the 21st century: A statement for healthcare professionals from the American Heart Association/American Stroke Association. *Stroke* **2013**, *44*, 2064–2089. [CrossRef]
15. Wardlaw, J.M.; Smith, E.E.; Biessels, G.J.; Cordonnier, C.; Fazekas, F.; Frayne, R.; Lindley, R.I.; O'Brien, J.; Barkhof, F.; Benavente, O.R.; et al. Neuroimaging standards for research into small vessel disease and its contribution to ageing and neurodegeneration. *Lancet Neurol.* **2013**, *12*, 822–838. [CrossRef]
16. Mancuso, P.; Antoniotti, P.; Quarna, J.; Calleri, A.; Rabascio, C.; Tacchetti, C.; Braidotti, P.; Wu, H.-K.; Zurita, A.J.; Saronni, L.; et al. Validation of a Standardized Method for Enumerating Circulating Endothelial Cells and Progenitors: Flow Cytometry and Molecular and Ultrastructural Analyses. *Clin. Cancer Res.* **2009**, *15*, 267–273. [CrossRef]
17. Ruszkowska-Ciastek, B.; Sokup, A.; Leszcz, M.; Drela, E.; Stankowska, K.; Boinska, J.; Haor, B.; Ślusarz, R.; Lisewska, B.; Gadomska, G.; et al. The number of circulating endothelial progenitor cells in healthy individuals—Effect of some anthropometric and environmental factors (a pilot study). *Adv. Med. Sci.* **2015**, *60*, 58–63. [CrossRef]
18. Lyden, P. Using the National Institutes of Health Stroke Scale. *Stroke* **2017**, *48*, 513–519. [CrossRef]
19. Quinn, T.J.; Dawson, J.; Walters, M.R.; Lees, K.R. Variability in modified Rankin scoring across a large cohort of international observers. *Stroke* **2008**, *39*, 2975–2979. [CrossRef]

20. Yip, H.-K.; Chang, L.-T.; Chang, W.-N.; Lu, C.-H.; Liou, C.-W.; Lan, M.-Y.; Liu, J.S.; Youssef, A.A.; Chang, H.-W. Level and Value of Circulating Endothelial Progenitor Cells in Patients After Acute Ischemic Stroke. *Stroke* **2008**, *39*, 69–74. [CrossRef] [PubMed]
21. Meamar, R.; Nikyar, H.; Dehghani, L.; Talebi, M.; Dehghani, M.; Ghasemi, M.; Ansari, B.; Saadatnia, M. The role of endothelial progenitor cells in transient ischemic attack patients for future cerebrovascular events. *J. Res. Med. Sci.* **2016**, *21*, 47. [CrossRef] [PubMed]
22. Regueiro, A.; Cuadrado-Godia, E.; Bueno-Betí, C.; Diaz-Ricart, M.; Oliveras, A.; Novella, S.; Gené, G.G.; Jung, C.; Subirana, I.; Ortiz-Pérez, J.T.; et al. Mobilization of endothelial progenitor cells in acute cardiovascular events in the PROCELL study: Time-course after acute myocardial infarction and stroke. *J. Mol. Cell. Cardiol.* **2015**, *80*, 146–155. [CrossRef]
23. Paczkowska, E.; Gołąb-Janowska, M.; Bajer-Czajkowska, A.; Machalinska, A.; Ustianowski, P.; Rybicka, M.; Kłos, P.; Dziedziejko, V.; Safranow, K.; Nowacki, P.; et al. Increased circulating endothelial progenitor cells in patients with haemorrhagic and ischaemic stroke: The role of Endothelin-1. *J. Neurol. Sci.* **2013**, *325*, 90–99. [CrossRef]
24. Leone, A.M.; Rutella, S.; Bonanno, G.; Abbate, A.; Rebuzzi, A.G.; Giovannini, S.; Lombardi, M.; Galiuto, L.; Liuzzo, G.; Andreotti, F.; et al. Mobilization of bone marrow-derived stem cells after myocardial infarction and left ventricular function. *Eur. Hear. J.* **2005**, *26*, 1196–1204. [CrossRef]
25. Roberts, N.; Jahangiri, M.; Xu, Q. Progenitor cells in vascular disease. *J. Cell. Mol. Med.* **2005**, *9*, 583–591. [CrossRef]
26. Ghani, U.; Shuaib, A.; Salam, A.; Nasir, A.; Shuaib, U.; Jeerakathil, T.; Sher, F.; O'Rourke, F.; Nasser, A.M.; Schwindt, B.; et al. Endothelial Progenitor Cells During Cerebrovascular Disease. *Stroke* **2005**, *36*, 151–153. [CrossRef] [PubMed]
27. Deng, Y.; Wang, J.; He, G.; Qu, F.; Zheng, M. Mobilization of endothelial progenitor cell in patients with acute ischemic stroke. *Neurol. Sci.* **2017**, *39*, 437–443. [CrossRef] [PubMed]
28. Zhou, W.-J.; Zhu, D.-L.; Yang, G.-Y.; Zhang, Y.; Wang, H.-Y.; Ji, K.-D.; Lu, Y.-M.; Gao, P.-J.; Zhou, D.-L.Z.W.-J. Circulating endothelial progenitor cells in Chinese patients with acute stroke. *Hypertens. Res.* **2009**, *32*, 306–310. [CrossRef] [PubMed]
29. Taguchi, A.; Matsuyama, T.; Moriwaki, H.; Hayashi, T.; Hayashida, K.; Nagatsuka, K.; Todo, K.; Mori, K.; Stern, D.M.; Soma, T.; et al. Circulating CD34-Positive Cells Provide an Index of Cerebrovascular Function. *Circulation* **2004**, *109*, 2972–2975. [CrossRef] [PubMed]
30. Martí-Fàbregas, J.; Crespo, J.; Delgado-Mederos, R.; Martínez-Ramírez, S.; Peña, E.; Marín, R.; Dinia, L.; Jiménez-Xarrié, E.; Fernández-Arcos, A.; Pérez-Pérez, J.; et al. Endothelial progenitor cells in acute ischemic stroke. *Brain Behav.* **2013**, *3*, 649–655. [CrossRef] [PubMed]
31. Sobrino, T.; Hurtado, O.; Moro, M.A.; Rodríguez-Yáñez, M.; Castellanos, M.; Brea, D.; Moldes, O.; Blanco, M.; Arenillas, J.F.; Leira, R.; et al. The increase of circulating endothelial progenitor cells after acute ischemic stroke is associated with good outcome. *Stroke* **2007**, *38*, 2759–2764. [CrossRef] [PubMed]
32. Pías-Peleteiro, J.; Pérez-Mato, M.; López-Arias, E.; Rodríguez-Yáñez, M.; Blanco, M.; Campos, F.; Castillo, J.; Sobrino, T. Increased Endothelial Progenitor Cell Levels are Associated with Good Outcome in Intracerebral Hemorrhage. *Sci. Rep.* **2016**, *6*, 28724. [CrossRef]
33. Sobrino, T.; Arias, S.; Pérez-Mato, M.; Agulla, J.; Brea, D.; Rodríguez-Yáñez, M.; Castillo, J. Cd34+progenitor cells likely are involved in the good functional recovery after intracerebral hemorrhage in humans. *J. Neurosci. Res.* **2011**, *89*, 979–985. [CrossRef] [PubMed]
34. Bogoslovsky, T.; Chaudhry, A.; Latour, L.; Maric, D.; Luby, M.; Spatz, M.; Frank, J.; Warach, S. Endothelial progenitor cells correlate with lesion volume and growth in acute stroke. *Neurology* **2010**, *75*, 2059–2062. [CrossRef]
35. Park, D.-H.; Eve, D.J.; Musso, J.; Klasko, S.K.; Cruz, E.; Borlongan, C.V.; Sanberg, P.R. Inflammation and Stem Cell Migration to the Injured Brain in Higher Organisms. *Stem Cells Dev.* **2009**, *18*, 693–702. [CrossRef] [PubMed]
36. Tajiri, N.; Duncan, K.; Antoine, A.; Pabon, M.; Acosta, S.A.; De La Peña, I.C.; Hernadez-Ontiveros, D.G.; Shinozuka, K.; Ishikawa, H.; Kaneko, Y.; et al. Stem cell-paved biobridge facilitates neural repair in traumatic brain injury. *Front. Syst. Neurosci.* **2014**, *8*, 116. [CrossRef]

37. Chen, J.; Chopp, M. Neurorestorative treatment of stroke: Cell and pharmacological approaches. *NeuroRX* **2006**, *3*, 466–473. [CrossRef]
38. Morancho, A.; Ma, F.; Barcelo, V.; Giralt, D.; Montaner, J.; Rosell, A. Impaired vascular remodeling after endothelial progenitor cell transplantation in MMP9-deficient mice suffering cortical cerebral ischemia. *J. Cereb. Blood Flow Metab.* **2015**, *35*, 1547–1551. [CrossRef]

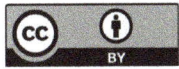

© 2020 by the authors. Licensee MDPI, Basel, Switzerland. This article is an open access article distributed under the terms and conditions of the Creative Commons Attribution (CC BY) license (http://creativecommons.org/licenses/by/4.0/).

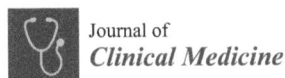

Article

Timing of Transfusion, not Hemoglobin Variability, Is Associated with 3-Month Outcomes in Acute Ischemic Stroke

Chulho Kim [1,2,*], Sang-Hwa Lee [1], Jae-Sung Lim [3], Mi Sun Oh [3], Kyung-Ho Yu [3], Yerim Kim [4], Ju-Hun Lee [4], Min Uk Jang [5], San Jung [6] and Byung-Chul Lee [3,*]

1. Department of Neurology, Chuncheon Sacred Heart Hospital, Chuncheon 24253, Korea; neurolsh@hallym.or.kr
2. Chuncheon Translational Research Center, Hallym University College of Medicine, Chuncheon 24252, Korea
3. Department of Neurology, Hallym University Sacred Heart Hospital, Anyang 14068, Korea; jaesunglim@hallym.or.kr (J.-S.L.); iyyar@hallym.or.kr (M.S.O.); ykh1030@hallym.or.kr (K.-H.Y.)
4. Department of Neurology, Kangdong Sacred Heart Hospital, Seoul 05355, Korea; brainyrk@kdh.or.kr (Y.K.); leejuhun@kdh.or.kr (J.-H.L.)
5. Department of Neurology, Dongtan Sacred Heart Hospital, Hwaseong 18450, Korea; mujang@hallym.or.kr
6. Department of Neurology, Kangnam Sacred Heart Hospital, Seoul 07440, Korea; neurojs@hallym.or.kr
* Correspondence: gumdol52@hallym.or.kr (C.K.); ssbrain@hallym.ac.kr (B.-C.L.); Tel.: +82-33-240-5255 (C.K.); +82-31-380-3741 (B.-C.L.); Fax: +82-33-255-6244 (C.K.); +82-31-381-4659 (B.-C.L.)

Received: 5 May 2020; Accepted: 20 May 2020; Published: 21 May 2020

Abstract: Objectives: This study aimed to investigate whether transfusions and hemoglobin variability affects the outcome of stroke after an acute ischemic stroke (AIS). Methods: We studied consecutive patients with AIS admitted in three tertiary hospitals who received red blood cell (RBC) transfusion (RBCT) during admission. Hemoglobin variability was assessed by minimum, maximum, range, median absolute deviation, and mean absolute change in hemoglobin level. Timing of RBCT was grouped into two categories: admission to 48 h (early) or more than 48 h (late) after hospitalization. Late RBCT was entered into multivariable logistic regression model. Poor outcome at three months was defined as a modified Rankin Scale score ≥3. Results: Of 2698 patients, 132 patients (4.9%) received a median of 400 mL (interquartile range: 400–840 mL) of packed RBCs. One-hundred-and-two patients (77.3%) had poor outcomes. The most common cause of RBCT was gastrointestinal bleeding (27.3%). The type of anemia was not associated with the timing of RBCT. Late RBCT was associated with poor outcome (odd ratio (OR), 3.55; 95% confidence interval (CI), 1.43–8.79; p-value = 0.006) in the univariable model. After adjusting for age, sex, Charlson comorbidity index, and stroke severity, late RBCT was a significant predictor (OR, 3.37; 95% CI, 1.14–9.99; p-value = 0.028) of poor outcome at three months. In the area under the receiver operating characteristics curve comparison, addition of hemoglobin variability indices did not improve the performance of the multivariable logistic model. Conclusion: Late RBCT, rather than hemoglobin variability indices, is a predictor for poor outcome in patients with AIS.

Keywords: anemia; cerebral infarction; blood transfusion; red blood cells; outcome assessment

1. Introduction

Anemia is an independent predictor for mortality and cardiovascular disease in the general population [1]. The incidence of anemia in acute ischemic stroke (AIS) is 20–30%, and both extreme of admission hemoglobin has a U-shaped association with poor clinical outcomes [1,2]. Cerebral autoregulation enables the brain to maintain sufficient oxygenation in the blood when the cerebral perfusion pressure decreases [3]. However, this autoregulatory response to brain ischemia is already impaired in ischemic penumbra. Thus, anemia can have harmful effects on infarct growth or poor outcome [4,5].

As the erythropoietin trial has failed to validate the efficacy of outcomes in patients with AIS [6], red blood cell transfusion (RBCT) is the only way to normalize hemoglobin in patients with anemia. However, RBCT is associated with increased blood viscosity and a proinflammatory/prothrombotic state related with stored RBC and its additives [7,8]. The impact of hemoglobin status and RBCT on acute ischemic stroke is controversial [1]. In several studies, low hemoglobin status was associated with poor outcomes in patients with AIS; however, these studies focused on admission hemoglobin level and did not assess whether RBCT was performed during the admission [1]. There are several reports on the association between RBCT and AIS outcome. Moman et al. have reported that RBCT is associated with a longer hospital stay in patients with AIS with no difference in mortality [9]. They used propensity score matching to evaluate the impact of transfusion; however, they did not assess the hemoglobin status in all participants. Kellert et al. studied the association between RBCT and mortality and 3-month outcomes in patients with AIS admitted to a neurologic intensive care unit [10]. They reported that RBCT was not associated with mortality or 3-month outcomes. Further, they did not show variation in hemoglobin levels based on RBCT. In addition, one systematic review has suggested that anemia increases the mortality rate in patients with acute stroke; however, the association between RBCT and change in hemoglobin level were not evaluated [1]. Optimal hemoglobin management in acute stroke care should not only consider admission hemoglobin levels, but also the change in hemoglobin levels and RBCT during the hospitalization. Therefore, our aim is to assess the effect of type of anemia, timing of RBCT, and hemoglobin variability index during admission on the 3-month outcomes in patients with AIS, who received RBCT.

2. Material and Methods

2.1. Study Population

This retrospective observational study included prospectively collected stroke registry patients. Three tertiary teaching hospitals, part of the Clinical Research Center to Stroke—5 database and all laboratory data and clinical outcomes were prospectively collected, and central queries were revised bimonthly [11]. This study was approved by the Hallym University Hospital IRB (No. 2017-43), and an informed consent for registry enrollment and prospective outcome capture was given by all participants or next of kin. Our stroke registry included information of consecutive patients admitted within 7 days of the onset of stroke symptom. We screened patients diagnosed with AIS between January 2015 and December 2017. AIS was diagnosed if focal neurologic deficits persisted for more than 24 h and relevant lesions were confirmed by diffusion MRI. Patients without prospective outcome capture or relevant laboratory and clinical variables were excluded from this study.

2.2. Data Collection

The prospective registry data contained only admission hemoglobin level; therefore, all sequential hemoglobin levels during the hospital admission were extracted using the clinical data warehouse. The hemoglobin level was monitored according to the 2013 American Heart Association/American Stroke Association guideline. We used hemoglobin variability index as minimum, maximum, range (maximum-minimum), standard deviation (SD), coefficient of variance (CoV), median absolute deviation (MAD), and mean absolute change (MAC). Of these variability indices, MAC reflects a more temporal variation of the parameter than other variability indices [12]. Anemia was defined as a hemoglobin level of <13.0 g/dL for men and <12.0 g/dL for women according to World Health Organization criteria.

Whether the patient received RBCT was validated by filtering of the clinical data warehouse and retrospective chart review. We did not assess the administration of other blood products such as platelet concentrate or fresh frozen plasma. The criteria for determining the RBCT might vary from case to case, but they are commonly performed when hemoglobin falls below 8 g/dL. The timing of RBCT was divided into two categories—admission to 48 h (early) and >48 h after admission (late) [13]. The reason for RBCT was classified into five categories—gastrointestinal (GI) bleeding, cancer-related anemia, iron-deficiency anemia (IDA)/anemia of chronic disorder (ACD), surgery/procedure-related anemia, and others. GI bleeding was defined as the bleeding from the GI tract with an evidence of bleeding on endoscopy [14]. IDA was defined as an anemia with biochemical evidence of iron deficiency. ACD was defined as an anemia associated with chronic inflammatory, infectious disease, or malignancies [15]. Anemia associated with chronic kidney disease was also classified into this category. Cancer-related anemia was defined as anemia accompanied by a newly diagnosed, active, or metastatic cancer [16]. The determination of IDA/ACD or cancer-related anemia was mutually exclusive. For example, when the patient being treated with active cancer showed the IDA/ACD pattern, it was defined as cancer-related anemia. Surgery/procedure-related anemia was defined as newly developed anemia within 24 h after surgery or procedure without evidence of the other cause [17]. Finally, anemia without obvious causes was classified as other types of anemia (Figure 1).

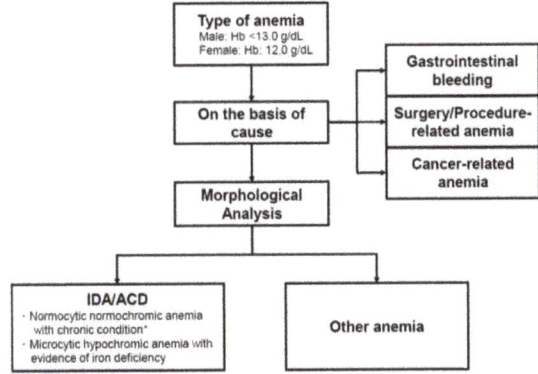

Figure 1. Type of anemia according to cause of anemia or morphological analysis of erythrocytes. * Patients with anemia of chronic disease were classified as cancer-related anemia when they had active cancer. Hb: hemoglobin; IDA: iron-deficiency anemia; ACD: anemia of chronic disease. We included the additional laboratory results that can affect the hemoglobin levels and anemia status: white blood cell (WBC) and platelet counts; blood urea nitrogen, creatinine, and blood glucose levels; international normalized ratio; and blood pressure. The functional outcome was assessed by modified Rankin Scale (mRS) score at 3 months [18], and stroke severity was measured using the National Institute of Health Stroke Scale (NIHSS) score at admission [19]. The primary outcome was poor outcome at 3 months, which was defined the mRS score of 3–6 [20]. Secondary analysis was performed to assess the significance of each hemoglobin variability parameters during admission in poor outcome prediction.

2.3. Statistical Analysis

We compared the baseline characteristics of patients who received early and late RBC transfusion. The patients were divided into the good (mRS 0–2) and poor (mRS 3–6) group according to the 3-month outcome. Baseline demographic and clinical characteristics were compared using the χ2 or t-test (Mann–Whitney U test) as appropriate. Univariable logistic regression analysis was performed to assess the predictors for poor outcome. The multivariable logistic regression model was used for independent variables with a p-value of <0.05 in the univariable model or with the clinical relevance. We used four different multivariable models: model 1 adjusting for age and sex; model 2 adjusting for age, sex, and the Charlson comorbidity index (CCI); model 3 adjusting for age, sex, CCI, and NIHSS; and model 4 adjusting for age, sex, CCI, NIHHS, WBC count, and fasting blood glucose. For assessing the significance of hemoglobin variability parameters, model performance for each multivariable logistic regression analysis was performed using the area under the receiver operating characteristics curve (AUROC). Significant statistical differences among independent variables were considered with a *p*-value of 0.05 in multivariable models. All statistical analyses were performed using R (Foundation for Statistical Computing, Vienna, Austria, http://www.R-project.org).

3. Results

3.1. Baseline Characteristics

Among the 2698 patients with AIS, 592 (21.9%) were anemic at the time of admission and 132 (4.9%) received RBCT during the admission (Table S1). Patients who received RBCT were older, more likely to be male, had history of previous stroke and smoking, and a higher stroke severity and cardioembolic cause of stroke than those who did not receive RBCT. The number of patients taking anticoagulants was higher in the RBCT group, but there was no difference in the previous use of antiplatelet agents before the index stroke between the two groups.

In total, 63 of 132 (47.7%) patients received early RBCT (Table 1). The mean age of patients who received RBCT during admission was the mean (± standard deviation) of 71.6 (±13.5) years, and 46.2% patients were men. Patients who received early RBCT were less likely to have previous strokes than those who received late RBCT. CCI and NIHSS score were not different between the early and late RBCT group. The proportion of patients with poor outcome (mRS >2) at 3 months was less in the early RBCT group than in the late RBCT group.

Table 1. Baseline characteristics of the participants.

Parameters	Early Transfusion (n = 63)	Late Transfusion (n = 69)	p
Age, years	68.6 ± 16.3	74.4.1 ± 9.7	0.450
Male	30 (47.6%)	31 (44.9%)	0.893
Past medical history			
Stroke	16 (25.4%)	30 (43.5%)	0.002
Hypertension	41 (65.1%)	52 (75.4%)	0.270
Diabetes	17 (27.0%)	23 (33.3%)	0.546
Hyperlipidemia	18 (28.6%)	20 (29.0%)	0.985
Current smoking	19 (30.2%)	12 (17.4%)	0.128
Charlson comorbidity index	5.0 (3.0–7.0)	5.0 (4.0–7.0)	0.221
Stroke subtype			0.116
Cardioembolic	14 (22.2%)	25 (36.2%)	
Non-cardioembolic	49 (77.8%)	44 (63.8%)	
NIHSS score	9.0 (2.5–16.0)	13.0 (6.0–18.0)	0.091
Thrombolysis	9 (14.3%)	6 (8.7%)	0.461
Onset to visit time, hour	3.7 (1.2–30.0)	4.9 (1.0–30.5)	0.879
Laboratory parameter			
WBC, $10^3/\mu L$	9.1 ± 4.5	9.4 ± 4.3	0.660
Platelet, $10^3/\mu L$	280 ± 152	234 ± 111	0.050
BUN, mg/dL	22.2 ± 15.6	22.5 ± 16.9	0.926
Creatinine, mg/dL	1.2 ± 1.3	1.3 ± 1.2	0.614
Total cholesterol, mg/dL	147.0 ± 49.7	160.0 ± 48.3	0.130
TG, mg/dL	95.5 ± 55.2	113.0 ± 55.5	0.078
HDL, mg/dL	45.6 ± 13.2	42.0 ± 11.8	0.108
LDL, mg/dL	90.3 ± 41.2	92.6 ± 42.9	0.759
FBS, mg/dL	133.0 ± 57.3	139.0 ± 55.9	0.574
INR	1.2 ± 0.7	1.3 ± 0.9	0.816
Systolic BP, mmHg	140 ± 25	140 ± 28	0.997
Diastolic BP, mmHg	81.8 ± 13.7	78.9 ± 17.3	0.284
History of antithrombotics usage	23 (36.5%)	34 (49.3%)	0.193
Poor outcome (mRS >2)	43 (68.3%)	61 (88.4%)	0.009

Categorical variables are represented by the number (column percent), and continuous variable are represented by mean (± standard deviation) or median (interquartile range) as appropriate. SD: standard deviation; iqr: interquartile range; NIHSS: National Institute of Health Stroke Scale; WBC: white blood cell, BUN: blood urea nitrogen; TG: triglycerides; HDL: high-density lipoprotein; LDL: low-density lipoprotein; FBS: fasting blood sugar; INR: international normalized ratio; BP: blood pressure; mRS: modified Rankin Scale.

Patients who had poor outcomes had more severe stroke, shorter onset to admission time, and had a higher WBC count and fasting blood glucose level than those with good outcomes. Patients who received intravenous thrombolysis and RBCT were in the poor outcome group (Table 2).

Table 2. The comparison of clinical and laboratory parameters between good and poor outcome group.

Parameters	Poor (n = 104)	Good (n = 28)	p
Age, years	70.1 ± 14.9	72.0.1 ± 13.2	0.514
Male	43 (41.3%)	18 (64.3%)	0.051
Past medical history			
Stroke	39 (37.5%)	7 (25.0%)	0.313
Hypertension	75 (72.1%)	18 (64.3%)	0.567
Diabetes	34 (32.7%)	6 (21.4%)	0.358
Hyperlipidemia	29 (27.9%)	9 (32.1%)	0.836
Current smoking	21 (20.2)	10 (35.7)	0.142
Stroke subtype			0.718
Cardioembolic	32 (30.8%)	7 (25.0%)	
Non-cardioembolic	70 (68.6%)	23 (76.7%)	
NIHSS, score	13.0 (7.0–18.0)	3.0 (1.0–4.5)	<0.001
Thrombolysis	15 (14.4%)	0 (0.0%)	0.072
onset to visit time, hour	3.2 (0.9–26.0)	12.9 (3.2–61.7)	0.012
Laboratory parameter			
WBC, $10^3/\mu L$	9.7 ± 4.6	7.4 ± 2.7	0.011
Platelet, $10^3/\mu L$	246 ± 127	292 ± 152	0.102
BUN, mg/dL	21.5 ± 14.8	25.8 ± 20.6	0.211
Creatinine, mg/dL	1.2 ± 1.3	1.3 ± 0.9	0.878
Total cholesterol, mg/dL	157.0 ± 50.2	142.0 ± 44.3	0.178
TG, mg/dL	103.0 ± 53.5	109.0 ± 63.4	0.558
HDL, mg/dL	44.5 ± 12.1	40.3 ± 13.7	0.120
LDL, mg/dL	93.6 ± 43.5	84.0 ± 35.5	0.290
FBS, mg/dL	143.0 ± 58.7	110.0 ± 37.5	0.006
INR	1.3 ± 0.9	1.1 ± 0.1	0.274
Systolic BP, mmHg	143.0 ± 26.6	132.0 ± 24.4	0.058
Diastolic BP, mmHg	81.2 ± 16.2	77.0 ± 13.4	0.211
History of antithrombotics usage	46 (44.2%)	11 (39.3%)	0.780
Number of Hb measure	13.0 (6.0–23.5)	8.0 (5.8–19.3)	0.309
Admission Hb, g/dL	9.7 ± 2.6	8.8 ± 2.5	0.129
Hb variability parameter			
Mean, g/dL	10.2 ± 1.5	9.4 ± 1.2	0.012
Median, g/dL	10.2 ± 1.5	9.5 ± 1.2	0.018
Minimum, g/dL	8.0 ± 1.8	7.2 ± 1.4	0.025
Maximum, g/dL	12.2 ± 1.9	11.3 ± 1.7	0.026
IQR, g/dL	1.6 ± 0.9	1.6 ± 0.9	0.806
Range, g/dL	4.2 ± 1.9	4.1 ± 1.6	0.889
SD, g/dL	1.3 ± 0.5	1.4 ± 0.5	0.640
MAD, g/dL	1.1 ± 0.7	1.2 ± 0.7	0.529
CoV, %	12.9 ± 4.8	14.4 ± 4.5	0.134
MAC, g/dL	0.7 ± 0.4	0.8 ± 0.2	0.165
Type of anemia			0.164
GI bleeding	24 (23.1)	12 (42.9)	
Cancer-related	18 (17.3)	2 (7.1)	
IDA or ACD	24 (23.1)	8 (28.6)	
Surgery/Procedure-related	23 (22.1)	4 (14.3)	
Others	15 (14.4)	2 (7.1)	
Transfusion amount, mL	400 (400–800)	800 (400–1140)	0.337
Timing of transfusion			0.009
Early (≤ 48 h)	43 (41.3%)	20 (71.4%)	
Late (> 48 h)	61 (58.7%)	8 (28.6%)	

Categorical variables are represented by the number (column percent) and continuous variable are represented by mean (± standard deviation) or median (interquartile range) as appropriate. NIHSS: National Institute of Health Stroke Scale; WBC: white blood cell; BUN: blood urea nitrogen; TG: triglycerides; HDL: high-density lipoprotein; LDL: low-density lipoprotein; FBS: fasting blood sugar; INR: international normalized ratio; BP: blood pressure; Hb: hemoglobin; IQR: interquartile range; SD: standard deviation; MAD: median absolute deviation; CoV: coefficient of variation; MAC: mean absolute change; GI: gastrointestinal; IDA: iron deficiency anemia; ACD: anemia of chronic disorder.

3.2. Type of Anemia, RBC Transfusion and Hemoglobin Variability

GI bleeding (27.3%) was the most common cause of RBCT, followed by IDA/ACD (24.2%), surgery/procedure-related anemia (20.5%), and cancer-related anemia (15.2%). Most RBCT was performed within seven days of hospitalization (Figure 2a). The type of anemia was not associated with poor outcomes (*p* = 0.164 for chi-square, Table 2) and the timing of RBCT (Figure 2b and Table 3). However, patients with poor outcomes were found to have received RBCT later than those with good outcomes (*p* = 0.009 for chi-square, Table 2). The amount of RBCT showed left-shifted distribution and was higher in the good outcome group than in the poor outcome group, but it was not statistically significant (*p* = 0.337 for Wilcoxon signed-rank test).

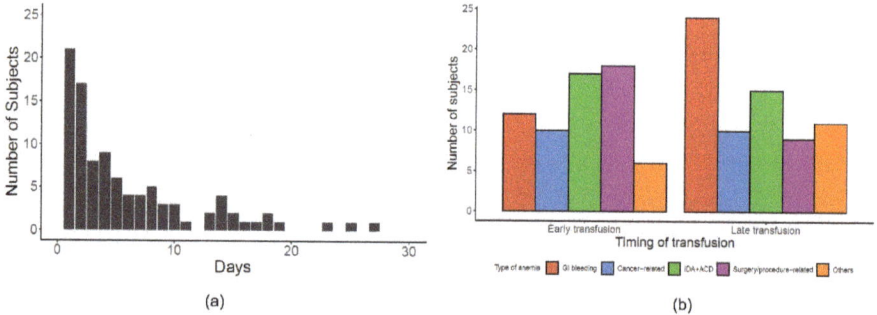

Figure 2. The timing of red blood cell transfusion and the relationship of type of anemia between early and late red blood cell transfusion: (**a**) The frequency of red blood cell transfusion performed after hospitalization (X-axis means the timing (days) of RBCT after admission; Y-axis means the number of subjects who received red blood cell transfusion). (**b**) The differences of proportion in type of anemia according to the timing of the red blood cell transfusion (early vs. late).

Table 3. The comparison of hemoglobin variability parameters and type of anemia between early and late transfusion group.

Parameters	Early Transfusion (*n* = 63)	Late Transfusion (*n* = 69)	Total (*n* =132)	*p*
Number of Hb measure, number	7.0 (4.0–14.0)	19.0 (10.0–30.0)	13.0 (6.0–23.0)	<0.001
Admission Hb, mg/dL	9.4 ± 2.7	9.6±2.5	9.5 ± 2.6	0.639
Hb variability parameter				
Mean, mg/dL	10.1 ± 1.8	9.9 ± 1.1	10.0 ± 1.5	0.391
Median, mg/dL	10.3 ± 1.9	9.9 ± 1.1	10.1 ± 1.5	0.109
Minimum, mg/dL	8.2 ± 2.1	7.6 ± 1.3	7.9 ± 1.7	0.065
Maximum, mg/dL	11.7 ± 1.9	12.3 ± 1.8	12.0 ± 1.9	0.052
IQR, mg/dL	1.3 ± 0.8	1.8 ± 1.0	1.9 ± 0.6	0.004
Range, mg/dL	3.5 ± 1.6	4.7 ± 1.8	4.1 ± 1.8	<0.001
SD, mg/dL	1.3 ± 0.5	1.4 ± 0.5	1.3 ± 0.5	0.292
MAD, mg/dL	1.0 ± 0.7	1.3 ± 0.7	0.5 ± 0.5	0.025
CoV, %	12.6 ± 4.8	13.7 ± 4.7	13.2 ± 4.8	0.212
MAC, mg/dL	0.8 ± 0.4	0.6 ± 0.3	0.4 ± 0.3	0.004
Type of anemia				0.080
GI bleeding	12 (19.0)	24 (34.8)	36 (27.3)	
Cancer-related	10 (15.9)	10 (14.5)	20 (15.2)	
IDA or ACD	17 (27.0)	15 (21.7)	32 (24.2)	
Surgery/Procedure-related	18 (28.6)	9 (13.0)	27 (20.5)	
Others	6 (9.5)	11 (16.0)	17 (12.9)	
Transfusion amount, mL	400 (400–800)	640 (400–1120)	400 (400–840)	0.448

Categorical variables are represented by the number (column percent) and continuous variable are represented by mean (± standard deviation) or median (interquartile range) as appropriate. Hb: hemoglobin; IQR: interquartile range; SD: standard deviation; MAD: median absolute deviation; CoV: coefficient of variation; MAC: mean absolute change; GI: gastrointestinal; IDA: iron deficiency anemia; ACD: anemia of chronic disorder.

During hospitalization, 2359 hemoglobin measurements were performed for the 132 patients receiving RBCT (Table 3). The median (interquartile range (IQR)) of hemoglobin measurements in each patient with RBCT was 13 (6–13) and the number of hemoglobin measurement was more frequent in the late RBCT group than in the early RBCT group (p <0.001). Among the hemoglobin variability parameters, IQR, range, and median absolute deviation (MAD) hemoglobin levels were lower and the mean absolute change (MAC) hemoglobin levels was higher in the early RBCT group than in the late RBCT group (Table 3). Mean, median, minimum, and maximum hemoglobin levels were higher in patients with poor outcomes than in those with good outcomes (Table 2). Other hemoglobin variability parameters including IQR, range, standard deviation (SD), MAD, coefficient of variation (CoV), and MAC hemoglobin were not different between the two groups.

3.3. Predictors for Poor Outcome

The proportion of patients with poor outcomes was 78.8% (104/132). In the univariable analysis, higher NIHSS score, late RBCT was associated with poor outcomes (odds ratio (OR), 3.55; 95% confidence interval (CI), 1.43–8.79) in univariable analysis. When we adjusted age, sex, CCI, NIHSS score, WBC count, and fasting blood sugar level, late RBCT was a significant predictor for poor outcomes (OR, 3.37; 95% CI, 1.14–9.99, Table 4).

Because of the high correlation between the hemoglobin variability parameters (Figure S1), the statistical significances of hemoglobin variability indices were compared to identify if the AUROC value indicating the model performance increased significantly when the hemoglobin variability parameters were added into the original logistic regression model. The performance of the original multivariable logistic regression was AUROC (0.883; 95% CI, 0.821–0.936, p <0.001). Figure 3 shows the model performance of each logistic regression model, which additionally included each hemoglobin variability parameter in the original model. However, there were no additional improvements in model performance when the hemoglobin variability indices were included in the original model.

Table 4. The predictors of poor outcome in multivariable logistic regression analysis according to the timing of the transfusion.

	Crude Model		Model 1		Model 2		Model 3		Model 4	
	OR (95% CI)	p	OR (95% CI)	p	OR (95% CI)	p	OR (95% CI)	p	OR (95% CI)	p
Late transfusion	3.55 (1.43–8.79)	0.006	3.61 (1.42–9.19)	0.007	3.65 (1.43–9.29)	0.007	3.21 (1.14–9.09)	0.028	3.37 (1.14–9.99)	0.028
Age			1.00 (0.97–1.03)	0.983	1.00 (0.96–1.03)	0.806	0.99 (0.95–1.04)	0.694	0.98 (0.93–1.03)	0.403
Male			0.38 (0.16–0.93)	0.035	0.38 (0.15–0.92)	0.033	0.43 (0.16–1.17)	0.099	0.42 (0.15–1.21)	0.109
CCI					1.04 (0.86–1.27)	0.677	1.06 (0.84–1.35)	0.629	1.07 (0.83–1.39)	0.592
NIHSS							1.22 (1.11–1.34)	<0.001	1.19 (1.08–1.31)	<0.001
WBC, $10^3/\mu L$									1.16 (0.98–1.37)	0.089
FBS, mg/dL									1.01 (1.00–1.02)	0.189

Model 1 adjusted for age and sex; Model 2 included variables in Model 1 plus Charlson comorbidity index; Model 3 included variables in Model 2 plus National Institute of Health Stroke Scale score; Model 4 included variables in Model 3 plus white blood cell count and fasting blood sugar. OR: odds ratio; CI: confidence interval; CCI: Charlson comorbidity index; NIHSS: National Institute of Health Stroke Scale; WBC: white blood cell; FBS: fasting blood sugar.

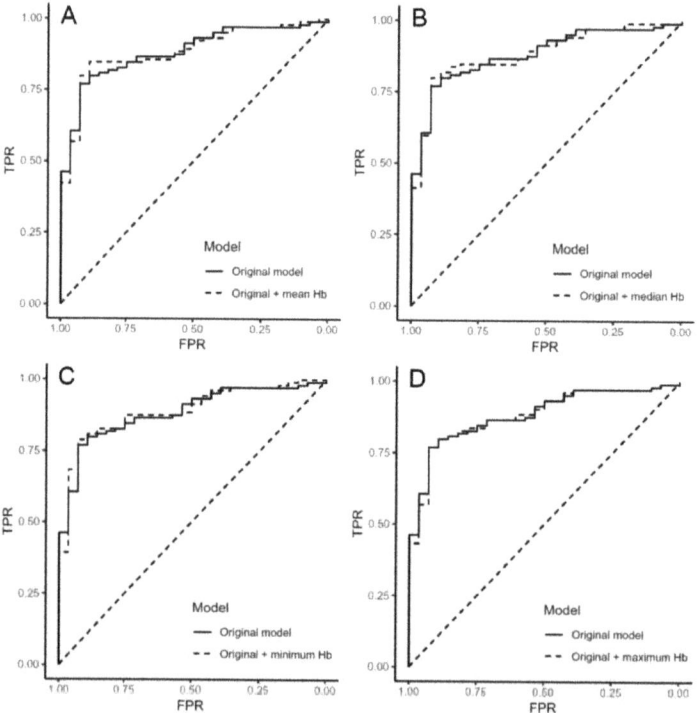

Figure 3. Receiver operating characteristics curve showing performances of original logistic regression model and the other models with hemoglobin variability parameter. The original model was the final logistic regression model in Table 4. The area under the curve of the Receiver Operating Characteristic (AUROC) of the original model was 0.883. AUROC of mean (**A**), median (**B**), minimum (**C**), and maximum (**D**) hemoglobin-adjusted models were 0.884, 0.885, 0.889, and 0.882, respectively. TPR: true positive rate; FPR: false positive rate; Hb: hemoglobin.

4. Discussion

In this study, 21.9% patients with AIS were anemic at admission and 4.9% had received RBCT during hospitalization. Approximately 79% patients who received RBCT had a poor outcome at three months. The mean, median, minimum, and maximum hemoglobin levels were higher in patients with poor outcomes than in those with good outcomes. However, differences in hemoglobin variability indices, including IQR, range, SD, CoV, MAD, and MAC, did not differ between the two groups. Late RBCT was a significant predictor for poor outcome in patients with AIS in the multivariable model. However, hemoglobin variability indices were not associated with functional outcome in patients with AIS and RBCT.

We found that 5% AIS had received RBCT during hospitalization, and more than two-thirds of those had a poor outcome at three months. Additionally, late transfusion, rather than hemoglobin variability indices during hospitalization, was a significant predictor for poor outcome. Our study included all hemoglobin measurements performed during the hospital stay and differs from previous studies as we only investigated patients with AIS who had received RBCT. When analyzing the effect of hemoglobin on the AIS outcome, RBCT should be stratified RBCT or by analyzing only patients who had received RBCT.

Limited studies have assessed the relationship between the type of anemia and the functional outcome in patients with AIS. Ogata et al. have investigated the effect of GI bleeding in patients with

AIS during hospitalization. Using the Fukuoka Stroke Registry, they showed that GI bleeding occurred most commonly within 1 week after the onset of stroke and was associated with poor outcome [21]. In our study, GI bleeding occurred in 38.8% patients, even after 7 days of hospitalization. As the antiplatelet agent regimen in AIS was changed and the characteristics of the patients varied in each study, there is a possibility that the prevalent period of GI bleeding may be different. However, RBCT performed to correct various causes of anemia not only during hospitalization but also at admission. In the retrospective observational study by Sharma et al., 28% of patients without anemia on admission developed anemia during admission [22]. In prospectively collected UK Regional Stroke Register data, hypochromic microcytic or normochromic normocytic anemia were associated with poor clinical outcomes in patients with AIS [23]. They concluded that the type of anemia is a salient indicator of comorbidity burden. Therefore, we suggest that the type of anemia or timing of RBCT could be an important predictor of functional outcome in patients with AIS.

In general, low or high hemoglobin levels adversely affect stroke outcomes [2,22,23]. The reason that our results did not show the U-shaped relationship between hemoglobin levels and stroke outcomes was due to the difference in patient population. The previous reports have assessed admission hemoglobin levels for all patients admitted with AIS, and this study only included patients with AIS who received RBCT during the hospital stay. Likewise, when analyzing only patients who had received RBCT, we can hypothesize that the other variables, including the type of anemia, had more impact on stroke outcome than the initial hemoglobin level.

RBCT had a poorer outcome than those with early RBCT due to admission hemoglobin level not differing between early and late RBCT group; however, the IQR and range hemoglobin were higher in late transfusion group than in early RBCT group in our report. Furthermore, the number of hemoglobin measurements performed during the hospital stay was an average of 7 times in early RBCT group, but an average of 19 measurements in late RBCT group. Based on these observations, the change in hemoglobin status was higher and more abrupt in the late transfusion group than in the early RBCT group, and it can be expected that more frequent hemoglobin measurements in late RBCT group were made to monitor this rapid change. The autoregulatory mechanism for maintaining cerebral blood flow is already lost in infarct core, and that mechanism is already maximized in the penumbral area [24]. Therefore, the rapid drop in hemoglobin may further exacerbate the oligemia and cause infarct growth in penumbral area. In a study by Bellwald et al., decreased hemoglobin level after hospital arrival was associated with the amount and velocity of infarct growth in patients with AIS [25]. We did not assess infarct growth of our participants; rapid alteration of hemoglobin status in the late RBCT group may have a worse effect on the cerebral autoregulatory mechanism, which can exacerbate stroke outcome. Second, although the type of anemia was not statistically different between early and late RBCT group ($p = 0.080$) in our data, different cause of RBCT may affect stroke outcome. Surgery/procedure-related anemia was higher in the early RBCT group, and GI bleeding was higher in the late RBCT group in our study. However, our study did not include a large number of patients who received RBCT (only 5% in total AIS population), it should be reassessed in a larger prospective study whether this type of anemia affected stroke outcome.

In general population, history of RBCT is associated with 1.6-fold increase in the risk of ischemic stroke [26]. This association is explained by the fact that stored RBC increases blood viscosity, and decreases nitric oxide concentration, vasoconstriction, and platelet activation [1]. On the other hand, low hemoglobin is inversely correlated with initial infarct volume or infarct growth, and the author suggested that RBCT would be beneficial for recovery of stroke [1]. However, restrictive transfusion strategy in patients of cardiovascular diseases was not inferior compared to liberal strategy in two systematic review [1]. In our data, transfusion amount did change between the good and poor outcome group, though those with good outcome had low mean, median, minimum, and maximum hemoglobin compared to those with poor outcome. Our study did not directly assess the exact transfusion strategy because the study design was retrospective in nature. However, we suggested that restrictive transfusion strategies can reduce the thrombotic complication and maximize the beneficial effect by RBCT compared to the liberal strategy in AIS patients.

In our study, hemoglobin variability indices did not affect the functional outcome in patients with AIS. In the previous report, minimum or maximum hemoglobin level was associated with worse outcome [1]. However, these hemoglobin parameters did not affect the stroke outcome in our study. Kellert et al. studied the impact of low hemoglobin level and transfusion in neurologic intensive care unit patients and found that hemoglobin parameters were not associated with in-hospital mortality or 90-day functional outcomes, but they were associated with length of intensive care unit length of stay and duration of mechanical ventilation [10]. The author suggested that the impact of hemoglobin parameters in neurologically severe patients might be reduced by the important predictors such as stroke severity. In our study, patients with RBCT had more severe stroke than those without RBCT (median NIHSS score 13 vs. 3). Our study also suggests that stroke severity, rather than hemoglobin parameters, is an important predictor for poor outcome in patients with severe ischemic stroke. However, as our study and Kellert's study had a small sample size, larger prospective studies are needed to confirm these associations.

Our study had some limitations. First, our study was a small sampled-sized retrospective observation, and therefore there is a chance of selection bias and residual confounding. However, the incidence of anemia and the proportion who had received RBCT during hospitalization were comparable to other studies on patients with AIS [1]. Second, the effect of RBCT on functional outcome was likely to be underestimated because we only collected RBCT data, which were performed only during hospitalization. However, anemia usually developed 2–11 days following admission in patients with AIS [27]. Therefore, only several patients would receive RBCT after discharge.

Despite these limitations, our study had several strengths. First, we minimized residual confounding by including information such as stroke severity, type of anemia, and timing and amount of RBCT. Second, the characteristics of patients with AIS who received RBCT differ significantly compared to those who did not receive RBCT. If the rare event (such as patients with RBCT; ~5% of all AIS patients) is evaluated with logistic regression method, the results may be vulnerable to biases [28]. We solved this problem by analyzing the binary outcome only in patients with RBCT and minimized the interaction between anemia and RBCT transfusion. Third, cerebral perfusion can be changed dynamically depending on the degree of anemia and whether the RBCT is performed or not. We evaluated all hemoglobin measurements during the hospitalization. In addition, we analyzed the overall hemoglobin parameters such as SD, CoV, and MAD, and temporal variation parameter such as MAC. In addition, we identified all bleeding events during hospitalization and reflected them in the type of anemia variable.

5. Conclusions

Late RBCT was associated with 3-month poor outcome in patients with AIS. To verify this, a larger prospective study is needed for assessing the type of anemia and cause of RBCT, and the fluctuation of hemoglobin status during the admission.

Supplementary Materials: The following are available online at http://www.mdpi.com/2077-0383/9/5/1566/s1, Table S1: The comparison between patients with and without red blood cell transfusion during admission, Figure S1: The correlation between hemoglobin variability parameters.

Author Contributions: Conceptualization, B.-C.L.; Data curation, M.U.J.; Formal analysis, C.K., S.-H.L., J.-S.L., and M.S.O.; Funding acquisition, C.K.; Methodology, S.-H.L., Y.K., and J.-H.L.; Resources, Y.K. and S.J.; Supervision, K.-H.Y., J.-H.L., and B.-C.L.; Visualization, J.-S.L. and M.U.J.; Writing—original draft, C.K. and B.-C.L.; Writing—review & editing, M.S.O., K.-H.Y., and S.J. All authors have read and agreed to the published version of the manuscript.

Funding: This research was funded by the National Research Fund of Korea (NRF-2019R1G1A1097707), the Hallym University Research Fund (HURF-2019-54), and a grant from the CJ healthcare Corp (2018-12-031). The funders had no role in the study design, data collection and analysis, decision to publish, or preparation of the manuscript.

Conflicts of Interest: The authors declare no conflicts of interest.

References

1. Sarnak, M.J.; Tighiouart, H.; Manjunath, G.; MacLeod, B.; Griffith, J.; Salem, D.; Levey, A.S. Anemia as a risk factor for cardiovascular disease in the atherosclerosis risk in communities (ARIC) study. *J. Am. Coll. Cardiol.* **2002**, *40*, 27–33.
2. Wei, C.C.; Zhang, S.T.; Tan, G.; Zhang, S.H.; Liu, M. Impact of anemia on in-hospital complications after ischemic stroke. *Eur. J. Neurol.* **2018**, *25*, 768–774.
3. Powers, W.J. Cerebral hemodynamics in ischemic cerebrovascular disease. *Ann. Neurol.* **1991**, *29*, 231–240.
4. Tsai, C.F.; Yip, P.K.; Chen, C.C.; Yeh, S.J.; Chung, S.T.; Jeng, J.S. Cerebral infarction in acute anemia. *J. Neurol.* **2010**, *257*, 2044–2051.
5. Kellert, L.; Herweh, C.; Sykora, M.; Gussmann, P.; Martin, E.; Ringleb, P.A.; Steiner, T.; Bösel, J. Loss of penumbra by impaired oxygen supply? Decreasing Hemoglobin levels predict infarct growth after acute ischemic stroke. *Cerebrovasc. Dis. Extra* **2012**, *2*, 99–107.
6. Ehrenreich, H.; Weissenborn, K.; Prange, H.; Schneider, D.; Weimar, C.; Wartenberg, K.; Schellinger, P.D.; Bohn, M.; Becker, H.; Wegrzyn, M.; et al. Recombinant human erythropoietin in the treatment of acute ischemic stroke. *Stroke* **2009**, *40*, e647–e656.
7. Goel, R.; Patel, E.U.; Cushing, M.M.; Frank, S.M.; Ness, P.M.; Takemoto, C.M.; Vasovic, L.V.; Sheth, S.; Nellis, M.E.; Shaz, B.; et al. Association of perioperative red blood cell transfusions with venous thromboembolism in a North American registry. *JAMA. Surg.* **2018**, *153*, 826–833.
8. Byrnes, J.R.; Wolberg, A.S. Red blood cells in thrombosis. *Blood* **2017**, *130*, 1795–1799.
9. Moman, R.N.; Kor, D.J.; Chandran, A.; Hanson, A.C.; Schroeder, D.R.; Rabinstein, A.A.; Warner, M.A. Red blood cell transfusion in acute brain injury subtypes: An observational cohort study. *J. Crit. Care* **2019**, *50*, 44–49.
10. Kellert, L.; Schrader, F.; Ringleb, P.; Steiner, T.; Bösel, J. The impact of low hemoglobin levels and transfusion on critical care patients with severe ischemic stroke STroke: Relevant impact of HemoGlobin, Hematocrit and Transfusion (STRAIGHT)—An observational study. *J. Crit. Care* **2014**, *29*, 236–240.
11. Kim, J.Y.; Kang, K.; Kang, J.; Koo, J.; Kim, D.H.; Kim, B.J.; Kim, W.J.; Kim, E.G.; Kim, J.G.; Kim, J.M.; et al. Executive summary of stroke statistics in Korea 2018: A report from the epidemiology research council of the Korean stroke society. *J. Stroke* **2019**, *21*, 42–59.
12. Kohnert, K.D.; Heinke, P.; Fritzsche, G.; Vogt, L.; Augstein, P.; Salzsieder, E. Evaluation of the mean absolute glucose change as a measure of glycemic variability using continuous glucose monitoring data. *Diabetes Technol. Ther.* **2013**, *15*, 448–454.
13. Chelemer, S.B.; Prato, B.S.; Cox Jr., P.M.; O'Connor, G.T.; Morton, J.R. Association of bacterial infection and red blood cell transfusion after coronary artery bypass surgery. *Ann. Thorac. Surg.* **2002**, *73*, 138–142.
14. Raju, G.S.; Gerson, L.; Das, A.; Lewis, B.; American Gastroenterological Association (AGA). Institute medical position statement on obscure gastrointestinal bleeding. *Gastroenterology* **2007**, *133*, 1694–1696.
15. Weiss, G.; Goodnough, L.T. Anemia of chronic disease. *N. Engl. J. Med.* **2005**, *352*, 1011–1023.
16. Ludwig, H.; Van, B.S.; Barrett-Lee, P.; Birgegård, G.; Bokemeyer, C.; Gascón, P.; Kosmidis, P.; Krzakowski, M.; Nortier, J.; Olmi, P.; et al. The European Cancer Anaemia Survey (ECAS): A large, multinational, prospective survey defining the prevalence, incidence, and treatment of anaemia in cancer patients. *Eur. J. Cancer* **2004**, *40*, 2293–2306.
17. Valeri, C.R.; Dennis, R.C.; Ragno, G.; Macgregor, H.; Menzoian, J.O.; Khuri, S.F. Limitations of the hematocrit level to assess the need for red blood cell transfusion in hypovolemic anemic patients. *Transfusion* **2006**, *46*, 365–371.
18. Sulter, G.; Steen, C.; De Keyser, J.D. Use of the Barthel index and modified Rankin Scale in acute stroke trials. *Stroke* **1999**, *30*, 1538–1541.
19. Wityk, R.J.; Pessin, M.S.; Kaplan, R.F.; Caplan, L.R. Serial assessment of acute stroke using the NIH Stroke Scale. *Stroke* **1994**, *25*, 362–365.
20. Jansen, I.G.; Mulder, M.J.; Goldhoorn, R.-J.B. Endovascular treatment for acute ischaemic stroke in routine clinical practice: Prospective, observational cohort study (MR CLEAN registry). *BMJ.* **2018**, *360*, k949.
21. Ogata, T.; Kamouchi, M.; Matsuo, R.; Kuroda, J.; Ago, T.; Sugimori, H.; Inoue, T.; Kitazono, T.; Fukuoka Stroke Registry. Gastrointestinal bleeding in acute ischemic stroke: Recent trends from the Fukuoka stroke registry. *Cerebrovasc. Dis. Extra* **2014**, *4*, 156–164.

22. Sharma, K.; Johnson, D.J.; Johnson, B.; Frank, S.M.; Stevens, R.D. Hemoglobin concentration does not impact 3-month outcome following acute ischemic stroke. *BMC. Neurol.* **2018**, *18*, 78.
23. Barlas, R.S.; McCall, S.J.; Bettencourt-Silva, J.H.; Clark, A.B.; Bowles, K.M.; Metcalf, A.K.; Mamas, M.A.; Potter, J.F.; Myint, P.K. Impact of anaemia on acute stroke outcomes depends on the type of anaemia: Evidence from a UK stroke register. *J. Neurol. Sci.* **2017**, *383*, 26–30.
24. Yamada, S.; Koizumi, A.; Iso, H.; Wada, Y.; Watanabe, Y.; Date, C.; Yamamoto, A.; Kikuchi, S.; Inaba, Y.; Kondo, T.; et al. History of blood transfusion before 1990 is a risk factor for stroke and cardiovascular diseases: The Japan collaborative cohort study (JACC study). *Cerebrovasc. Dis.* **2005**, *20*, 164–171.
25. Jordan, J.D.; Powers, W.J. Cerebral autoregulation and acute ischemic stroke. *Am. J. Hypertens.* **2012**, *25*, 946–950.
26. Bellwald, S.; Balasubramaniam, R.; Nagler, M.; Burri, M.S.; Fischer, S.D.A.; Hakim, A.; Dobrocky, T.; Yu, Y.; Scalzo, F.; Heldner, M.R.; et al. Association of anemia and hemoglobin decrease during acute stroke treatment with infarct growth and clinical outcome. *PLoS ONE* **2018**, *13*, e0203535.
27. Abe, A.; Sakamoto, Y.; Nishiyama, Y.; Suda, S.; Suzuki, K.; Aoki, J.; Kimura, K. Decline in Hemoglobin during hospitalization may be associated with poor outcome in acute stroke patients. *J. Stroke Cerebrovasc. Dis.* **2018**, *27*, 1646–1652.
28. Bradburn, M.J.; Deeks, J.J.; Berlin, J.A.; Russell Localio, A. Much ado about nothing: A comparison of the performance of meta-analytical methods with rare events. *Stat. Med.* **2007**, *26*, 53–77.

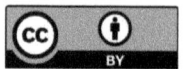

© 2020 by the authors. Licensee MDPI, Basel, Switzerland. This article is an open access article distributed under the terms and conditions of the Creative Commons Attribution (CC BY) license (http://creativecommons.org/licenses/by/4.0/).

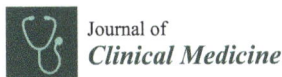

Article

Predicting Stroke Outcomes Using Ankle-Brachial Index and Inter-Ankle Blood Pressure Difference

Minho Han [1], Young Dae Kim [1,2], Jin Kyo Choi [1], Junghye Choi [1], Jimin Ha [1], Eunjeong Park [3], Jinkwon Kim [4], Tae-Jin Song [5], Ji Hoe Heo [1,2] and Hyo Suk Nam [1,2,*]

1. Department of Neurology, Yonsei University College of Medicine, Seoul 03722, Korea; umsthol18@yuhs.ac (M.H.); neuro05@yuhs.ac (Y.D.K.); JKSNAIL85@yuhs.ac (J.K.C.); hye07@yuhs.ac (J.C.); jiminha@yuhs.ac (J.H.); jhheo@yuhs.ac (J.H.H.)
2. Integrative Research Center for Cerebrovascular and Cardiovascular Diseases, Seoul 03722, Korea
3. Cardiovascular Research Institute, Yonsei University College of Medicine, Seoul 03722, Korea; EUNJEONG-PARK@yuhs.ac
4. Department of Neurology, Yongin Severance Hospital, Yonsei University College of Medicine, Yongin-si 16995, Korea; ANTITHROMBUS@yuhs.ac
5. Department of Neurology, Seoul Hospital, Ewha Womans University College of Medicine, Seoul 07804, Korea; knstar@ewha.ac.kr
* Correspondence: hsnam@yuhs.ac; Tel.: +82-2-2228-1617; Fax: +82-2-393-0705

Received: 17 March 2020; Accepted: 13 April 2020; Published: 15 April 2020

Abstract: Background: This study investigated the association of high ankle-brachial index difference (ABID) and systolic inter-ankle blood pressure difference (IAND) with short- and long-term outcomes in acute ischemic stroke patients without peripheral artery disease (PAD). Methods: Consecutive patients with acute ischemic stroke who underwent ankle-brachial index (ABI) measurement were enrolled. ABID was calculated as |right ABI-left ABI|. IAND and systolic inter-arm blood pressure difference (IAD) were calculated as |right systolic blood pressure − left systolic blood pressure|. Poor functional outcome was defined as modified Rankin Scale score ≥3 at 3 months. Major adverse cardiovascular events (MACEs) were defined as stroke recurrence, myocardial infarction, or death. Results: A total of 2901 patients were enrolled and followed up for a median of 3.1 (interquartile range, 1.6–4.7) years. Among them, 2643 (84.9%) patients did not have PAD. In the logistic regression analysis, ABID ≥ 0.15 and IAND ≥ 15 mmHg were independently associated with poor functional outcome (odds ratio (OR), 1.970, 95% confidence interval (CI), 1.175-3.302; OR, 1.665, 95% CI, 1.188-2.334, respectively). In Cox regression analysis, ABID ≥0.15 and IAND ≥ 15 mmHg were independently associated with MACEs (hazard ratio (HR), 1.514, 95% CI, 1.058-2.166; HR, 1.343, 95% CI, 1.051-1.716, respectively) and all-cause mortality (HR, 1.524, 95% CI, 1.039-2.235; HR, 1.516, 95% CI, 1.164-1.973, respectively) in patients without PAD. Conclusion: High ABID and IAND are associated with poor short-term outcomes, long-term MACE occurrence, and all-cause mortality in acute ischemic stroke without PAD.

Keywords: ankle-brachial index difference; inter-ankle blood pressure difference; stroke; peripheral artery disease; outcome

1. Introduction

Blood pressure (BP) ratios and differences between the four limbs can be simultaneously obtained and calculated with ankle-brachial index (ABI) measurement [1]. Among the ratios and differences, ABI difference (ABID), systolic inter-ankle blood pressure difference (IAND), and systolic inter-arm BP difference (IAD) have been reported to be useful in predicting the prognosis in patients with cardiovascular disease, high-risk populations, and the general population [2,3].

Lower extremity peripheral artery disease (PAD) is defined by a low ABI, calculated by dividing the ankle systolic BP by the arm systolic BP. ABI has high specificity and sensitivity for the diagnosis of PAD [4], and ABI may also provide information beyond PAD. A previous study showed that ABID ≥ 0.15 was an independent risk factor for overall mortality in patients undergoing hemodialysis [5]. However, the prognostic value of ABID in patients with ischemic stroke remains uncertain.

IAD is strongly associated with increased cardiovascular and all-cause mortality [6]. Previous studies showed that IAND provided additional information to estimate stroke incidence and cardiovascular mortality beyond IAD [1,3]. To the best of our knowledge, no study has reported the prognostic impact of IAND on the outcomes of patients with acute ischemic stroke.

A previous study showed that the prevalence of PAD in patients with ischemic stroke was 32% and the rate of asymptomatic PAD in patients with stroke was 68% [7]. Another study showed that stroke patients with asymptomatic PAD had an increased risk of recurrent vascular events, including stroke [8]. Therefore, the prognostic significance needs to be separately assessed in ischemic stroke patients without PAD.

In this regard, we hypothesized that ABID and IAND are associated with poor short-term functional outcomes, major adverse cardiovascular events (MACEs), and all-cause mortality in patients with acute ischemic stroke. Whether the prognostic values of these parameters are valid in acute ischemic stroke patients without PAD was also investigated.

2. Materials and Methods

2.1. Patients and Evaluation

A hospital-based, retrospective observational study using prospectively collected stroke registry data was conducted. The Yonsei Stroke Registry collected the data of patients with acute cerebral infarction or transient ischemic attack (TIA) who presented to the emergency department within 7 days of symptom onset between January 1, 2007 and June 30, 2013 [9]. Acute cerebral infarction was defined as sudden onset of acute neurological deficits of presumed vascular etiology lasting 24 h or evidence of acute infarction on brain computed tomography (CT) or magnetic resonance imaging (MRI). TIA was diagnosed when a patient had transient (<24 h) neurologic dysfunction of vascular origin and did not show acute lesions on CT or MRI. Among these candidates, only patients with available four-limb BPs measured by ABI examination and a cerebral angiographic evaluation using either CT angiography, MR angiography, or digital subtraction angiography performed during the admission period were included. Patients were treated by standard treatment protocols based on the guidelines for acute ischemic stroke [10–13]. Stroke classifications were determined during weekly conferences. Based on a consensus of three stroke neurologists, stroke subtypes were classified according to the Trial of ORG 10172 in Acute Stroke Treatment (TOAST) classification [14].

2.2. Demographic Characteristics and Risk Factors

We collected data on baseline characteristics, including sex, age, and neurological deficit (National Institutes of Health Stroke Scale (NIHSS) score) upon admission; presence of risk factors; and laboratory data (glucose, high-density lipoprotein (HDL), and low-density lipoprotein (LDL)). Hypertension was defined as resting systolic blood pressure (SBP) of ≥140 mmHg or diastolic blood pressure (DBP) of ≥90 mmHg after repeated measurements during hospitalization or currently taking antihypertensive medication. Diabetes mellitus was defined as fasting plasma glucose levels of ≥7 mmol/L or taking an oral hypoglycemic agent or insulin. Current smoking was defined as having smoked a cigarette within 1 year prior to admission. Congestive heart failure was determined from the history of heart failure diagnosis, treatment with loop diuretics, and ejection fraction of ≤35% on echocardiography. Coronary artery disease (CAD) was diagnosed when a patient had a previous history of CAD (acute myocardial infarction, unstable angina, coronary artery bypass graft, or percutaneous coronary artery stent/angioplasty) or the presence of significant stenosis (≥50%) in any of the three main coronary arteries on multi-slice CT coronary angiography upon admission. Cerebral artery atherosclerosis (CAA) was defined as occlusion or significant stenosis (≥50%) of any intracranial or extracranial cerebral artery. PAD was determined if a patient had an ABI of <0.9 or a history of angiographically confirmed PAD.

2.3. ABI and Brachial-Ankle Pulse Wave Velocity Measurement

ABI and brachial-ankle pulse wave velocity (baPWV) were measured in the supine position using an automatic device (VP-1000; Colin Co., Ltd., Komaki, Japan), which has been validated previously [6,15]. This device automatically and simultaneously measures four-limb pulse wave forms and BP using the oscillometric method. Right ABI was calculated by the ratio of the right ankle SBP divided by the higher SBP of the arms. Left ABI was calculated by the ratio of the left ankle SBP divided by the higher SBP of the arms. ABID was calculated as |right ABI-left ABI|. IAND was extracted as BPs from both legs and calculated as |right ankle SBP-left ankle SBP|. IAD was extracted as BPs from arms and calculated as |right brachial SBP-left brachial SBP|. BaPWV on each side was automatically calculated as the transmission distance divided by the transmission time and expressed in centimeters per second. Transmission distance from the arm to each ankle was automatically calculated according to the patient's height. Transmission time was defined as the time interval between the initial increase of brachial and tibial waveforms. The higher values of baPWV on both sides were used for analysis.

2.4. Follow-Up and Outcome Measures

Patients were followed up in the outpatient clinic or by a structured telephone interview at 3 months and yearly after discharge. Short-term functional outcomes at 3 months were determined by a structured interview using the modified Rankin Scale (mRS). Poor outcome was defined as an mRS of ≥3. Deaths among participants from January 1, 2007 to December 31, 2013, were confirmed by matching the information in the death records and identification numbers assigned to the participants at birth [16]. We obtained data for the date and causes of death from the Korean National Statistical Office, which were identified based on death certificates. MACEs were defined as any stroke recurrence, myocardial infarction occurrence, or death.

2.5. Statistical Analysis

SPSS for Windows (version 23, SPSS, Chicago, IL, USA) was used for the statistical analysis. Intergroup statistical analyses were performed to compare the demographic characteristics and risk factors in the whole study population. The statistical significance of intergroup differences was assessed using the χ^2 or Fisher's exact test for categorical variables and independent two-sample t-test or Mann–Whitney U-test for continuous variables. Data were expressed as means ± standard deviations or medians (interquartile ranges (IQRs)) for continuous variables and numbers (%) for categorical variables. Cutoff values for IAND and IAD were based on those used in the previous study [3]. In elderly people, IAND of ≥15 mmHg and IAD of ≥15 mmHg were cutoff values that could predict mortality [3]. The cutoff value of ABID of ≥0.15 mmHg was based on a study wherein ABID predicted the mortality of patients with chronic hemodialysis [5]. Multivariable logistic regression analysis was performed after adjusting for sex, age, cardiovascular risk factors (hypertension, diabetes mellitus, hypercholesterolemia, current smoking, congestive heart failure, CAD, CAA, and PAD), and variables that exhibited a p value of <0.05 in the univariate analysis, to investigate the association of ABID, IAND, or IAD with short-term functional outcomes. Survival curves were generated according to the Kaplan–Meier method and compared using the log-rank test. Multivariable Cox proportional hazard regression was performed to determine independent factors associated with survival after an ischemic stroke. Subgroup analysis was also performed to confirm that the associations between short- and long-term outcomes and BP differences were valid in patients without PAD. We analyzed the diastolic IAND and diastolic IAD separately as supplemental data. All P values were two-tailed, and differences were considered significant at $p < 0.05$.

2.6. Standard Protocol Approval, Registration, and Patient Consent

The Institutional Review Board of Severance Hospital, Yonsei University Health System, approved this study and waived the need for informed consent because of the retrospective design and observational nature of this study (approval date: 2020-01-16; approval number: 4-2019-1196).

2.7. Data availability Statement

De-identified participant data are available upon reasonable request.

3. Results

3.1. Patient Demographic and Clinical Characteristics

A total of 3822 patients with acute ischemic stroke or TIA were recruited during the study period. After exclusions (follow-up loss (n = 154), no ABI measurements (n = 729), hemodialysis of one arm (n = 16), and TIA (n = 22)), 2901 patients were finally enrolled in this study (Figure 1).

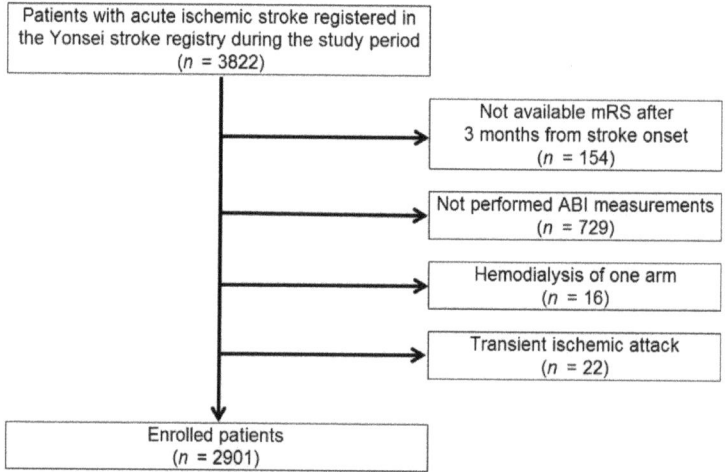

Figure 1. Flowchart of participants according to inclusion and exclusion criteria. ABI, ankle brachial index; mRS; modified Rankin Scale score.

A total of 258 (8.9%) patients had PAD. The mean age was 65.4 ± 12.2 years, and 61.8% were men. Among them, 582 (20.1%) had poor outcomes (Table 1). Compared with patients with good outcomes, those with poor outcomes were older, were more likely to be women, had more severe initial stroke severity, were less likely to be current smokers, and were more likely to have CAA, PAD, and a stroke subtype of large artery atherosclerosis (all p values <0.05). For four-limb BP profiles, both ankle SBP and ABI were lower in patients with poor outcomes than in those with good outcomes (all p values <0.001). All BP differences including ABID, IAND, and IAD were higher in patients with poor outcomes than in those with good outcomes (all p values <0.001). Compared with the included patients, excluded patients were older, were more likely to be women, had higher NIHSS score, were more likely to have congestive heart failure, and were less likely to be current smokers or have CAD (Supplementary Table S1).

Table 1. Patient demographic and clinical characteristics.

	Total (n = 2901)	Good Outcomes (mRS of 0-2; n = 2319)	Poor Outcomes (mRS of 3-6; n = 582)	p Value
Age, y	65.4 ± 12.2	64.0 ± 12.0	71.0 ± 11.4	<0.001
Men	1793 (61.8)	1489 (64.2)	304 (52.2)	<0.001
NIHSS score at admission	3.0 (1.0, 6.0)	2.0 (1.0, 4.0)	8.0 (4.0, 15.0)	<0.001
Risk factors				
Hypertension	2164 (74.6)	1712 (73.8)	452 (77.7)	0.057
Diabetes mellitus	920 (31.7)	728 (31.4)	192 (33.0)	0.459
Hypercholesterolemia	622 (21.4)	486 (21.0)	136 (23.4)	0.205
Current smoking	717 (24.7)	622 (26.8)	95 (16.3)	<0.001
Congestive heart failure	119 (4.1)	92 (4.0)	27 (4.6)	0.465
Coronary artery disease	686 (23.6)	549 (23.7)	137 (23.5)	0.946
Cerebral artery atherosclerosis	1727 (59.5)	1292 (55.7)	435 (74.7)	<0.001
Peripheral artery disease	258 (8.9)	152 (6.6)	106 (18.2)	<0.001
Laboratory findings				
Glucose, mg/dL	143.5 ± 63.9	142.7 ± 63.2	1468 ± 66.0	0.168
HDL, mg/dL	42.8 ± 11.0	42.6 ± 10.8	43.4 ± 11.6	0.127
LDL, mg/dL	114.5 ± 38.6	114.7 ± 37.5	113.8 ± 42.5	0.651
Stroke subtype				<0.001
LAA	587 (20.2)	440 (19.0)	147 (25.3)	
CE	754 (26.0)	600 (25.9)	154 (26.5)	
SVO	261 (9.0)	232 (10.0)	29 (5.0)	
OC	72 (2.5)	58 (2.5)	14 (2.4)	
UE	1227 (42.3)	989 (42.6)	238 (40.9)	
Arm BP, mmHg				
Right SBP	146.3 ± 23.5	146.7 ± 23.2	145.1 ± 24.6	0.147
Left SBP	145.3 ± 23.8	145.6 ± 23.6	144.0 ± 24.6	0.129
IAD	4.90 ± 6.51	4.71 ± 6.45	5.77 ± 7.15	0.001
Ankle BP, mmHg				
Right SBP	164.5 ± 31.3	166.3 ± 30.1	157.7 ± 35.1	<0.001
Left SBP	163.6 ± 31.3	165.2 ± 30.4	157.2 ± 34.6	<0.001
IAND	9.23 ± 11.94	8.42 ± 10.82	12.65 ± 15.87	<0.001
ABI				
Right ABI	1.111 ± 0.132	1.122 ± 0.118	1.071 ± 0.170	<0.001
Left ABI	1.105 ± 0.130	1.114 ± 0.118	1.069 ± 0.171	<0.001
ABID	0.063 ± 0.083	0.058 ± 0.077	0.086 ± 0.104	<0.001
Right ABI >1.30	58 (2.0)	44 (1.9)	14 (2.4)	0.434
Left ABI >1.30	44 (1.5)	31 (1.3)	13 (2.2)	0.113
Both ABI >1.30	18 (0.6)	14 (0.6)	4 (0.7)	0.818

Data are expressed as means ± standard deviations, medians [interquartile ranges], or numbers (%). ABI, ankle brachial index; ABID, ankle brachial index difference; BP, blood pressure; CE, cardioembolism; DBP, diastolic blood pressure; HDL, high density lipoprotein; IAD, systolic inter-arm blood pressure difference; IAND, systolic inter-ankle blood pressure difference; LAA, large artery atherosclerosis; LDL, low density lipoprotein; mRS, modified Rankin Scale; NIHSS, National Institutes of Health Stroke Scale; OC, other cause; SBP, systolic blood pressure; SVO, small vessel occlusion; and UE, undetermined etiology.

In all study patients, 236 (8.1%) patients showed ABID ≥0.15, 450 (15.5%) had IAND ≥15 mmHg, and 116 (4.0%) had IAD ≥15 mmHg. Among atherosclerotic diseases, CAA and PAD were independent determinants of ABID ≥0.15 (CAA: odds ratio (OR), 1.718, 95% confidence interval (CI), 1.211-2.437; PAD: OR, 22.124, 95% CI, 15.844-30.894) and IAND ≥15 mmHg (CAA: OR, 1.646, 95% CI, 1.281-2.114; PAD: OR, 13.328, 95% CI, 9.876-17.987). However, only PAD was an independent determinant of IAD ≥15 mmHg (PAD: OR, 3.044, 95% CI, 1.890-4.904) (Table 2).

Table 2. Determinants of IAD ≥15 mmHg, IAND ≥15 mmHg, and ABID ≥0.15.

	ABID ≥0.15		IAND ≥15 mmHg		IAD ≥15 mmHg	
	OR (95% CI)	p value *	OR (95% CI)	p value *	OR (95% CI)	p value *
CAD	1.290 (0.954-1.745)	0.098	0.957 (0.752-1.217)	0.718	0.912 (0.580-1.434)	0.689
CAA	1.718 (1.211-2.437)	0.002	1.646 (1.281-2.114)	<0.001	1.451 (0.926-2.274)	0.104
PAD	22.124 (15.844-30.894)	<0.001	13.328 (9.876-17.987)	<0.001	3.044 (1.890-4.904)	<0.001

Data were derived from the multivariable logistic regression analysis. ABID, ankle brachial index difference; CAD, coronary artery disease; CAA, cerebral artery atherosclerosis; CI, confidence interval; IAD, systolic inter-arm blood pressure difference; IAND, systolic inter-ankle blood pressure difference; NIHSS, National Institutes of Health Stroke Scale; OR, odds ratio; and PAD, peripheral artery disease. *adjusted for sex, age, NIHSS score at admission, hypertension, diabetes mellitus, hypercholesterolemia, current smoking, congestive heart failure, and stroke subtype.

ABID ≥0.15 and IAND ≥15 mmHg were more likely to have ABI >1.30 (all p values <0.001), but not IAD ≥15 mmHg (Table 3). BaPWVs were well correlated with ABID, IAND, and IAD (with ABID, $r = 0.139, p < 0.001$; with IAND, $r = 0.207, p < 0.001$; and with IAD, $r = 0.121, p < 0.001$) (Supplementary Table S2).

Table 3. Relationship between IAD, IAND, ABID, and ABI >1.30.

	Right ABI >1.30		Left ABI >1.30		Both ABI >1.30	
	n (%)	p value	n (%)	p value	n (%)	p value
ABID						
ABID <0.15	45 (1.7)	0.001	30 (1.1)	<0.001	18 (0.7)	0.392
ABID ≥0.15	13 (5.5)		14 (5.9)		0 (0.0)	
IAND						
IAND <15 mmHg	36 (1.5)	<0.001	27 (1.1)	<0.001	16 (0.7)	1.000
IAND ≥15 mmHg	22 (4.9)		17 (3.8)		2 (0.4)	
IAD						
IAD <15 mmHg	55 (2.0)	0.503	42 (1.5)	0.695	17 (0.6)	0.521
IAD ≥15 mmHg	3 (2.6)		2 (1.7)		1 (0.9)	

ABI, ankle brachial index; ABID, ankle brachial index difference; IAD, systolic inter-arm blood pressure difference; and IAND, systolic inter-ankle blood pressure difference.

3.2. Poor Functional Outcome

All patients with ($n = 2901$) and without PAD ($n = 2643$) were separately analyzed. In all study patients, poor outcome was independently associated with ABID (OR, 5.289, 95% CI, 1.723-16.236) and cutoff of ABID ≥0.15 (OR, 1.920, 95% CI, 1.361-2.708). Poor outcome was also independently associated with IAND (OR, 1.015, 95% CI, 1.007-1.023) and cutoff of IAND ≥15 mmHg (OR, 1.818, 95% CI, 1.389-2.381). In patients without PAD, the cutoff of ABID ≥0.15 was independently associated with poor outcomes (OR, 1.970, 95% CI, 1.175-3.302). IAND and cutoff of IAND ≥15 mmHg were also independently associated with poor outcomes (IAND: OR, 1.025, 95% CI, 1.009-1.041; IAND ≥15 mmHg: OR, 1.665, 95% CI, 1.188-2.334). Conversely, IAD ≥15 mmHg was associated with poor outcomes in the whole population (OR, 1.623, 95% CI, 1.011-2.605) but was not associated with poor outcomes in patients without PAD (Table 4).

Table 4. Predictors of poor outcome at 3 months.

	All Patients (n = 2901)		Patients without PAD (n = 2643)	
	OR (95% CI)	p value*	OR (95% CI)	p value*
ABI				
ABID	5.289 (1.723-16.236)	0.004	5.774 (0.948-35.151)	0.057
ABID ≥0.15	1.920 (1.361-2.708)	<0.001	1.970 (1.175-3.302)	0.010
Ankle BP, mmHg				
IAND	1.015 (1.007-1.023)	<0.001	1.025 (1.009-1.041)	0.002
IAND ≥15 mmHg	1.818 (1.389-2.381)	<0.001	1.665 (1.188-2.334)	0.003
Arm BP, mmHg				
IAD	1.009 (0.995-1.024)	0.190	1.009 (0.991-1.027)	0.329
IAD ≥15 mmHg	1.623 (1.011-2.605)	0.045	1.337 (0.758-2.360)	0.316

Data were derived from the multivariable logistic regression analysis. ABI, ankle brachial index; ABID, ankle brachial index difference; BP, blood pressure; CI, confidence interval; IAD, systolic inter-arm blood pressure difference; IAND, systolic inter-ankle blood pressure difference; NIHSS, National Institutes of Health Stroke Scale; OR, odds ratio; and PAD, peripheral artery disease. *adjusted for sex, age, NIHSS score at admission, hypertension, diabetes mellitus, hypercholesterolemia, current smoking, congestive heart failure, coronary artery disease, cerebral artery atherosclerosis, and stroke subtype.

3.3. All-Cause Mortality and MACEs

Study patients were followed up for a median of 3.1 (IQR, 1.6–4.7) years. A total of 622 patients had MACEs (21.4%) including 496 all-cause deaths (17.1%) during the study period. In Kaplan–Meier survival curves (Figure 2), higher all-cause mortality and MACEs (log-rank test; $p < 0.001$) were found in patients with ABID ≥0.15 or IAND ≥15 mmHg (log-rank test; all $p < 0.001$). Higher all-cause mortality (log-rank test; $p = 0.007$) and MACEs (log-rank test; $p = 0.008$) were also found in patients with IAD ≥15 mmHg.

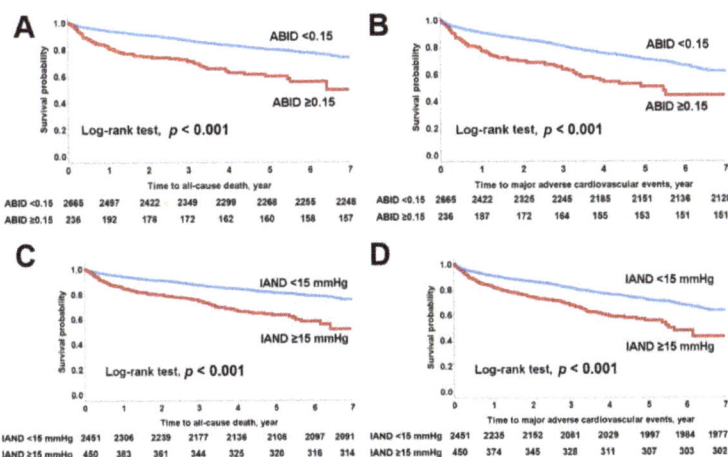

Figure 2. Kaplan–Meier survival analysis. (A) All-cause mortality; (B) major adverse cardiovascular event according to ABID ≥0.15. (C) All-cause mortality; (D) major adverse cardiovascular event according to IAND ≥15 mmHg. ABID; ankle-brachial index difference; IAND, systolic inter-ankle blood pressure difference.

In multivariable Cox regression analysis, ABID and ABID ≥0.15 were independently associated with all-cause mortality (ABID: hazard ratio (HR), 6.221, 95% CI, 2.973-13.018; ABID ≥0.15: HR, 1.567, 95% CI, 1.223-2.009) and MACEs (ABID: HR, 3.926, 95% CI, 1.906-8.087; ABID ≥0.15: HR, 1.416, 95% CI, 1.117-1.794). IAND and IAND ≥15 mmHg were also independently associated with all-cause mortality

(IAND: HR, 1.013, 95% CI, 1.007-1.019; IAND ≥15 mmHg: HR, 1.616, 95% CI, 1.317-1.982) and MACEs (IAND: HR, 1.010, 95% CI, 1.005-1.015; IAND ≥15 mmHg: HR, 1.380, 95% CI, 1.139-1.672).

In patients without PAD, ABID and ABID ≥0.15 were independently associated with all-cause mortality (ABID: HR, 9.221, 95% CI, 3.013-28.220; ABID ≥0.15: HR, 1.524, 95% CI, 1.039-2.235) and MACEs (ABID: HR, 6.605, 95% CI, 2.281-19.124; ABID ≥0.15: HR, 1.514, 95% CI, 1.058-2.166). IAND and IAND ≥15 mmHg were also independently associated with all-cause mortality (IAND: HR, 1.017, 95% CI, 1.004-1.030; IAND ≥15 mmHg: HR, 1.516, 95% CI, 1.164-1.973) and MACEs (IAND: HR, 1.015, 95% CI, 1.004-1.027; IAND ≥15 mmHg: HR, 1.343, 95% CI, 1.051-1.716). Meanwhile, IAD was associated only with the long-term occurrence of MACEs in all patients (HR, 1.010, 95% CI, 1.001-1.019), but not in those without PAD (HR, 1.006, 95% CI, 0.993-1.018, $p = 0.374$) (Table 5).

Table 5. Predictors of long-term outcome.

	All Patients (n = 2901)			
	All-Cause Mortality		MACE	
	HR (95% CI)	p value*	HR (95% CI)	p value*
ABI				
ABID	6.221 (2.973-13.018)	<0.001	3.926 (1.906-8.087)	<0.001
ABID ≥0.15	1.567 (1.223-2.009)	<0.001	1.416 (1.117-1.794)	0.004
Ankle BP, mmHg				
IAND	1.013 (1.007-1.019)	<0.001	1.010 (1.005-1.015)	<0.001
IAND ≥15 mmHg	1.616 (1.317-1.982)	<0.001	1.380 (1.139-1.672)	0.001
Arm BP, mmHg				
IAD	1.009 (0.999-1.019)	0.068	1.010 (1.001-1.019)	0.027
IAD ≥15 mmHg	1.176 (0.810-1.708)	0.395	1.151 (0.820-1.617)	0.417
	Patients without PAD (n = 2643)			
	All-Cause Mortality		MACE	
	HR (95% CI)	p value*	HR (95% CI)	p value*
ABI				
ABID	9.221 (3.013-28.220)	<0.001	6.605 (2.281-19.124)	0.001
ABID ≥0.15	1.524 (1.039-2.235)	0.031	1.514 (1.058-2.166)	0.023
Ankle BP, mmHg				
IAND	1.017 (1.004-1.030)	0.010	1.015 (1.004-1.027)	0.010
IAND ≥15 mmHg	1.516 (1.164-1.973)	0.002	1.343 (1.051-1.716)	0.019
Arm BP, mmHg				
IAD	1.007 (0.993-1.021)	0.333	1.006 (0.993-1.018)	0.374
IAD ≥15 mmHg	1.075 (0.681-1.697)	0.755	1.032 (0.682-1.563)	0.881

Data were derived from the cox proportional hazards regression analysis. ABI, ankle brachial index; ABID, ankle brachial index difference; BP, blood pressure; CI, confidence interval; HR, hazard ratio; IAD, systolic inter-arm blood pressure difference; IAND, systolic inter-ankle blood pressure difference; MACE, major adverse cardiovascular event; NIHSS, National Institutes of Health Stroke Scale; and PAD, peripheral artery disease. *adjusted for sex, age, NIHSS score at admission, hypertension, diabetes mellitus, hypercholesterolemia, current smoking, congestive heart failure, coronary artery disease, cerebral artery atherosclerosis, and stroke subtype.

4. Discussion

We demonstrated that higher ABID and IAND were independently associated with poor short-term functional outcomes, long-term MACE occurrence, and all-cause mortality in patients with acute ischemic stroke. In particular, higher ABID and IAND had prognostic effects even in patients without PAD. Meanwhile, IAD was associated with poor short-term outcomes and MACEs in all patients, but not in those without PAD. These findings suggest that higher ABID and IAND have prognostic value for both poor short- and long-term outcomes of acute ischemic stroke and are more sensitive than IAD for predicting outcomes in acute ischemic stroke patients without PAD.

Primarily, increased ABID and IAND are attributable to the presence of PAD [17]. PAD affects approximately 200 million people worldwide and is the third most common cause of atherosclerotic cardiovascular death after CAD and stroke [18]. Traditional cardiovascular risk factors (smoking, hypertension, diabetes mellitus, and hypercholesterolemia) and advanced aging are important determinants of PAD. Therefore, patients with PAD often have concomitant atherosclerosis on the cerebral and coronary artery. In the Reduction of Atherothrombosis for Continued Health registry involving 44 countries worldwide, 39% of patients with PAD had CAD, 10% had cerebral artery disease, and 13% had both [19]. Accumulated systemic atherosclerosis worsens stroke prognosis [20]. Among the atherosclerotic burdens, ABID and IAND were associated with CAA and PAD. In contrast, IAD was only associated with PAD. It can be assumed that stroke patients with large ABID and IAND are more likely to have additional cerebral atherosclerotic burden and may have a poorer prognosis.

To the best of our knowledge, no study has previously evaluated ABID as a prognosis predictor in patients with acute ischemic stroke. ABI measurement is a well-established method to identify patients with PAD. Low ABI is commonly defined as ABI <0.9 and provides good sensitivity (80%) and excellent specificity (95%) to detect PAD [4]. ABI is also associated with poor initial stroke severity [21] and predicts poor prognosis and mortality in patients with stroke [2]. However, several previous studies have shown that low ABI was not sensitive enough to detect asymptomatic PAD in the general population [22]. To detect PAD and predict stroke prognosis accurately, novel parameters besides ABI should be developed. We found that ABID and IAND were independent and strong predictors of MACEs and all-cause mortality in patients with acute ischemic stroke. Interestingly, ABID and IAND remained to be significantly associated with poor short- and long-term outcomes in patients without PAD. This finding suggests that ABID and IAND may provide additional information for patients with subclinical or mild PAD. The strength of ABID might be related to the consideration of IAND and arm BP simultaneously. In addition, ABID and IAND can be obtained and easily calculated during ABI measurement in routine clinical practice.

In patients with stroke, IAD has been demonstrated to be associated with recurrent stroke [23], poor prognosis [24], and mortality [6]. However, some patients undergo dialysis with one arm because of end-stage renal disease, making it difficult to measure IAD. In addition, IAD (and ABI) may be "pseudonormal" when a patient has severe stenosis in both arms and in one leg. In contrast, IAND can be calculated without BP measurement in the arm and provide consistent data [3]. Several studies showed the increased usefulness of IAND and ABI relative to IAD. One study showed that IAND could better predict both overall and cardiovascular mortality than IAD in elderly patients [3]. ABI exhibits better association with cardiovascular outcomes than IAD in patients with type 2 diabetes [25]. However, no study has reported the comparison between IAND and IAD in patients with acute ischemic stroke.

Because lower limbs are more prone to be affected by PAD than upper limbs, IAND could be a better predictor of PAD than IAD [26]. High IAND was associated with increased left ventricular mass index [27] and arterial stiffness [28] and also predicted mortality in the elderly people [3]. Similarly, large ABID provided the prognostic value for mortality in patients undergoing chronic hemodialysis [5]. These findings suggest that the cardiovascular risk was higher in patients with lower extremity PAD than in those with upper extremity PAD [29]. Therefore, the circulatory burden assumed from the heart to the ankles may be greater than that from the heart to the arms.

Endothelial dysfunction [26], calcification burden [30], and arterial stiffness [27] are more frequent in the lower extremities than in the upper extremities. The degree of endothelial dysfunction in leg circulation is related to PAD severity. Endothelial dysfunction of leg circulation may occur before the impairment of forearm circulation in PAD [26]. Our data showed that high ABID and IAND were more likely to have ABI >1.30 than IAD. High ABI (i.e., ABI >1.30) is generally believed to occur because of medial arterial calcification and may be a marker for vascular stiffness [4]. High ABI was associated with an increase in both overall and cardiovascular mortality in patients with chronic kidney disease undergoing hemodialysis [31] and in the general population [32]. PWV and ABI are both atherosclerotic markers. ABI reflects stenosis or peripheral artery obstruction, whereas PWV represents arterial stiffness [5]. ABID, IAND, and IAD was positively correlated with baPWV.

The correlation coefficient was highest in IAND, followed by ABID and IAD. In patients undergoing hemodialysis, high PWV and low ABI are significantly associated with mortality [33]. Therefore, ABID and IAND could be more influenced by endothelial dysfunction, systemic atherosclerosis, calcification burden, and arterial stiffness than IAD, which may be related to more frequent PAD in the lower extremities [25,26,28,29].

This study has several limitations. First, radiological studies to detect atherosclerosis in the lower extremities were not routinely performed. A correlation study between apparent atherosclerosis and IAND or ABID might be helpful for better understanding [4,17]. Second, multiple, automatic, and simultaneous assessments are recommended for accurate BP difference measurement rather than single, manual, and sequential evaluation methods [34]. We used an automatic and simultaneous measurement device, but BP difference was investigated only once during the ABI measurement, and additional follow-up data were limited. Third, BP differences in this study focused on SBP, rather than DBP. Additional analysis was performed with DBP data, which found that the prognostic effect of DBP was not different from that of SBP (Supplementary Tables S3 and S4). Fourth, our findings may not be generalized to other populations or cohorts because our study population is limited to Korean patients. Fifth, the stroke standard treatment guidelines were updated and changed several times during the study period. Lastly, a total of 921 patients were excluded from the analysis. Among them, patients who did not undergo ABI measurements were mostly excluded. Therefore, the possibility of selection bias exists because of the retrospective study design; however, consecutive patients were included, and a relatively large sample size was analyzed.

5. Conclusions

This study suggests that high ABID and IAND are associated with poor short-term outcomes, long-term MACE occurrence, and all-cause mortality in patients with acute ischemic stroke. In addition, ABID and IAND predict post-stroke outcomes, even in patients without PAD. Therefore, ABID and IAND can be simple and reliable methods for identifying patients with an increased risk of poor short- and long-term outcomes in acute ischemic stroke.

Supplementary Materials: The following are available online at http://www.mdpi.com/2077-0383/9/4/1125/s1, Table S1. Comparison of acute stroke patients during the study period who were included and excluded in this study, Table S2. Correlations between IAD, IAND, ABID, and baPWV in all patients (n = 2901), Table S3. Predictors of short-term outcome, Table S4. Predictors of long-term outcome.

Author Contributions: Conceptualization, M.H. and H.S.N.; methodology, M.H. and H.S.N.; formal analysis, M.H.; investigation, M.H. and H.S.N.; writing—original draft preparation, M.H. and H.S.N.; writing—review and editing, M.H., J.K., T.-J.S. and H.S.N.; data curation, M.H., J.K.C., J.C., J.H. and E.P.; supervision, Y.D.K., J.H.H. and H.S.N.; funding acquisition, H.S.N. All authors have read and agreed to the published version of the manuscript.

Funding: This study was supported by the National Research Foundation of Korea (NRF) grant funded by the Korean government (MSIT) (2019R1H1A1079907) and by a faculty research grant of Yonsei University College of Medicine (6-2019-0065, 6-2019-0170).

Acknowledgments: We thank Kangsik Seo, MT, for his small consideration in the course of writing the paper.

Conflicts of Interest: The authors declare no conflict of interest.

References

1. Guo, H.; Sun, F.; Dong, L.; Chang, H.; Gu, X.; Zhang, H.; Sheng, L.; Tian, Y. The Association of Four-Limb Blood Pressure with History of Stroke in Chinese Adults: A Cross-Sectional Study. *PLoS ONE* **2015**, *10*, e0139925. [CrossRef] [PubMed]
2. Milionis, H.; Vemmou, A.; Ntaios, G.; Makaritsis, K.; Koroboki, E.; Papavasileiou, V.; Savvari, P.; Spengos, K.; Elisaf, M.; Vemmos, K. Ankle-brachial index long-term outcome after first-ever ischaemic stroke. *Eur. J. Neurol.* **2013**, *20*, 1471–1478. [CrossRef] [PubMed]
3. Sheng, C.-S.; Liu, M.; Zeng, W.-F.; Huang, Q.-F.; Li, Y.; Wang, J.-G. Four-limb blood pressure as predictors of mortality in elderly Chinese. *Hypertension* **2013**, *61*, 1155–1160. [CrossRef] [PubMed]

4. Aboyans, V.; Criqui, M.H.; Abraham, P.; Allison, M.A.; Creager, M.A.; Diehm, C.; Fowkes, F.G.; Hiatt, W.R.; Jonsson, B.; Lacroix, P.; et al. Measurement and interpretation of the ankle-brachial index: A scientific statement from the American Heart Association. *Circulation* **2012**, *126*, 2890–2909. [CrossRef] [PubMed]
5. Lin, C.Y.; Leu, J.G.; Fang, Y.W.; Tsai, M.H. Association of interleg difference of ankle brachial index with overall and cardiovascular mortality in chronic hemodialysis patients. *Ren. Fail.* **2015**, *37*, 88–95. [CrossRef] [PubMed]
6. Kim, J.; Song, T.J.; Song, D.; Lee, H.S.; Nam, C.M.; Nam, H.S.; Kim, Y.D.; Heo, J.H. Interarm blood pressure difference and mortality in patients with acute ischemic stroke. *Neurology* **2013**, *80*, 1457–1464. [CrossRef]
7. Huttner, H.B.; Kohrmann, M.; Mauer, C.; Lucking, H.; Kloska, S.; Doerfler, A.; Schwab, S.; Schellinger, P.D. The prevalence of peripheral arteriopathy is higher in ischaemic stroke as compared with transient ischaemic attack and intracerebral haemorrhage. *Int. J. Stroke* **2010**, *5*, 278–283. [CrossRef]
8. Sen, S.; Lynch, D.R., Jr.; Kaltsas, E.; Simmons, J.; Tan, W.A.; Kim, J.; Beck, J.; Rosamond, W. Association of asymptomatic peripheral arterial disease with vascular events in patients with stroke or transient ischemic attack. *Stroke* **2009**, *40*, 3472–3477. [CrossRef]
9. Han, M.; Kim, Y.D.; Park, H.J.; Hwang, I.G.; Choi, J.; Ha, J.; Heo, J.H.; Nam, H.S. Prediction of functional outcome using the novel asymmetric middle cerebral artery index in cryptogenic stroke patients. *PLoS ONE* **2019**, *14*, e0208918. [CrossRef]
10. Sacco, R.L.; Adams, R.; Albers, G.; Alberts, M.J.; Benavente, O.; Furie, K.; Goldstein, L.B.; Gorelick, P.; Halperin, J.; Harbaugh, R.; et al. Guidelines for prevention of stroke in patients with ischemic stroke or transient ischemic attack: A statement for healthcare professionals from the American Heart Association/American Stroke Association Council on Stroke: Co-sponsored by the Council on Cardiovascular Radiology and Intervention: The American Academy of Neurology affirms the value of this guideline. *Stroke* **2006**, *37*, 577–617. [CrossRef]
11. Adams, R.J.; Albers, G.; Alberts, M.J.; Benavente, O.; Furie, K.; Goldstein, L.B.; Gorelick, P.; Halperin, J.; Harbaugh, R.; Johnston, S.C.; et al. Update to the AHA/ASA recommendations for the prevention of stroke in patients with stroke and transient ischemic attack. *Stroke* **2008**, *39*, 1647–1652. [CrossRef] [PubMed]
12. Furie, K.L.; Kasner, S.E.; Adams, R.J.; Albers, G.W.; Bush, R.L.; Fagan, S.C.; Halperin, J.L.; Johnston, S.C.; Katzan, I.; Kernan, W.N.; et al. Guidelines for the prevention of stroke in patients with stroke or transient ischemic attack: A guideline for healthcare professionals from the american heart association/american stroke association. *Stroke* **2011**, *42*, 227–276. [CrossRef] [PubMed]
13. Jauch, E.C.; Saver, J.L.; Adams, H.P., Jr.; Bruno, A.; Connors, J.J.; Demaerschalk, B.M.; Khatri, P.; McMullan, P.W., Jr.; Qureshi, A.I.; Rosenfield, K.; et al. Guidelines for the early management of patients with acute ischemic stroke: A guideline for healthcare professionals from the American Heart Association/American Stroke Association. *Stroke* **2013**, *44*, 870–947. [CrossRef] [PubMed]
14. Adams, H.P., Jr.; Bendixen, B.H.; Kappelle, L.J.; Biller, J.; Love, B.B.; Gordon, D.L.; Marsh, E.E., 3rd. Classification of subtype of acute ischemic stroke. Definitions for use in a multicenter clinical trial. TOAST. Trial of Org 10172 in Acute Stroke Treatment. *Stroke* **1993**, *24*, 35–41. [CrossRef]
15. Han, M.; Kim, Y.D.; Park, H.J.; Hwang, I.G.; Choi, J.; Ha, J.; Heo, J.H.; Nam, H.S. Brachial-ankle pulse wave velocity for predicting functional outcomes in patients with cryptogenic stroke. *J. Clin. Neurosci.* **2019**, *69*, 214–219. [CrossRef]
16. Nam, H.S.; Kim, H.C.; Kim, Y.D.; Lee, H.S.; Kim, J.; Lee, D.H.; Heo, J.H. Long-term mortality in patients with stroke of undetermined etiology. *Stroke* **2012**, *43*, 2948–2956. [CrossRef]
17. Herraiz-Adillo, A.; Soriano-Cano, A.; Martinez-Hortelano, J.A.; Garrido-Miguel, M.; Mariana-Herraiz, J.A.; Martinez-Vizcaino, V.; Notario-Pacheco, B. Simultaneous inter-arm and inter-leg systolic blood pressure differences to diagnose peripheral artery disease: A diagnostic accuracy study. *Blood Press.* **2018**, *27*, 121–122. [CrossRef]
18. Fowkes, F.G.; Rudan, D.; Rudan, I.; Aboyans, V.; Denenberg, J.O.; McDermott, M.M.; Norman, P.E.; Sampson, U.K.; Williams, L.J.; Mensah, G.A.; et al. Comparison of global estimates of prevalence and risk factors for peripheral artery disease in 2000 and 2010: A systematic review and analysis. *Lancet* **2013**, *382*, 1329–1340. [CrossRef]
19. Bhatt, D.L.; Steg, P.G.; Ohman, E.M.; Hirsch, A.T.; Ikeda, Y.; Mas, J.L.; Goto, S.; Liau, C.S.; Richard, A.J.; Rother, J.; et al. International prevalence, recognition, and treatment of cardiovascular risk factors in outpatients with atherothrombosis. *JAMA* **2006**, *295*, 180–189. [CrossRef]

20. Hoshino, T.; Sissani, L.; Labreuche, J.; Ducrocq, G.; Lavallee, P.C.; Meseguer, E.; Guidoux, C.; Cabrejo, L.; Hobeanu, C.; Gongora-Rivera, F.; et al. Prevalence of systemic atherosclerosis burdens and overlapping stroke etiologies and their associations with long-term vascular prognosis in stroke with intracranial atherosclerotic disease. *JAMA Neurol.* **2018**, *75*, 203–211. [CrossRef]
21. Lee, D.H.; Kim, J.; Lee, H.S.; Cha, M.J.; Kim, Y.D.; Nam, H.S.; Nam, C.M.; Heo, J.H. Low ankle-brachial index is a predictive factor for initial severity of acute ischaemic stroke. *Eur. J. Neurol.* **2012**, *19*, 892–898. [CrossRef] [PubMed]
22. Zhang, Z.; Ma, J.; Tao, X.; Zhou, Y.; Liu, X.; Su, H. The prevalence and influence factors of inter-ankle systolic blood pressure difference in community population. *PLoS ONE* **2013**, *8*, e70777. [CrossRef] [PubMed]
23. Chang, Y.; Kim, J.; Kim, Y.J.; Song, T.J. Inter-arm blood pressure difference is associated with recurrent stroke in non-cardioembolic stroke patients. *Sci. Rep.* **2019**, *9*, 12758. [CrossRef] [PubMed]
24. Chang, Y.; Kim, J.; Kim, M.H.; Kim, Y.J.; Song, T.J. Interarm Blood Pressure Difference is Associated with Early Neurological Deterioration, Poor Short-Term Functional Outcome, and Mortality in Noncardioembolic Stroke Patients. *J. Clin. Neurol.* **2018**, *14*, 555–565. [CrossRef]
25. Yan, B.P.; Zhang, Y.; Kong, A.P.; Luk, A.O.; Ozaki, R.; Yeung, R.; Tong, P.C.; Chan, W.B.; Tsang, C.C.; Lau, K.P.; et al. Borderline ankle-brachial index is associated with increased prevalence of micro- and macrovascular complications in type 2 diabetes: A cross-sectional analysis of 12,772 patients from the Joint Asia Diabetes Evaluation Program. *Diab. Vasc. Dis. Res.* **2015**, *12*, 334–341. [CrossRef]
26. Sanada, H.; Higashi, Y.; Goto, C.; Chayama, K.; Yoshizumi, M.; Sueda, T. Vascular function in patients with lower extremity peripheral arterial disease: A comparison of functions in upper and lower extremities. *Atherosclerosis* **2005**, *178*, 179–185. [CrossRef]
27. Su, H.M.; Lin, T.H.; Hsu, P.C.; Lee, W.H.; Chu, C.Y.; Chen, S.C.; Lee, C.S.; Voon, W.C.; Lai, W.T.; Sheu, S.H. Association of interankle systolic blood pressure difference with peripheral vascular disease and left ventricular mass index. *Am. J. Hypertens.* **2014**, *27*, 32–37. [CrossRef]
28. Su, H.M.; Lin, T.H.; Hsu, P.C.; Lee, W.H.; Chu, C.Y.; Chen, S.C.; Lee, C.S.; Voon, W.C.; Lai, W.T.; Sheu, S.H. Association of bilateral brachial-ankle pulse wave velocity difference with peripheral vascular disease and left ventricular mass index. *PLoS ONE* **2014**, *9*, e88331. [CrossRef]
29. Lin, L.Y.; Hwu, C.M.; Chu, C.H.; Won, J.G.S.; Chen, H.S.; Chang, L.H. The ankle brachial index exhibits better association with cardiovascular outcomes than interarm systolic blood pressure difference in patients with type 2 diabetes. *Medicine (Baltimore)* **2019**, *98*, e15556. [CrossRef]
30. Aboyans, V.; Ho, E.; Denenberg, J.O.; Ho, L.A.; Natarajan, L.; Criqui, M.H. The association between elevated ankle systolic pressures and peripheral occlusive arterial disease in diabetic and nondiabetic subjects. *J. Vasc. Surg.* **2008**, *48*, 1197–1203. [CrossRef]
31. Chen, S.C.; Chang, J.M.; Hwang, S.J.; Tsai, J.C.; Liu, W.C.; Wang, C.S.; Lin, T.H.; Su, H.M.; Chen, H.C. Ankle brachial index as a predictor for mortality in patients with chronic kidney disease and undergoing haemodialysis. *Nephrology (Carlton)* **2010**, *15*, 294–299. [CrossRef] [PubMed]
32. Resnick, H.E.; Lindsay, R.S.; McDermott, M.M.; Devereux, R.B.; Jones, K.L.; Fabsitz, R.R.; Howard, B.V. Relationship of high and low ankle brachial index to all-cause and cardiovascular disease mortality: The Strong Heart Study. *Circulation* **2004**, *109*, 733–739. [CrossRef]
33. Chen, S.C.; Chang, J.M.; Tsai, Y.C.; Tsai, J.C.; Su, H.M.; Hwang, S.J.; Chen, H.C. Association of interleg BP difference with overall and cardiovascular mortality in hemodialysis. *Clin. J. Am. Soc. Nephrol.* **2012**, *7*, 1646–1653. [CrossRef] [PubMed]
34. Verberk, W.J.; Kessels, A.G.; Thien, T. Blood pressure measurement method and inter-arm differences: A meta-analysis. *Am. J. Hypertens.* **2011**, *24*, 1201–1208. [CrossRef] [PubMed]

© 2020 by the authors. Licensee MDPI, Basel, Switzerland. This article is an open access article distributed under the terms and conditions of the Creative Commons Attribution (CC BY) license (http://creativecommons.org/licenses/by/4.0/).

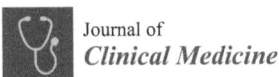

Article

Interhemispheric Functional Connectivity in the Primary Motor Cortex Assessed by Resting-State Functional Magnetic Resonance Imaging Aids Long-Term Recovery Prediction among Subacute Stroke Patients with Severe Hand Weakness

Yu-Sun Min [1,2,3,†], Jang Woo Park [4,†], Eunhee Park [1,2], Ae-Ryoung Kim [1,2], Hyunsil Cha [4], Dae-Won Gwak [2], Seung-Hwan Jung [2], Yongmin Chang [4,5,6,*] and Tae-Du Jung [1,2,*]

1. Department of Rehabilitation Medicine, School of Medicine, Kyungpook National University, Daegu 41944, Korea; ssuni119@naver.com (Y.-S.M.); ehmdpark@naver.com (E.P.); ryoung20@hanmail.net (A.-R.K.)
2. Department of Rehabilitation Medicine, Kyungpook National University Hospital, Daegu 41944, Korea; eodnjs108@naver.com (D.-W.G.); pyromyth@naver.com (S.-H.J.)
3. Department of Biomedical Engineering, Seoul National University College of Medicine, Seoul 03080, Korea
4. Department of Medical & Biological Engineering, Kyungpook National University, Daegu 41944, Korea; giantstar.jw@gmail.com (J.W.P.); hscha1002@daum.net (H.C.)
5. Department of Radiology, Kyungpook National University Hospital, Daegu 41944, Korea
6. Department of Molecular Medicine, School of Medicine, Kyungpook National University, Daegu 41944, Korea
* Correspondence: ychang@knu.ac.kr (Y.C.); teeed0522@hanmail.net (T.-D.J.); Tel.: +82-53-420-5471 (Y.C.); +82-53-200-2167 (T.-D.J.)
† Contributed equally to this work.

Received: 25 February 2020; Accepted: 30 March 2020; Published: 1 April 2020

Abstract: This study aimed to evaluate the usefulness of interhemispheric functional connectivity (FC) as a predictor of motor recovery in severe hand impairment and to determine the cutoff FC level as a clinically useful parameter. Patients with stroke ($n = 22$; age, 59.9 ± 13.7 years) who presented with unilateral severe upper-limb paresis and were confirmed to elicit no motor-evoked potential responses were selected. FC was measured using resting-state functional magnetic resonance imaging (rsfMRI) scans at 1 month from stroke onset. The good recovery group showed a higher FC value than the poor recovery group ($p = 0.034$). In contrast, there was no statistical difference in FC value between the good recovery and healthy control groups ($p = 0.182$). Additionally, the healthy control group showed a higher FC value than that shown by the poor recovery group ($p = 0.0002$). Good and poor recovery were determined based on Brunnstrom stage of upper-limb function at 6 months as the standard, and receiver operating characteristic curve indicated that a cutoff score of 0.013 had the greatest prognostic ability. In conclusion, interhemispheric FC measurement using rsfMRI scans may provide useful clinical information for predicting hand motor recovery during stroke rehabilitation.

Keywords: functional magnetic resonance imaging; neuronal plasticity; recovery of function; stroke; motor cortex

1. Introduction

Stroke is the leading cause of adult disability worldwide, accounting for a majority of patients with upper-limb impairment. The degrees of spontaneous improvement vary according to the severity of upper-limb paresis. In patients with mild-to-moderate upper-limb paresis, spontaneous recovery, as reflected by improvements in clinical parameters including Fugl-Meyer assessment of the upper extremity (FMA-UE) scores, is mainly restricted to the first 4 weeks post-stroke [1].There is evidence in the literature that in stroke patients with mild-to-moderate impairment, the degree of initial deficits predicts outcome. In contrast to mildly impaired patients, it is relatively difficult to predict the spontaneous recovery pattern of upper-limb motor function in severely impaired patients. Clinical data alone cannot accurately predict arm recovery, particularly in patients with initial severe upper-limb impairment [2–4]. High inter-individual variability associated with recovery makes it difficult to predict arm recovery. However, very few severely impaired patients show late-onset motor recovery of the upper-limb [5]. Therefore, a prognostic biomarker reflecting functional long-term motor recovery is urgently required to decide the manner in which rehabilitation treatment strategies, including goal setting and effective treatment duration, for upper-limb recovery in severe hemiplegic stroke patients can be modified.

Recently, we reported that initial power spectral density (PSD) analysis of resting-state functional magnetic resonance imaging (rsfMRI) data can provide a sensitive prognostic predictor for patients with subacute stroke combined with severe hand disability [6]. PSD is measured as resting-state intrinsic neuronal activity in the frequency domain. In contrast to PSD, functional connectivity (FC) analysis is another approach to measure the resting-state intrinsic neuronal activity in the time domain using rsfMRI. Changes in FC value in the interhemispheric motor cortex (M1) after stroke are reportedly reflective of long-term recovery, and patients with good functional outcomes have greater FC values than patients with poor outcomes [7–9]. However, a recent study reported that differences in FC value in the interhemispheric M1 did not change over time with recovery [10]. Therefore, whether motor recovery after stroke can be predicted by the change in interhemispheric FC still remains controversial.

This study aimed to evaluate whether interhemispheric FC is useful for predicting upper-limb motor recovery among patients with severe hand impairment for whom it was difficult to predict the recovery pattern based on an initial clinical parameter. Therefore, addition of FC as a prognostic parameter for patients with severe hand deficits may eventually be useful for setting individualized therapeutic goals and strategies as well as for selecting patients for future trials.

2. Materials and Methods

2.1. Subjects

Twenty-two patients (59.9 ± 13.7 years; 9 males and 13 females) and 12 healthy subjects (60.2 ± 6.8 years; 8 males, 4 females) were included in this study. They were all right-handed. The inclusion criteria for patients were as follows: (1) unilateral ischemic stroke in the middle cerebral artery (MCA) territory confirmed by MRI, (2) first stroke, (3) age over 20, (4) hemiplegic motor deficit less than Gr 1 by manual muscle test present at the time of admission (Table 1). Patients with unstable medical conditions and those lost to follow-up were excluded.

All patients underwent resting functional magnetic resonance imaging about 1 month (27.8 ± 8.4) from stroke onset. We used Brunnstrom stage (hand score) as a parameter to assess clinical outcome at 1 month and 6 months after stroke onset. We included the patients with Brunnstrom stage 1 (flaccidity or absence of an active finger movement) but without any motor-evoked potential (MEP) responses of the affected hand at 1 month after stroke. Patients with severely impaired cognitive function [Mini-Mental State Examination (MMSE) < 24], severe visual or perceptual impairment, previous musculoskeletal abnormality, or damaged upper-limbs were excluded. All patients received individual physiotherapy training as well as cognitive training every day. The physiotherapy treatments comprised 30-min sessions two times per day for five days a week and included walking and balance training as well as individual exercise. Informed consent was provided to all patients according to OO University Institutional Review Board (2012-05-023).

Table 1. Demographics and baseline characteristics of enrolled patients.

Subject	Group	Sex	Age	Lesion Territory	Total Lesion Volume (cc)	Lesion Volume (CST-Overlapped) (cc)	BS-Hand (Pre)	BS-Hand (Post)	Hand Dominance	BDI	MMSE	NIHSS
1	Good	F	57	MCA	4.8	0.247	1	4	Rt	10	28	8
2	Good	F	67	MCA	58.3	0.359	1	4	Rt	12	25	3
3	Good	F	70	MCA	13.1	0.439	1	4	Rt	22	27	9
4	Good	F	32	MCA	75	0.683	1	4	Rt	12	30	9
5	Good	F	80	MCA	4.7	0.226	1	4	Rt	10	27	5
6	Good	M	67	MCA	11.2	0.177	1	5	Rt	16	28	7
7	Good	F	75	MCA	7.1	0.241	1	4	Rt	24	26	9
8	Good	F	75	MCA	2.1	0.305	1	4	Rt	16	23	4
9	Good	M	40	MCA	9.0	0.216	1	4	Rt	23	27	9
10	Good	M	57	MCA	7.5	0.189	1	4	Rt	8	18	6
11	Good	M	44	MCA	130.4	0.544	1	5	Rt	5	14	7
12	Poor	F	66	MCA	84.5	0.522	1	1	Rt	33	5	16
13	Poor	M	42	MCA	273.8	0.246	1	1	Rt	20	24	7
14	Poor	M	59	MCA	268.7	0.680	1	2	Rt	4	24	9
15	Poor	F	75	MCA	78.3	0.291	1	1	Rt	29	-	13
16	Poor	F	75	MCA	25.0	0.257	1	1	Rt	13	25	13
17	Poor	M	68	MCA	23.6	0.247	1	1	Rt	5	21	15
18	Poor	M	40	MCA	334.2	0.442	1	1	Rt	-	-	21
19	Poor	F	69	MCA	121.4	0.683	1	1	Rt	15	24	14
20	Poor	F	44	MCA	164.4	0.571	1	1	Rt	-	-	12
21	Poor	M	53	MCA	5.1	0.302	1	2	Rt	2	30	6
22	Poor	F	64	MCA	5.3	0.245	1	3	Rt	28	30	11

CST, CorticoSpinal Tract; BS, Brunnstrom stage; BDI, Beck Depression Inventory; MMSE, Mini Mental State Examination; NIHSS, National Institutes of Health Stroke Scale MCA, Middle Cerebral Artery.

2.2. Motor Task Functional Magnetic Resonance Imaging

Region of interest (ROI) of M1 for each participant was defined using motor task functional magnetic resonance imaging (fMRI). Motor task fMRI alternatively comprised three active periods and three rest periods, and each period was 30-s long. A light touch on the leg or hand was used to give a start signal at the start point of each period. Participants performed the motor task twice with the right and left hands and repeated flexion–extension during scanning. If any of the participants could not move their hand, they received assistance to perform passive movement.

To perform motor task fMRI data acquisition, T2-weighted echo-planar imaging sequences were used with the following parameters: TE (echo time) = 40 ms, TR (repetition time) = 3000 ms, Flip Angle (FA) = 90°, FOV (field-of-view) = 21 cm, acquisition matrix = 64 × 64, 4-mm thickness with no gap, and total scan time = 4 min and 12 s, with four dummy scans.

2.3. Resting-State fMRI

All fMRI data were obtained on a Signa Exite 3.0-T scanner (GE Healthcare, Milwaukee, WI, USA). All applicants were instructed to lie down comfortably and close their eyes during MRI scanning, but not fall asleep. The rsfMRI data were obtained using T2-weighted echo-planar imaging sequences using the following parameters: TE = 40 ms, TR = 2000 ms, FA = 90°, FOV = 22 cm, acquisition matrix = 64 × 64, 4-mm thickness with no gap, and total scan time = 8 min and 12 s, with six dummy scans.

Three-dimensional-fast spoiled gradient echo sequence [repetition time (TR) = 7.8 ms; echo time (TE) = 3 ms; inversion time = 450 ms; flip angle = 20; matrix = 256 × 256; field-of-view (FOV) = 24 mm; 1.3 mm thickness] was used for the acquisition of T1-weighted high-resolution anatomical images.

2.4. fMRI Data Analysis

Image preprocessing and statistical analyses of fMRI data were conducted using the statistical parametric mapping software SPM12 (http://www.fil.ion.ucl.ac.uk/spm/), implemented in MATLAB (Mathworks, Inc., Sherborn, MA, USA). By slice-timing, realignment, co-registration, and normalization, functional images were preprocessed into the Montreal Neurological Institute (MNI) template based on a standard stereotaxic coordinate system and spatial smoothing with 8-mm full-width at half-maximum (FWHM) Gaussian kernel. FMRI data are superimposed onto MNI space. The seed MNI coordinates for the patients were summarized in Table S1 (Supplementary Materials).

2.5. Rest State Functional Connectivity

The seed-based method was used to determine resting-state functional connectivity (rsFC). In brief, FC CONN15 toolbox (http://web.mit.edu/swg/software.htm) was used to show a strong temporal correlation between bilateral M1 and supplementary motor area (SMA). The contralesion and ipsilesion (namely M1 and SMA; spheres of 5-mm radius) were identified using MarsBar ROI tool (http://marsbar.sourceforge.net/) on MNI coordinates. Four ROI positions (spheres of 5 mm radius), namely contralesional M1, ipsilesional M1, contralesional SMA, and ipsilesional SMA, were selected based on individual motor task results. Noise, cerebrospinal fluid, white matter, and motion parameters were used to correct time fluctuations in blood-oxygen-level-dependent (BOLD) signals as nuisance covariates, and a band-pass filter (range, 0.008 Hz–0.09 Hz) was used. FC scores between pairs of ROIs on each subject were calculated using the FC SPM12 toolbox.

2.6. Lesion Volume Analysis

The lesion volume associated with hand motor function in the stroke area was calculated based on the overlapping area of the lesion mask between the T1-weighted images and the template of the corticospinal tract (CST). T1-weighted images were taken by preprocessing, which involves co-registration and normalization to a T1-weighted template using the SPM12 software package. A stroke physiatrist, who was blinded to the study, manually drew the lesions by using MRIcro (http:

//www.mccauslandcenter.sc.edu/crnl/mricro). The CST template was constructed using a previously reported method of probabilistic tractography [11,12]. Probabilistic tractography was conducted for 26 healthy controls to reconstruct CST. The seed, target, waypoint, and exclusion mask were drawn as follows. Individual seed masks for each hemisphere were placed in the hand knob area of M1 (MNI coordinates (37, −25, 62); (−37, −25, 62)), and each participant used an established semi-automated pipeline. The target masks were basis pontis. The waypoint masks included the posterior limb of the internal capsules and cerebral peduncles. For CST, a mask covering trajectories at the tegmentum pontis was added to the mid-sagittal and basal ganglia exclusion masks as an additional exclusion mask. A total of 50,000 streamlines were sent from M1 to the spinal target masks in the ventral medulla oblongata. Three different thresholds at 0.5%, 1%, and 2% were established for CST output distributions. The average of each tract was calculated for each of the three thresholds by summing all individual threshold- and subject-specific trajectories.

2.7. Statistical Analysis

To assess differences in FC scores between the three groups for each pair of ROIs, an ANOVA F-test was performed; subsequently, post-hoc two-sample t-tests were conducted for carrying out further comparisons. All statistical analyses were performed using the Statistical Package for the Social Sciences (SPSS, Chicago, IL, USA). A p value of <0.05 was considered to be statistically significant.

Receiver-operating characteristic (ROC) curve analysis was performed to determine the cutoff value for the prognostic model of upper-limb stroke recovery by using the difference in FC score between ipsilesional and contralesional M1 at 1 month.

True-positive rate (sensitivity) and false-positive rate (1-specificity) were computed and plotted as ROC curves. In an ROC space, a diagonal line corresponds to random discrimination. The area under the ROC curve (AUC) is commonly used to quantify classifier discriminability, with a value of 0.5 corresponding to random classification and a value of 1 corresponding to perfect classification.

3. Results

At 6 months after stroke onset, 11 patients (60.3 ± 15.9 years; seven males, four females) with Brunnstrom stage 4 (lateral prehension with release by thumb movement or semi-voluntary finger extension of a small range of motion) or 5 (palmar prehension or cylindrical/spherical grasp with limited function or voluntary mass finger extension of variable range) were categorized into the good recovery group and 11 patients (59.5 ± 12.9 years; six males, five females) with Brunnstrom stage 1, 2, and 3 were categorized into the poor recovery group. There were no age and sex-based differences between the good recovery and the poor recovery groups and the healthy control group (p = 0.986 and p = 0.827, respectively). Additionally, there was no statistical difference (p = 0.158) in lesion overlap volume between the good recovery group (0.33 ± 0.15 cc) and the poor recovery group (0.40 ± 0.17 cc). However, there was statistical difference (p = 0.019) in total lesion volume between the good recovery group (29.37 ± 41.31 cc) and the poor recovery group (125 ± 118.73 cc) (Figure 1). The demographic and clinical characteristics of 22 patients with stroke are summarized in Table 1.

Among the three groups, ANOVA F-test results reveal a statistically significant difference in FC between ipsilesional M1–contralesional M1 (p = 0.00039) (Figure 2). Post-hoc two-sample t-tests were performed for comparing the three groups further. The good recovery group showed a higher FC than that of the poor recovery group (p = 0.034). Contrastingly, the good recovery group showed no statistical difference in FC when compared with the healthy control group (p = 0.182), but the latter had a higher FC than that of the poor recovery group (p = 0.0002).

Moreover, according to the ANOVA F-test, the FC between ipsilesional SMA and contralesional SMA was significantly different among the three groups (p = 0.003) (Figure 1). In the post-hoc two-sample t-test, the FC between ipsilesional SMA and contralesional SMA was higher in the healthy control group compared with that in the good recovery group and the poor recovery group (p = 0.019

and $p = 0.004$, respectively), but there was no difference in the FC value between the good recovery group and the poor recovery group ($p = 0.804$).

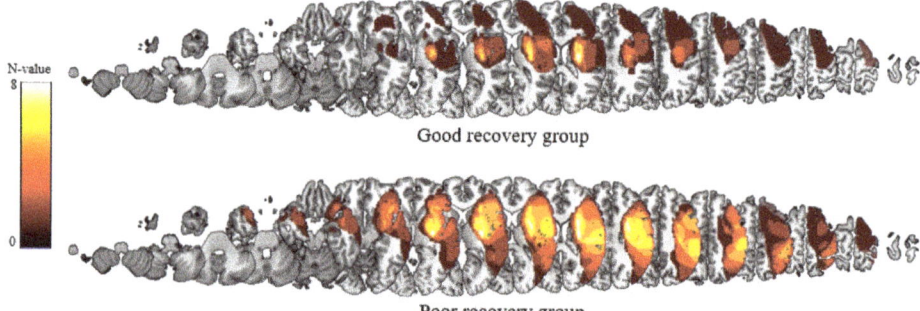

Figure 1. Total lesion overlay maps for the good recovery group and the poor recovery group.

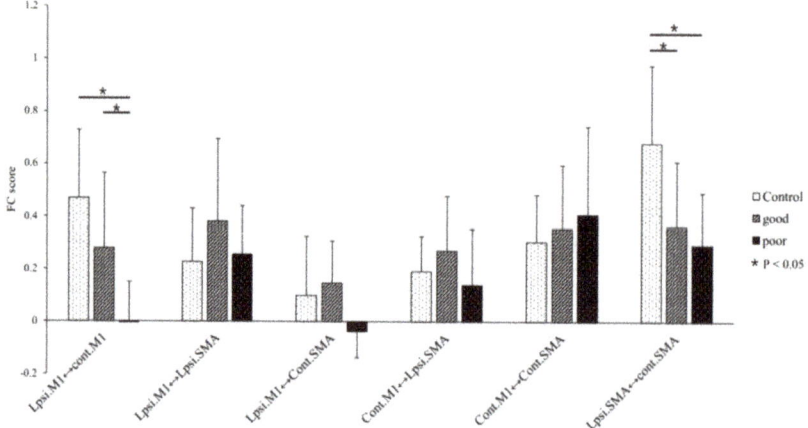

Figure 2. ANOVA F-tests showed significant differences in functional connectivity (FC) between ipsilesional M1-contralesional M1 among the three groups ($p = 0.00039$). Post-hoc two-sample t-tests were performed for further comparing between the groups. The good recovery group showed a higher FC than that shown by the poor recovery group ($p = 0.034$). In contrast, no significant difference in FC was seen between the good recovery and the healthy control groups ($p = 0.182$). Additionally, the healthy control group showed a higher FC than that of the poor recovery group ($p = 0.0002$).

Contrastingly, the ANOVA F-test result reveals no significant difference in FC among ipsilesional M1-SMA ($p = 0.318$), ipsilesional M1-contralesional SMA ($p = 0.056$), contralesional M1-ipsilesional SMA ($p = 0.297$), and contralesional M1-contralesional SMA ($p = 0.656$).

When the total lesion volume was included as a covariate in statistical analysis, ANOVA F-test results reveal a statistically significant difference in FC between ipsilesional M1–contralesional M1 among the three groups ($p = 0.018$) and in FC between ipsilesional M1–contralesional SMA among the three groups ($p = 0.015$). In the post-hoc two-sample t-test, however, there was no difference in the FC value between the good recovery group and poor recovery group ($p = 0.232$).

FC between ipsilesional and contralesional M1 positively correlated with hand function prognosis, as evaluated by Brunnstrom motor stages (BMS) ($r = 0.581$ and $p = 0.005$, respectively) (Figure 3). However, FC between ipsilesional and contralesional SMA did not correlate with hand function prognosis, as evaluated by BMS ($r = -0.006$, $p = 0.979$).

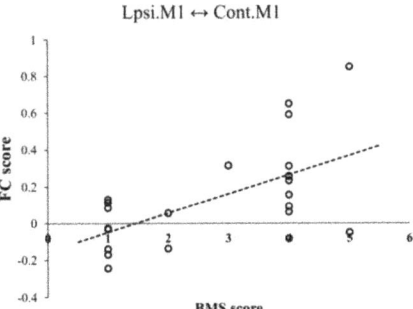

Figure 3. FC between ipsilesional and contralesional M1 is positively correlated with prognosis of hand function, as evaluated by Brunnstrom motor stages (BMS) (r = 0.581, p = 0.005).

Good and poor recovery outcomes based on the Brunnstrom stage of upper-limb function at 6 months were determined as the standard, and the ROC curve indicated that a cutoff score of 0.013 had the greatest prognostic ability (maximum sensitivity and specificity) (Figure 4). The sensitivity of this model for predicting good recovery was 81.8% and the specificity was 63.6%. AUC value was 0.793, which is a fair level.

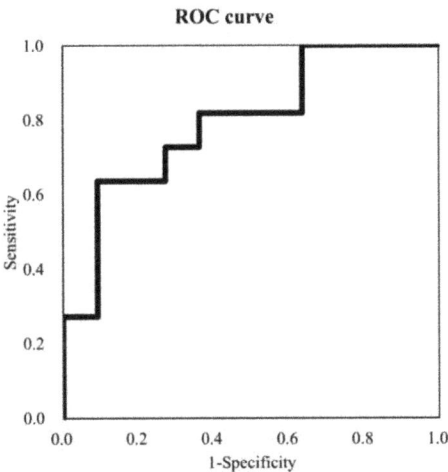

Figure 4. Good and poor recovery were determined based on Brunnstrom stage of upper-limb function at 6 months as the standard, and ROC (Receiver-operating characteristic) curve indicated that a cutoff score of 0.013 had the greatest prognostic ability (maximum sensitivity and specificity).

4. Discussion

Here, we demonstrated the predictive value of FC for long-term motor outcomes in subacute stroke patients with stroke, predominantly in the MCA territory. The FC between ipsilateral and contralateral M1 was lower in the poor recovery group compared with that in the good recovery and healthy control groups, and it was also well correlated with hand function prognosis, evaluated by BMS. Our study demonstrated that the interhemispheric FC score calculated at 1 month after stroke has a good predictive value for recovery over a 6-month period in patients with severe hand impairment. However, the total lesion volume showed a tendency to swallow a large amount of explanatory variance of the outcome parameter. We also suggested an FC cutoff score for discriminating the good recovery group from the poor recovery group with high sensitivity and specificity.

Previous rsfMRI studies on acute stroke demonstrated that patients with mild-to-moderate motor deficits showed low interhemispheric FC score between the motor cortices [8,9,13]. These studies also revealed that the low FC score gradually increased during the recovery process and finally restored to near-normal levels in a good recovery group, while the FC score in the poor recovery group continued to decrease. Our findings are in line with these previous studies, i.e., interhemispheric FC score is useful for assessing the stroke prognosis and recovery despite varying scanning times (e.g., 3 days vs. 4 weeks) and evaluation domains [7,14,15].

These results suggest that functional neuroadaptation (reorganization) may be occurring in the most severely injured brains. One possible explanation for this finding is the physiological balance in reciprocal inhibitory projections between both of the hemispheres [16]. This explanation suggests that an abnormal inhibitory influence of the undamaged contralesional motor cortex on the damaged ipsilesional motor cortex disturbs the balance between the hemispheres, which is important for voluntarily generating paretic hand movement in poor recovery patients [16–19]. Here, the patients in the good recovery group had a higher rsFC between the motor cortex, which enhanced motor ability in the paretic hand. Our findings are consistent with those of previous studies, which demonstrated that rsFC within either the ipsilesional primary sensorimotor cortex or contralesional primary sensorimotor cortex reduced at an early stage after stroke, after which, in those patients who showed an improvement in motor impairment, the rsFC gradually increased to near-normal levels during recovery.

However, Nijboer et al. reported that ipsilesional rsFC between motor areas was lower than the contralesional rsFC, but this difference did not change over time [10]; they demonstrated that no relations were observed between individual changes in rsFC and upper-limb motor recovery. In that study, patient population presented with mild upper-limb impairments as opposed to the patients in our study who had severe motor impairment at 4 weeks after stroke. The patients only showed a limited amount of improvement (i.e., ceiling effect) after the first 4 weeks. The changes in brain activation patterns (i.e., cerebral reorganization) might have a different impact on a mild patient population compared with that on a population comprising severely impaired patients [20]. Here, patients were completely motor deficit with no hand movement and MEP response.

Using rsfMRI, we elucidated the cutoff value of FC to be 0.013, and sensitivity and specificity rates for good recovery prediction were 81.8% and 63.6%, respectively. There have been many studies on modeling the prediction of function recovery after stroke. The representative models are the PREP algorithm and the proportional recovery model [2,21]. However, when the two models were validated, the predicted prognosis rate (sensitivity and specificity) remained around 73–88%. The reason is that fitting to that predictive model did not work well in patients with severe corticospinal tract damage early in the injury, clinically complete unilateral paralysis, and patients with no MEP response. That is, in the case of mild to moderate severity, the prediction through clinical data and infarction size fit well, but in severe cases, it was difficult to predict through the model, and these were called 'non-fitter'. In this study, we included relatively homogenous patients with MCA infarction, clinically no hand movement at all, and neurophysiologically no MEP response. Therefore, measuring interhemispheric functional connectivity in these patient populations can help predict prognosis. The prediction power associated with the use of only one parameter, namely interhemispheric rsFC, was comparable to the power associated with the multi-parameter model, without causing any compromise in sensitivity and specificity rates.

The present study had some limitations. First of all, our study is limited by small numbers in the patient population. Due to this limitation, stroke patients included only those with cortical and subcortical stroke, and we could not definitely determine the differential impact of lesion location and stroke severity on rsFC. Hence, from our results, we could not fully elucidate the mechanisms responsible for the reduction in rsFC after stroke as well as its influence on patient behavior. However, a more important clinical implication would be the establishment of the prognostic power of rsFC at an early stage. Therefore, larger sample size and longitudinal follow-up are warranted to confirm these relationships in future studies.

5. Conclusions

Interhemispheric FC estimated via rsfMRI provides useful clinical information and has a predictive value for hand motor recovery during stroke rehabilitation.

Supplementary Materials: The following are available online at http://www.mdpi.com/2077-0383/9/4/975/s1, Table S1: Individual ROI coordinates obtained from task-fMRI.

Author Contributions: Conceptualization, J.W.P.; Data curation, D.-W.G. and S.-H.J.; Formal analysis, E.P.; Funding acquisition, Y.C.; Investigation, A.-R.K.; Methodology, J.W.P.; Resources, H.C. and Y.C.; Software, J.W.P.; Supervision, T.-D.J.; Validation, E.P.; Visualization, J.W.P.; Writing—original draft, Y.-S.M.; Writing—review & editing, Y.C. All authors have read and agreed to the published version of the manuscript.

Funding: This work was supported by Biomedical Research Institute grant, Kyungpook National University Hospital (2015).

Conflicts of Interest: The authors declare no conflict of interest.

References

1. Kwakkel, G.; Kollen, B.J.; van der Grond, J.; Prevo, A.J.H. Probability of regaining dexterity in the flaccid upper limb: Impact of severity of paresis and time since onset in acute stroke. *Stroke* **2003**, *34*, 2181–2186. [CrossRef]
2. Byblow, W.D.; Stinear, C.M.; Barber, P.A.; Petoe, M.A.; Ackerley, S.J. Proportional recovery after stroke depends on corticomotor integrity. *Ann. Neurol.* **2015**, *78*, 848–859. [CrossRef]
3. Feng, W.; Wang, J.; Chhatbar, P.Y.; Doughty, C.; Landsittel, D.; Lioutas, V.A.; Kautz, S.A.; Schlaug, G. Corticospinal tract lesion load: An imaging biomarker for stroke motor outcomes. *Ann. Neurol.* **2015**, *78*, 860–870. [CrossRef] [PubMed]
4. Buch, E.R.; Rizk, S.; Nicolo, P.; Cohen, L.G.; Schnider, A.; Guggisberg, A.G. Predicting motor improvement after stroke with clinical assessment and diffusion tensor imaging. *Neurology* **2016**, *86*, 1924–1925. [CrossRef] [PubMed]
5. Jung, T.D.; Kim, J.Y.; Seo, J.H.; Jin, S.U.; Lee, H.J.; Lee, S.H.; Lee, Y.S.; Chang, Y. Combined information from resting-state functional connectivity and passive movements with functional magnetic resonance imaging differentiates fast late-onset motor recovery from progressive recovery in hemiplegic stroke patients: A pilot study. *J. Rehabil. Med.* **2013**, *45*, 546–552. [CrossRef] [PubMed]
6. Min, Y.S.; Park, J.W.; Jang, K.E.; Lee, H.J.; Lee, J.; Lee, Y.S.; Jung, T.D.; Chang, Y. Power Spectral Density Analysis of Long-Term Motor Recovery in Patients With Subacute Stroke. *Neurorehabil. Neural Repair* **2019**, *33*, 38–46. [CrossRef] [PubMed]
7. Puig, J.; Blasco, G.; Alberich-Bayarri, A.; Schlaug, G.; Deco, G.; Biarnes, C.; Navas-Martí, M.; Rivero, M.; Gich, J.; Figueras, J.; et al. Resting-State Functional Connectivity Magnetic Resonance Imaging and Outcome After Acute Stroke. *Stroke* **2018**, *49*, 2353–2360. [CrossRef] [PubMed]
8. Carter, A.R.; Shulman, G.L.; Corbetta, M. Why use a connectivity-based approach to study stroke and recovery of function? *Neuroimage* **2012**, *62*, 2271–2280. [CrossRef] [PubMed]
9. Golestani, A.M.; Tymchuk, S.; Demchuk, A.; Goodyear, B.G. VISION-2 Study Group Longitudinal evaluation of resting-state FMRI after acute stroke with hemiparesis. *Neurorehabil. Neural Repair* **2013**, *27*, 153–163. [CrossRef]
10. Nijboer, T.C.W.; Buma, F.E.; Winters, C.; Vansteensel, M.J.; Kwakkel, G.; Ramsey, N.F.; Raemaekers, M. No changes in functional connectivity during motor recovery beyond 5 weeks after stroke; A longitudinal resting-state fMRI study. *PLoS ONE* **2017**, *12*, e0178017. [CrossRef]
11. Schulz, R.; Koch, P.; Zimerman, M.; Wessel, M.; Bönstrup, M.; Thomalla, G.; Cheng, B.; Gerloff, C.; Hummel, F.C. Parietofrontal motor pathways and their association with motor function after stroke. *Brain* **2015**, *138*, 1949–1960. [CrossRef] [PubMed]
12. Schulz, R.; Park, C.H.; Boudrias, M.H.; Gerloff, C.; Hummel, F.C.; Ward, N.S. Assessing the integrity of corticospinal pathways from primary and secondary cortical motor areas after stroke. *Stroke* **2012**, *43*, 2248–2251. [CrossRef] [PubMed]

13. Carter, A.R.; Astafiev, S.V.; Lang, C.E.; Connor, L.T.; Rengachary, J.; Strube, M.J.; Pope, D.L.W.; Shulman, G.L.; Corbetta, M. Resting interhemispheric functional magn0065tic resonance imaging connectivity predicts performance after stroke. *Ann. Neurol.* **2010**, *67*, 365–375. [CrossRef] [PubMed]
14. Park, C.; Chang, W.H.; Ohn, S.H.; Kim, S.T.; Bang, O.Y.; Pascual-Leone, A.; Kim, Y.-H. Longitudinal changes of resting-state functional connectivity during motor recovery after stroke. *Stroke* **2011**, *42*, 1357–1362. [CrossRef]
15. Yin, D.; Song, F.; Xu, D.; Peterson, B.S.; Sun, L.; Men, W.; Yan, X.; Fan, M. Patterns in cortical connectivity for determining outcomes in hand function after subcortical stroke. *PLoS ONE* **2012**, *7*, e52727. [CrossRef]
16. Ward, N.S.; Brown, M.M.; Thompson, A.J.; Frackowiak, R.S.J. Neural correlates of outcome after stroke: A cross-sectional fMRI study. *Brain* **2003**, *126*, 1430–1448. [CrossRef]
17. Cramer, S.C.; Riley, J.D. Neuroplasticity and brain repair after stroke. *Curr. Opin. Neurol.* **2008**, *21*, 76–82. [CrossRef]
18. Buma, F.E.; Lindeman, E.; Ramsey, N.F.; Kwakkel, G. Functional neuroimaging studies of early upper limb recovery after stroke: A systematic review of the literature. *Neurorehabil. Neural Repair* **2010**, *24*, 589–608. [CrossRef]
19. Fan, Y.; Wu, C.; Liu, H.; Lin, K.; Wai, Y.; Chen, Y. Neuroplastic changes in resting-state functional connectivity after stroke rehabilitation. *Front. Hum. Neurosci.* **2015**, *9*. [CrossRef]
20. Xu, H.; Qin, W.; Chen, H.; Jiang, L.; Li, K.; Yu, C. Contribution of the Resting-State Functional Connectivity of the Contralesional Primary Sensorimotor Cortex to Motor Recovery after Subcortical Stroke. *PLoS ONE* **2014**, *9*, e84729. [CrossRef]
21. Stinear, C.M.; Barber, P.A.; Petoe, M.; Anwar, S.; Byblow, W.D. The PREP algorithm predicts potential for upper limb recovery after stroke. *Brain* **2012**, *135*, 2527–2535. [CrossRef] [PubMed]

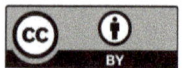

© 2020 by the authors. Licensee MDPI, Basel, Switzerland. This article is an open access article distributed under the terms and conditions of the Creative Commons Attribution (CC BY) license (http://creativecommons.org/licenses/by/4.0/).

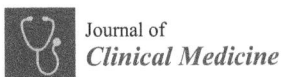

Article

The Prognostic Value of High Platelet Reactivity in Ischemic Stroke Depends on the Etiology: A Pilot Study

Adam Wiśniewski [1,*], Karolina Filipska [2], Joanna Sikora [3], Robert Ślusarz [2] and Grzegorz Kozera [4]

[1] Department of Neurology, Faculty of Medicine, Nicolaus Copernicus University in Toruń, Collegium Medicum in Bydgoszcz, 85-094 Bydgoszcz, Poland
[2] Department of Neurological and Neurosurgical Nursing, Faculty of Health Sciences, Nicolaus Copernicus University in Toruń, Collegium Medicum in Bydgoszcz, 85-821 Bydgoszcz, Poland; karolinafilipskakf@gmail.com (K.F.); robert_slu_cmumk@wp.pl (R.Ś.)
[3] Experimental Biotechnology Research and Teaching Team, Department of Transplantology and General Surgery, Nicolaus Copernicus University in Toruń, Collegium Medicum in Bydgoszcz, 85-094 Bydgoszcz, Poland; joanna.sikora@cm.umk.pl
[4] Medical Simulation Centre, Medical University of Gdańsk, Faculty of Medicine, 80-210 Gdańsk, Poland; gkozera1@wp.pl
* Correspondence: adam.lek@wp.pl; Tel.: +48-79-08-13513; Fax: +48-52-5854032

Received: 8 February 2020; Accepted: 19 March 2020; Published: 20 March 2020

Abstract: Background: Reduced aspirin response may result in a worse prognosis and a poor clinical outcome in ischemic stroke. The aim of this prospective pilot study was to assess the relationship between platelet reactivity and early and late prognosis, and the clinical and functional status in ischemic stroke, with the role of stroke etiology. Methods: The study involved 69 subjects with ischemic stroke, divided into large and small vessel etiological subgroups. Platelet function testing was performed with two aggregometric methods—impedance and optical—while the clinical condition was assessed using the National Institute of Health Stroke Scale (NIHSS) and the functional status was assessed using the modified Rankin Scale (mRS) on the first and eighth day (early prognosis) and the 90th day of stroke (late prognosis). Results: The initial platelet reactivity was found to be higher in patients with severe neurological deficits on the 90th day after stroke, than in the group with mild neurological deficits (median, respectively, 40 area under the curve (AUC) units vs. 25 AUC units, $p = 0.033$). In the large vessel disease group, a significant correlation between the platelet reactivity and the functional status on the first day of stroke was found (correlation coefficient (R) = 0.4526; $p = 0.0451$), the platelet reactivity was higher in the subgroup with a severe clinical condition compared to a mild clinical condition on the first day of stroke ($p = 0.0372$), and patients resistant to acetylsalicylic acid (aspirin) had a significantly greater possibility of a severe neurological deficit on the first day of stroke compared to those who were sensitive to aspirin (odds ratio (OR) = 14.00, 95% confidence interval (CI) 1.25–156.12, $p = 0.0322$). Conclusion: High on-treatment platelet reactivity in ischemic stroke was associated with a worse late prognosis regardless of the etiology. We demonstrated a significant relationship between high platelet reactivity and worse early prognosis and poor clinical and functional condition in the large vessel etiologic subgroup. However, due to the pilot nature of this study, its results should be interpreted with caution and further validation on a larger cohort is required.

Keywords: ischemic stroke; platelet reactivity; aspirin resistance; large vessel disease; carotid stenosis; clinical outcome; prognosis

1. Introduction

Stroke is a leading cause of disability and death worldwide and is associated with a worse quality of life [1]. Antiplatelet therapy is used to reduce the risk of recurrent ischemic stroke [2]. Acetylsalicylic acid (aspirin) is a primary antiplatelet agent; however, its effect can vary in different patients [3]. In some patients, a reduced aspirin response may be observed, resulting in a failure to inhibit the platelet reactivity [4]. Platelet function testing can evaluate the effectiveness of aspirin in decreasing platelet aggregation and activation. High on-treatment platelet reactivity or biochemical aspirin resistance is a multifactorial, negative feature that is associated with insufficient antiplatelet therapy [5].

One of the better-understood causes of cerebral ischemia is the pathology of large pre-cranial vessels, most often the internal carotid artery, which accounts for approximately 20–30% of all causes of stroke [6]. Our previous papers demonstrated the hyperaggregation and hyperactivation of platelets in this etiological subtype of ischemic stroke [7,8]. Furthermore, we hypothesize that it may be related to aspirin resistance and affect the clinical condition and prognosis due to the reduced inhibition of platelets. In the next step, we estimate the role of high on-treatment platelet reactivity for the clinical evaluation and prognosis of stroke patients.

Previous reports regarding the relationship between high platelet reactivity and clinical deterioration did not present clear conclusions [9–12]. The researchers did not focus on the potential role of stroke etiology for significant correlations in this field. The main objective of this study was to determine the relationship between platelet reactivity in the acute phase of ischemic strokes in patients treated with acetylsalicylic acid and the clinical and functional condition of patients, as well as early and late prognosis, with a particular emphasis on cerebral ischemic etiopathogenesis.

2. Materials and Methods

2.1. Study Population

The perspective, single-center, observational study was conducted at the Department of Neurology at the University Hospital No. 1 in Bydgoszcz. We consecutively enrolled 69 patients between February 2016 and December 2017 who underwent ischemic stroke according to the updated definition of stroke by the American Heart Association/American Stroke Association [13]. All subjects received a standard dose (150 mg) of acetylsalicylic acid based on the current guidelines. We divided the enrolled subjects into two subgroups considering the etiology of ischemic strokes. For the large vessel disease subgroup, we included patients with at least 50% of a carotid artery stenosis on the site correlated with clinical symptoms that were confirmed in an ultrasound examination [14]. The second etiological subgroup, small vessel disease, consisted of subjects with clinical and radiological features related to small vessel disease. We included patients with classic lacunar syndromes (pure motor or sensory stroke or ataxic hemiparesis) and typical neuroimaging markers (small subcortical infarcts <2 cm, hyperintensities in the white matter, lacunes < 15 mm, prominent perivascular spaces, microbleeds, and brain atrophy), where acute ischemic infarcts in neuroimaging were related to clinical symptoms of stroke [15]. The exclusion criteria were: a subject's inability to make an informed signature (speech disorders, or quantitative or qualitative disturbances of consciousness), an embolic background of ischemic stroke, a previous history of stroke, the chronic use of acetylsalicylic acid before stroke onset, gastrointestinal or urinary bleeding within the last 2 years, low platelet count <100,000/μL, anemia (hemoglobin <9 g/dL), or low hematocrit <35%, "silent" infarcts (infarcts in neuroimaging that are not related to clinical symptoms of stroke).

2.2. Clinical Outcome

Both the clinical status and functional status were assessed within 24 h after admission (first day) to the hospital, on the eighth day of hospitalization (early prognosis), and on the 90th (+/− 5 days) day (late prognosis) after the stroke onset. The clinical status and functional status were assessed using standardized research tools, the National Institute of Health Stroke Scale (NIHSS) and modified Rankin Scale (mRS), respectively. When analyzing the severity of the neurological deficit, two subgroups of patients with stroke were distinguished: a subgroup with a mild neurological deficit (0–5 points on the NIHSS) and a subgroup with moderate and severe neurological deficits (≥6 points on the NIHSS). Regarding the functional status of the patients, two subgroups of stroke patients were distinguished: a favorable prognosis (on the mRS 0–2 points) and an unfavorable prognosis (on the mRS 3–5 points). A comparison of the clinical and functional conditions in both etiological subgroups of the subjects is presented in Table 1.

Table 1. A comparison of the anthropometric data, platelet reactivity, clinical, and functional status in patients with stroke in both etiological subgroups.

Parameter	Large Vessel Disease $n = 20$	Small Vessel Disease $n = 49$	p-Value
Age median (range) *	67 (45–85)	68 (40–89)	0.7761
Male N, (%) **	14 (70%)	21 (42.9%)	0.0408
Platelet reactivity: optical aggregometry (AUC) median (range) *	17.1 (0–208.6)	20.4 (0–154.2)	0.7147
Platelet reactivity: impedance aggregometry (AUC) median (range) *	42 (9–101)	27.5 (6–108)	0.0622
NIHSS 1 day median (range) *	5 (2–17)	5 (1–17)	0.6770
NIHSS 8 day median (range) *	2 (0–10)	2 (0–10)	0.8324
NIHSS 90 day median (range) *	1 (0–8)	2 (0–10)	0.6625
mRS 1 day median (range) *	4 (1–5)	4 (1–5)	0.7304
mRS 8 day median (range) *	1 (0–5)	2 (0–4)	0.4999
mRS 90 day median (range) *	1 (0–4)	2 (0–4)	0.5740

* Mann–Whitney U test, ** Chi-squared calculation. AUC, area under the curve; NIHSS, National Institute of Health Stroke Scale; mRS, modified Rankin scale.

2.3. Ethics Statement

Written informed consent, after revision of the study protocol, was obtained from each participant. This study was approved by the Bioethics Committee of Nicolaus Copernicus University in Torun at Collegium Medicum of Ludwik Rydygier in Bydgoszcz (KB number 73/2016).

2.4. Platelet Function Testing

Aspirin-induced platelet function testing was measured using two methods: optical aggregometry and impedance aggregometry. Blood samples were collected from the participants within 24 h after the stroke onset. To standardize and to unify the time-points of measurements, most cases were performed between 18 and 24 h after the stroke onset, at the same time of day (10–12 AM). The optical aggregometry or light transmission aggregometry (LTA) was performed with an aggregometer (Chrono-Log Corp., Havertown, PA, USA) and the results were expressed as area under the curve (AUC) units. Values over 115 AUC units were defined as high on-treatment platelet reactivity or aspirin resistance. We performed impedance aggregometry using the Multiplate® platelet function analyzer (Roche Diagnostics, France) and its results were expressed as AUC units. For the aspirin-resistant group, we enrolled subjects with values over 40 AUC units. The procedures for performing platelet function testing were similar as described in the previous studies [16,17]. Of our 69 subjects, 43 underwent optical aggregometry measurements, and all 69 subjects underwent impedance aggregometry assessment.

2.5. Statistical Analysis

STATISTICA 13.1 (Dell Inc., Round Rock, TX, USA) was used to perform all statistical evaluations. The non-parametric Mann–Whitney U test was used to compare continuous variables. Categorical variables were compared with a Chi-squared test. Spearman's rank test was used to evaluate the correlations between the variables. The influence of platelet reactivity levels on stroke severity was performed with logistic regression analysis. In the present study, the statistical significance was defined as $p < 0.05$.

3. Results

3.1. All Subjects

There was no correlation between the platelet reactivity, assessed by Multiplate® and LTA methods, and the severity of the neurological deficit assessed using the NIHSS and functional status of the patients assessed on the mRS in the whole study group (Table 2). The comparison of the severity of neurological deficit (NIHSS) in patients with stroke assessed on the first, eighth, and 90th day after the stroke onset did not show significant differences between the subgroups of patients resistant and sensitive to aspirin (on the first day $p = 0.8663$, on the eighth day $p = 0.9234$, and on the 90th day $p = 0.8225$). There were no differences between the above groups regarding the functional status (mRS) of patients (on the first day $p = 0.9808$, on the eighth day $p = 0.4610$, and on the 90th day $p = 0.5892$).

In the present study, we found that the initial platelet reactivity assessed by Multiplate® was higher in patients with moderate/severe neurological deficits compared to a mild deficit on the 90th day after the stroke onset (median, respectively, 40 AUC units vs. 25 AUC units, $p = 0.033$) (Figure 1).

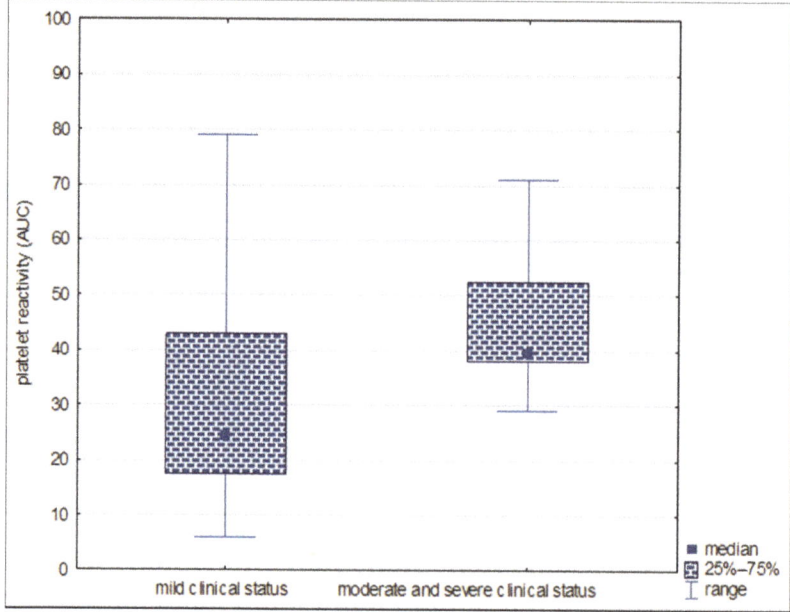

Figure 1. Comparison of platelet reactivity by Multiplate® (in area under the curve (AUC) units) in subgroups of patients with mild and moderate/severe neurological deficits on the 90th day in the general population of stroke patients.

However, there were no differences in the platelet reactivity between the groups distinguished on the basis of the severity of the deficit on the first and eighth day of stroke (on the first day $p = 0.6599$; on the eighth day $p = 0.3271$). The platelet reactivity assessed by Multiplate® did not differ between patients with a favorable and unfavorable prognosis on the first ($p = 0.6455$), eighth ($p = 0.6744$), and 90th day of the disease ($p = 0.7414$). The analysis of the relationship between the platelet reactivity in the LTA method and the clinical and functional status of stroke patients in the whole group of subjects showed no significant relationships ($p > 0.05$).

Logistic regression analysis showed that in the whole group of patients with stroke, aspirin-resistant subjects were 5.5 times more likely to have a severe neurological deficit on the 90th day of stroke than patients who were sensitive to aspirin; however, these differences did not reach statistical significance (odds ratio (OR) = 5.52, 95% confidence interval (CI) 0.54–56.86; $p = 0.1506$).

3.2. Two Etiological Subgroups

In the subgroups of patients with the pathology of large and small vessel disease, there were no statistically significant differences in the clinical and functional status of the stroke patients (NIHSS and mRS) (Table 1). In the subgroup of patients with large vessel disease, a significant correlation was found between the platelet reactivity assessed by Multiplate® and the functional status (mRS) on the first day of stroke (correlation coefficient (R) = 0.4526; $p = 0.0451$) (Figure 2, Table 2).

Table 2. Correlations of the clinical and functional conditions and platelet reactivity in both methods on individual days of stroke in the general population and in the subgroup of patients with large vessel disease.

	General Population				Large Vessel Disease			
	Multiplate®		LTA		Multiplate®		LTA	
	R	p	R	p	R	p	R	p
NIHSS 1 day	0.0713	0.5603	0.0010	0.9948	0.4908	0.0728	0.0010	0.9947
NIHSS 8 days	0.0473	0.6996	0.1472	0.3462	0.2636	0.2614	0.1472	0.3462
NIHSS 90 days	0.0781	0.5233	0.0859	0.5838	0.2801	0.2017	0.0859	0.5837
mRS 1 day	0.0273	0.8240	0.0170	0.9139	0.4526	0.0451	0.01698	0.9139
mRS 8 days	0.1233	0.3128	0.0781	0.6186	0.4068	0.0750	0.0781	0.6186
mRS 90 days	0.0968	0.4288	0.1099	0.4829	0.3676	0.1108	0.1099	0.4826

Spearman's rank correlation. R, correlation coefficient; LTA, light transmission aggregometry; NIHSS, National Institute of Health Stroke Scale; mRS, modified Rankin scale.

Assessing the relationship between the aspirin resistance groups and the severity of clinical deficit in patients with large vessel disease, we found that the aspirin-resistant patients did not differ in the NIHSS scores from aspirin-sensitive patients (on the first day $p = 0.06$, on the eighth day $p = 0.1167$, and on the 90th day $p = 0.0986$). Assessing the relationship with the functional status in patients with large vessel disease, we found that patients with aspirin resistance achieved a higher median of points on mRS on the eighth day of the disease than patients sensitive to aspirin ($p = 0.0352$) (Figure 3).

There were no differences in the mRS scores on the first and 90th day of stroke (respectively, $p = 0.0523$ for the first day, $p = 0.0631$ for the 90th day). In the subgroup of patients with the pathology of small vessels there were no significant differences in the severity of the clinical deficit and the functional status between the groups distinguished on the basis of the presence or absence of aspirin resistance ($p > 0.05$).

Comparing the platelet reactivity in patients with moderate/severe (NIHSS ≥6 points) and mild neurological deficits (NIHHS <6 points), we found that in the subgroup of patients with the pathology of large vessels, the median of platelet reactivity in the Multiplate® method was higher than in the subgroup of patients with severe neurological deficit compared to mild deficit on the first day of the disease (respectively, median 58.5 vs. 23.5 AUC units; $p = 0.0372$) (Figure 4); this did not differ on the eighth day ($p = 0.0762$), on the 90th day ($p = 0.0982$), or on particular days in the subgroup of patients with the pathology of small vessels ($p > 0.05$).

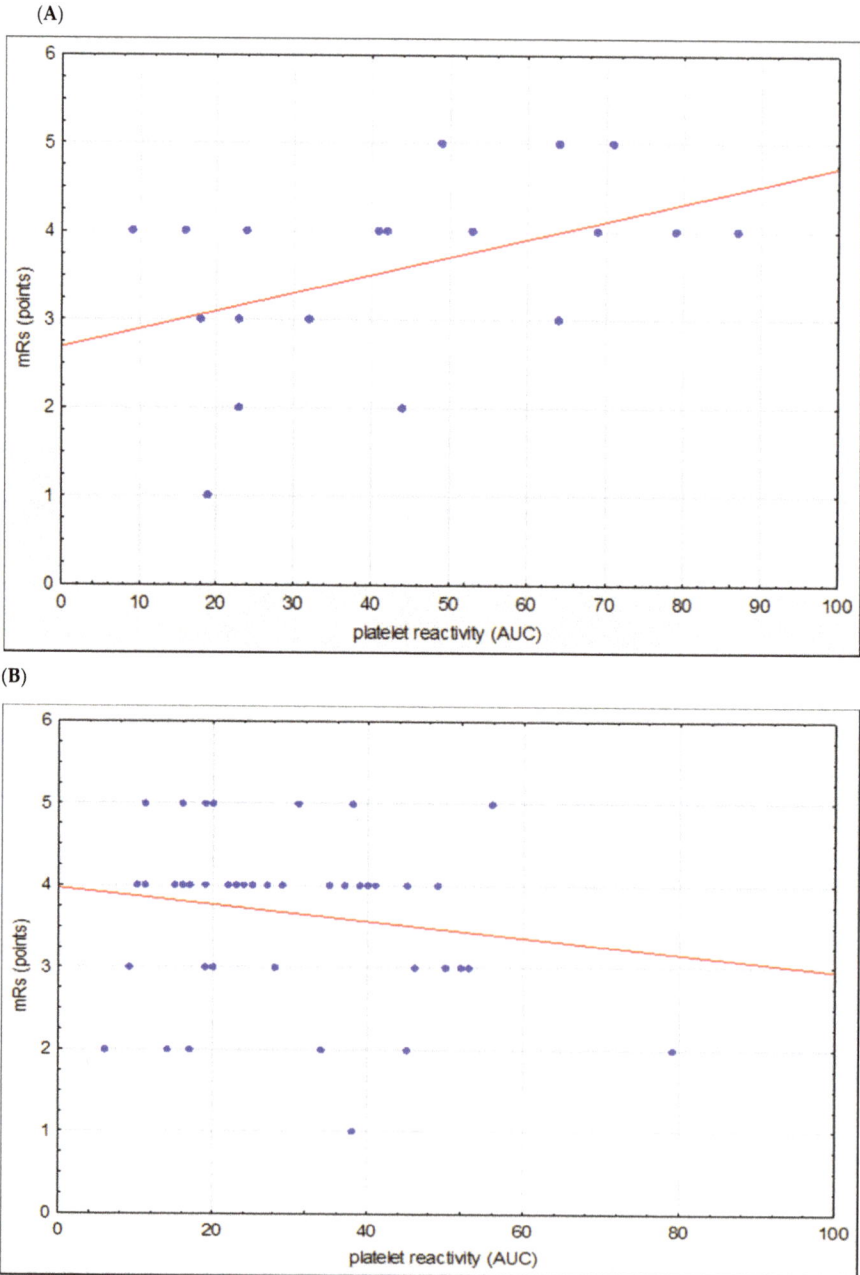

Figure 2. Correlation of platelet reactivity assessed by Multiplate® (in area under the curve (AUC) units) and functional status (modified Rankin scale (mRS) on the first day of stroke) in the subgroup of patients with large vessel disease (**A**) and small vessel disease (**B**).

Comparing the platelet reactivity in patients with favorable and unfavorable prognosis, the median of platelet reactivity in Multiplate® method did not differ between the above-mentioned groups both on the first, eighth, and 90th day of stroke in both subgroups ($p > 0.05$).

Logistic regression analysis showed that in the subgroup with large vessel disease, aspirin-resistant subjects had a 14 times greater probability of a severe neurological deficit on the first day of stroke than subjects sensitive to aspirin (OR = 14.00, 95% CI 1.25–156.12, $p = 0.0322$).

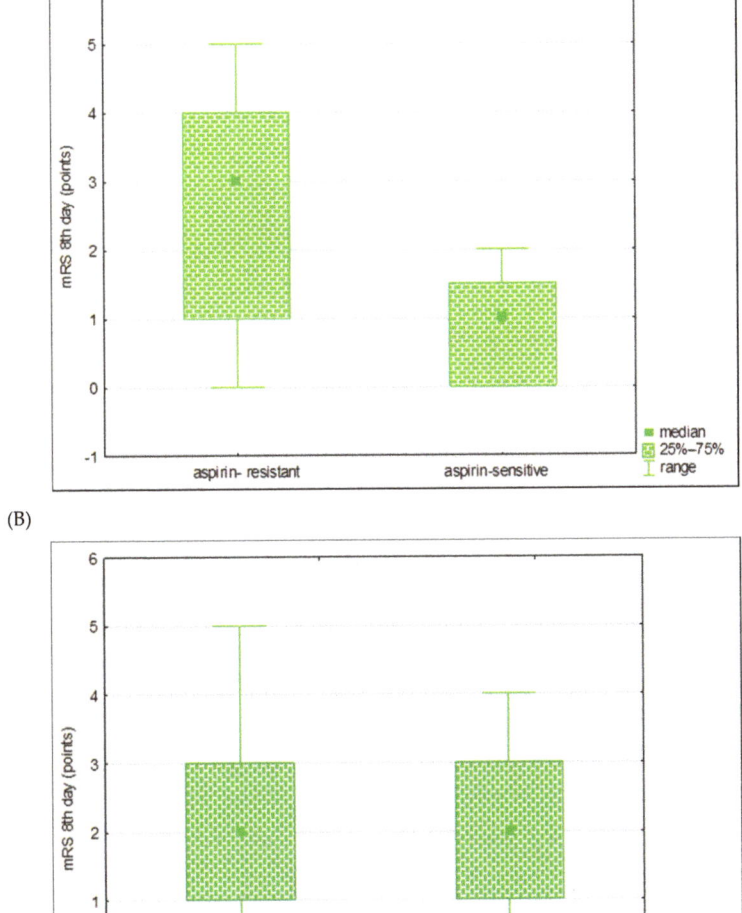

Figure 3. Comparison of the functional conditions (modified Rankin Scale (mRS)) on the eighth day of stroke in aspirin-resistant and aspirin-sensitive subjects in large vessel disease subgroup (**A**) and small vessel disease subgroup (**B**).

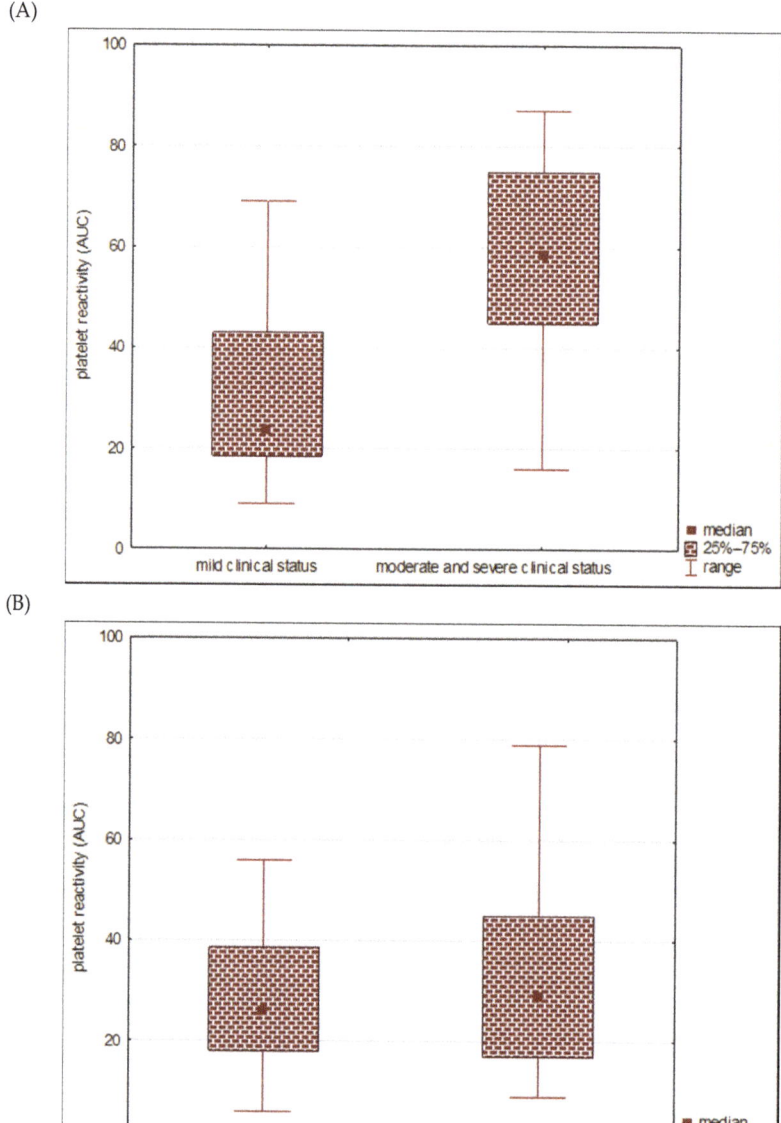

Figure 4. Comparison of platelet reactivity by Multiplate® (in AUC units) in the subgroup of patients with mild and moderate/severe neurological deficits on the first day of stroke in large vessel disease subgroup (**A**) and small vessel disease subgroup (**B**).

4. Discussion

In the present study, we demonstrated a significant role of ischemic stroke etiology for the prognostic value of high on-treatment platelet reactivity. We underline that the association between aspirin resistance and poor early clinical and functional conditions in ischemic stroke depends on the etiological subtype of the stroke. In the large vessel disease subgroup, we found a higher platelet reactivity in patients with severe neurological deficits on the first day of stroke, and that aspirin-resistant patients have a significantly higher probability of a severe clinical condition compared to aspirin-sensitive patients.

The division of patients according to the etiopathogenesis of stroke revealed a significant effect of platelet reactivity on the early functional condition. There was an average, though significant, correlation between platelet reactivity and functional status assessed on mRS on the first day of stroke, and patients resistant to aspirin had higher scores on the mRS (worse prognosis) on the eighth day of stroke than patients who were sensitive to aspirin. Both were present only in the large vessel disease subgroup. No similar results were demonstrated in the whole study population or in the small vessel disease subgroup.

These novel findings emphasize the great impact of stroke etiology on the association of high on-treatment platelet reactivity and poor early prognosis. However, it is difficult to refer the results of this research with other publications due to the heterogenous populations of the studied groups and different methodologies, and the lack of references in the literature on the impact of stroke etiopathogenesis on the relationship of platelet function testing with the prognosis of stroke subjects. Other authors did not assess the effect of stroke etiopathogenesis on the relationship of platelet reactivity with clinical and functional conditions.

In this study, there was no correlation between the platelet reactivity and the clinical condition in the whole group of subjects using the NIHSS on the first, eighth, and 90th day of stroke. In addition, the division into aspirin-resistant and -sensitive patients did not significantly differentiate the clinical status on particular days of the disease. Only the division of patients with mild to moderate/severe neurological deficits (according to the NIHSS score) revealed a significant effect on a higher initial platelet reactivity (within 24 h after onset) on the more severe clinical conditions, but this relationship was recorded only on the 90th day of stroke. Numerous authors showed that the aspirin-resistant group was characterized by a more severe early clinical condition, assessed on the NIHSS on the first day, than the group sensitive to aspirin [9–12]. Cheng et al. [12] indicated a significant correlation ($R = 0.56$) between platelet reactivity and the severity of neurological deficits assessed in the NIHSS. These results led to the conclusion that excessive platelet reactivity and aspirin resistance are associated with a worse clinical condition of patients in the acute phase of stroke. A different observation was demonstrated by Kim et al. [18] and Lai et al. [19], whose studies did not show the effect of platelet reactivity on the severity of the clinical condition assessed on the first day using the NIHSS. Similarly, Englyst et al. [20] did not find significant differences in the clinical status assessed on the NIHSS on the third day of stroke between the groups of patients resistant and sensitive to aspirin. The few literature reports on the long-term clinical conditions assessed on the 30th and 90th days of stroke showed contradictory results. Yip et al. [21] reported that aspirin-resistant patients were characterized by a worse clinical condition (NIHSS) both on the 30th and 90th days than patients sensitive to aspirin, while Lai et al. [19] did not find differences in the clinical condition (NIHSS) between these groups on the 90th day. We hypothesize that the contradictory conclusions from the presented studies may have resulted from omitting the important role of stroke etiology, as demonstrated in the current study.

The impact of platelet reactivity on the functional status of stroke patients is also debatable. Lai et al. [19] suggested a lack of relationship between platelet reactivity and early prognosis, as they did not reveal significant differences on the first day of stroke on mRS in the groups of patients sensitive and resistant to aspirin. On the other hand, Englyst et al. [20] showed a worse functional status of patients evaluated on mRS on the third day of stroke in aspirin-resistant patients compared to the aspirin-sensitive group (mRS median, respectively, 4 vs. 2, $p = 0.013$). Similar conclusions were reached by Sobol et al. [22] (mRS median 3 vs. 2, $p = 0.02$) assessing the functional status of patients on the 10th day of stroke. In our study, in the whole study population, there was no effect of platelet reactivity on the early prognosis—the functional status—on the first and eighth day of stroke or significant differences in the functional status of patients resistant and sensitive to aspirin. The differences in the results of this study from the data presented by other authors may be a result of including all etiological types of stroke (e.g., embolic) and other methodologies (Englyst et al., hemostatic thromboelastography; Sobol et al., Platelet Function Assay (PFA-100)). In addition, according to the results of Amy et al. [23] and Wilterdink et al. [24], aspirin administration before ischemic stroke onset results in a better prognosis of patients evaluated on mRS. Englyst et al. [20] assessed only patients treated with aspirin (for at least three days) before the incident. In the study by Sobol et al. [22], there is no information on whether patients with stroke had previously taken aspirin or only from the first day of stroke. In the only paper regarding late prognosis, Lai et al. [19] showed that on the 90th day of stroke, in the group with aspirin resistance, subjects with a worse functional status were more often reported, rated on mRS at 3–5 points, than in the group sensitive to aspirin ($p = 0.037$). However, the current study did not show any significant effects of platelet reactivity on the late functional status (even considering the etiopathogenesis of stroke). It is worth noting that Lai et al. evaluated the platelet reactivity with the PFA-100 method and recruited patients with stroke who received a dose of 100 mg of aspirin at least five days before platelet reactivity testing, which may have resulted in different functional outcomes than in this study.

The present study and previous reports, despite various methodologies and inclusion and exclusion criteria of the study population, underline that high on-treatment platelet reactivity may have a negative impact on early and late prognosis and a significant association with poor clinical and functional outcomes in stroke subjects. The novelty demonstrated in this research emphasizes that stroke etiology may be a key factor for the above dependencies.

According to the results obtained in this study, carotid artery stenosis appears to be an essential platelet activating factor. Tsai et al. [25], who assessed platelet function using flow cytometry, also demonstrated significantly higher platelet aggregation in patients with large vessel pathology compared to small vessel pathology. Importantly, the study was conducted on a similar population of patients with cerebral ischemia to this study (i.e., they excluded patients with stroke due to the embolic background. Similar results were presented by Zheng et al. [11], Kinsella et al. [26], and Dawson et al. [27], who demonstrated that platelet reactivity assessed by different methods is significantly elevated in patients with carotid artery stenosis. Kinsella et al. [28], using the PFA-100, reported that surgical treatment (e.g., stenting) in stroke subjects due to a carotid artery stenosis was associated with a significant reduction of platelet activation. These results were consistent with our current findings, highlighting the role of large vessel disease etiology for ischemic stroke in increasing platelet reactivity. These results indicate that platelet function monitoring may be useful for stroke subjects due to carotid artery stenosis. Additionally, platelet-function-guided individualized antiplatelet therapy can be essential to optimize clinical outcomes and to improve the functional status.

Unfortunately, both the American and European guidelines for the treatment and prevention of stroke do not distinguish between antiplatelet therapy and stroke pathomechanisms. Regardless of whether it is lacunar stroke or stroke due to a pathology of large extracranial vessels, aspirin administration is recommended for all patients with thrombotic stroke [2]. The current guidelines do not address the issue of aspirin resistance. It seems that this may be due to the lack of large, randomized clinical trials that could be used to develop clear guidelines.

As stroke in large extracranial pathology accounts for a fairly significant proportion of all strokes, and the results of current and previous studies highlight the significant impact of carotid artery pathology on platelet reactivity relationships with worse clinical conditions and prognoses, we recommend routinely determining platelet reactivity and detecting aspirin resistance, especially in cases of recurrent ischemic events. The authors believe that this would allow for personalized antiplatelet treatment based on platelet function testing, whose effectiveness for this group of patients is a priority.

The authors are aware that this study has several limitations. The evaluation of platelet function was performed only once and at different times during the first 24 h after the onset of stroke and at different times after the first dose of acetylsalicylic acid. It could have contributed to the variations in the measurements of platelet function. A single measurement with poorly validated methods in light of the marked variability of platelet reactivity that was previously demonstrated, may not be sufficient to properly assess the effect of high on-treatment platelet reactivity on the clinical condition and prognosis in ischemic stroke. More work is essential to sequentially determine platelet reactivity on successive days. Another limitation is that biochemical resistance does not always correspond with clinical resistance. The sample size in the study was small and imbalanced between the two etiological subgroups. The lack of recruitment of patients with severe stroke (especially those with impaired consciousness), due to the inability to obtain informed consent, constitutes a huge limitation of the study. Despite using stringent inclusion and exclusion criteria, in the face of low rates of in-hospital atrial fibrillation detection, there is a possibility that a small percentage of subjects may have had another etiology of stroke, such as embolism.

5. Conclusions

This pilot study demonstrated that high on-treatment platelet reactivity is associated with a worse late prognosis in ischemic stroke. In patients with large vessel disease, high platelet reactivity is associated with a worse early prognosis and clinical and functional condition of patients in the acute phase of stroke. The role of etiology demonstrated in this paper is novelty. However, due to the pilot nature of this study, the obtained results should be interpreted with caution. Further research, performed on larger sample size, is essential to validate and confirm our findings and to determine the optimal and personalized antiplatelet therapy.

Author Contributions: Conceptualization, A.W.; methodology, A.W., G.K., and J.S.; software, J.S.; validation, G.K.; formal analysis, A.W., K.F., and G.K.; investigation, A.W.; resources, J.S.; data curation, J.S..; writing—original draft preparation, A.W. and K.F.; writing—review and editing, A.W.; visualization, A.W.; supervision, G.K. and R.Ś.; project administration, A.W. and G.K. All authors have read and agreed to the published version of the manuscript.

Conflicts of Interest: The authors declare no conflicts of interest.

References

1. Naghavi, M.; Wang, H.; Lozano, R.; Davis, A.; Liang, X.; Zhou, M.; Vollset, S.E.; Ozgoren, A.A.; Abdalla, S.; Abd-Allah, F.; et al. Global, regional, and national age-sex specific all-cause and cause-specific mortality for 240 causes of death, 1990–2013: A systematic analysis for the Global Burden of Disease Study 2013. *Lancet* **2015**, *385*, 117–171.
2. Powers, W.J.; Rabinstein, A.A.; Ackerson, T.; Adeove, O.M.; Bambakidis, N.C.; Becker, K.; Biller, J.; Brwon, M.; Demaerschalk, B.M.; Hoh, B.; et al. 2018 Guidelines for the Early Management of Patients with Acute Ischemic Stroke: A Guideline for Healthcare Professionals from the American Heart Association/American Stroke Association. *Stroke* **2018**, *49*, e46–e110. [CrossRef] [PubMed]
3. Rondina, M.T.; Weyrich, A.S.; Zimmerman, G.A. Platelets as cellular effectors of inflammation in vascular diseases. *Circ. Res.* **2013**, *112*, 1506–1519. [CrossRef] [PubMed]
4. Linden, M.D.; Jackson, D.E. Platelets: Pleiotropic roles in atherogenesis and atherothrombosis. *Int. J. Biochem. Cell Biol.* **2010**, *42*, 1762–1766. [CrossRef] [PubMed]
5. Paniccia, R.; Priora, R.; Liotta, A.A.; Agatina, A. Platelet function tests: A comparative review. *Vasc. Health Risk Manag.* **2015**, *11*, 133–148. [CrossRef]
6. Marulanda-Londono, E.; Chaturvedi, S. Stroke due to large vessel atherosclerosis. *Neurol. Clin. Pract.* **2016**, *6*, 252–258. [CrossRef]
7. Wiśniewski, A.; Sikora, J.; Filipska, K.; Kozera, G. Assessment of the relationship between platelet reactivity, vascular risk factors and gender in cerebral ischaemia patients. *Neurol. Neurochir. Pol.* **2019**, *53*, 258–264. [CrossRef]
8. Wiśniewski, A.; Sikora, J.; Sławińska, A.; Filipska, K.; Karczmarska-Wódzka, A.; Serafin, Z.; Kozera, G. High On-Treatment Platelet Reactivity Affects the Extent of Ischemic Lesions in Stroke Patients Due to Large-Vessel Disease. *J. Clin. Med.* **2020**, *9*, 251. [CrossRef]
9. Oh, M.S.; Yu, K.H.; Lee, J.H.; Jung, S.; Kim, C.; Jang, M.U.; Lee, J.; Lee, B.C. Aspirin resistance is associated with increased stroke severity and infarct volume. *Neurology* **2016**, *86*, 1808–1817. [CrossRef]

10. Agayeva, N.; Topcuoglu, M.A.; Arsava, E.M. The Interplay between Stroke Severity, Antiplatelet Use, and Aspirin Resistance in Ischemic Stroke. *J. Stroke Cerebrovasc. Dis.* **2016**, *25*, 397–403. [CrossRef]
11. Zheng, A.S.; Churilov, L.; Colley, R.E.; Goh, C.; Davis, S.M.; Yan, B. Association of aspirin resistance with increased stroke severity and infarct size. *JAMA Neurol.* **2013**, *70*, 208–213. [CrossRef] [PubMed]
12. Cheng, X.; Xie, N.C.; Hu, H.L.; Chen, C.; Lian, Y.J. Biochemical aspirin resistance is associated with increased stroke severity and infarct volumes in ischemic stroke patients. *Oncotarget* **2017**, *8*, 77086–77095. [CrossRef] [PubMed]
13. Sacco, R.L.; Kasner, S.E.; Broderick, J.P.; Caplan, L.R.; Connors, J.J.; Culebras, A.; Elkind, M.S.; George, M.G.; Hamdan, A.D.; Higashida, R.T.; et al. An updated definition of stroke for the 21st century: A statement for healthcare professionals from the American Heart Association/American Stroke Association. *Stroke* **2013**, *44*, 2064–2089. [CrossRef] [PubMed]
14. Wojczal, J.; Tomczyk, T.; Luchowski, P. Standards in neurosonology. *J. Ultrason.* **2016**, *16*, 44–45. [CrossRef] [PubMed]
15. Wardlaw, J.M.; Smith, E.E.; Biessels, G.J.; Cordonnier, C.; Fazekas, F.; Frayne, R.; Lindley, R.I.; O'Brien, J.T.; Barkhof, F.; Benavente, O.R.; et al. Neuroimaging standards for research into small vessel disease and its contribution to ageing and neurodegeneration. *Lancet Neurol.* **2013**, *12*, 822–838. [CrossRef]
16. Sibbing, D.; Braun, S.; Jawansky, S.; Vogt, W.; Mehilli, J.; Schömig, A.; Kastrati, A.; von Beckerath, N. Assessment of ADP-induced platelet aggregation with light transmission aggregometry and multiplate electrode platelet aggregometry before and after clopidogrel treatment. *Thromb. Haemost.* **2008**, *99*, 121–126.
17. Tóth, O.; Calatzis, A.; Penz, S.; Losonczy, H.; Siess, W. Multiple electrode aggregometry: A new device to measure platelet aggregation in whole blood. *Thromb. Haemost.* **2006**, *96*, 781–788.
18. Kim, J.T.; Heo, S.H.; Lee, J.S.; Choi, M.J.; Choi, K.H.; Nam, T.S.; Lee, S.H.; Park, M.S.; Kim, B.C.; Kim, M.K.; et al. Aspirin resistance in the acute stages of acute ischemic stroke is associated with the development of new ischemic lesions. *PLoS ONE* **2015**, *10*, e0120743. [CrossRef]
19. Lai, P.T.; Chen, S.Y.; Lee, Y.S.; Ho, Y.P.; Chiang, Y.Y.; Hsu, H.Y. Relationship between acute stroke outcome, aspirin resistance, and humoral factors. *J. Chin. Med. Assoc.* **2012**, *75*, 513–518. [CrossRef]
20. Englyst, N.A.; Horsfield, G.; Kwan, J.; Byrne, C.D. Aspirin resistance is more common in lacunar strokes than embolic strokes and is related to stroke severity. *J. Cereb. Blood Flow Metab.* **2008**, *28*, 1196–1203. [CrossRef]
21. Yip, H.K.; Liou, C.W.; Chang, H.W.; Lan, M.Y.; Liu, J.S.; Chen, M.C. Link between platelet activity and outcomes after an ischemic stroke. *Cerebrovasc. Dis.* **2005**, *20*, 120–128. [CrossRef] [PubMed]
22. Sobol, A.B.; Mochecka, A.; Selmaj, K.; Loba, J. Is there a relationship between aspirin responsiveness and clinical aspects of ischemic stroke? *Adv. Clin. Exp. Med.* **2009**, *18*, 473–479.
23. Amy, Y.X.; Keezer, M.R.; Zhu, B.; Wolfson, C.; Côté, R. Pre-stroke use of antihypertensives, antiplatelets, or statins and early ischemic stroke outcomes. *Cerebrovasc. Dis.* **2009**, *27*, 398–402.
24. Wilterdink, J.L.; Bendixen, B.; Adams, H.P., Jr.; Woolson, R.F.; Clarke, W.R.; Hansen, M.D. Effect of prior aspirin use on stroke severity in the trial of Org 10172 in acute stroke treatment (TOAST). *Stroke* **2001**, *32*, 2836–2840. [CrossRef] [PubMed]
25. Tsai, N.W.; Chang, W.N.; Shaw, C.F.; Jan, C.R.; Chang, H.W.; Huang, C.R.; Chen, S.D.; Chuang, Y.C.; Lee, L.H.; Wang, H.C.; et al. Levels and value of platelet activation markers in different subtypes of acute non-cardio-embolic ischemic stroke. *Thromb. Res.* **2009**, *124*, 213–218. [CrossRef] [PubMed]
26. Kinsella, J.A.; Tobin, W.O.; Hamilton, G.; McCabe, D.J. Platelet activation, function, and reactivity in atherosclerotic carotid artery stenosis: A systematic review of the literature. *Int. J. Stroke* **2013**, *8*, 451–464. [CrossRef]
27. Dawson, J.; Quinn, T.; Lees, K.R.; Walters, M.R. Microembolic signals and aspirin resistance in patients with carotid stenosis. *Cardiovasc. Ther.* **2012**, *30*, 234–239. [CrossRef]
28. Kinsella, J.A.; Tobin, W.A.; Tierney, S. Assessment of 'on-treatment platelet reactivity' and relationship with cerebral micro-embolic signals in asymptomatic and symptomatic carotid stenosis. *J. Neurol. Sci.* **2017**, *376*, 133–139. [CrossRef]

© 2020 by the authors. Licensee MDPI, Basel, Switzerland. This article is an open access article distributed under the terms and conditions of the Creative Commons Attribution (CC BY) license (http://creativecommons.org/licenses/by/4.0/).

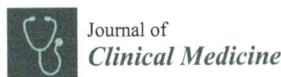

Article

To Treat or Not to Treat: Importance of Functional Dependence in Deciding Intravenous Thrombolysis of "Mild Stroke" Patients

Giovanni Merlino [1,*,†], Carmelo Smeralda [2,3,†], Simone Lorenzut [1], Gian Luigi Gigli [2,4], Andrea Surcinelli [2,3] and Mariarosaria Valente [2,3]

1. Stroke Unit, Department of Neuroscience, Udine University Hospital, Piazzale S. Maria della Misericordia 15, 33100 Udine, Italy; simone.lorenzut@asufc.sanita.fvg.it
2. Clinical Neurology, Udine University Hospital, 33100 Udine, Italy; carmelosmeralda@gmail.com (C.S.); gigli@uniud.it (G.L.G.); andsurcinelli@gmail.com (A.S.); mariarosaria.valente@uniud.it (M.V.)
3. Department of Medical Area (DAME), University of Udine, 33100 Udine, Italy
4. Department of Mathematics, Informatics and Physics (DMIF), University of Udine, 33100 Udine, Italy
* Correspondence: giovanni.merlino@asufc.sanita.fvg.it
† Drs. Merlino and Smeralda contributed equally as authors.

Received: 15 February 2020; Accepted: 10 March 2020; Published: 12 March 2020

Abstract: Intravenous thrombolysis (IVT) in patients with a low National Institutes of Health Stroke Scale (NIHSS) score of 0–5 remains controversial. IVT should be used in patients with mild but nevertheless disabling symptoms. We hypothesize that response to IVT of patients with "mild stroke" may depend on their level of functional dependence (FD) at hospital admission. The aims of our study were to investigate the effect of IVT and to explore the role of FD in influencing the response to IVT. This study was a retrospective analysis of a prospectively collected database, including 389 patients stratified into patients receiving IVT (IVT$^+$) and not receiving IVT (IVT$^-$) just because of mild symptoms. Barthel index (BI) at admission was used to assess FD, dividing subjects with BI score < 80 (FD$^+$) and with BI score ≥ 80 (FD$^-$). The efficacy endpoints were the rate of positive disability outcome (DO$^+$) (3-month mRS score of 0 or 1), and the rate of positive functional outcome (FO$^+$) (mRS score of zero or one, plus BI score of 95 or 100 at 3 months). At the multivariate analysis, IVT treatment was an independent predictor of DO$^+$ (OR 3.12, 95% CI 1.34–7.27, $p = 0.008$) and FO$^+$ (OR: 4.70, 95% CI 2.38–9.26, $p = 0.001$). However, FD$^+$ IVT$^+$ patients had a significantly higher prevalence of DO$^+$ and FO$^+$ than those FD$^+$ IVT$^-$. Differently, IVT treatment did not influence DO$^+$ and FO$^+$ in FD$^-$ patients. In FD$^+$ patients, IVT treatment represented the strongest independent predictor of DO$^+$ (OR 6.01, 95% CI 2.59–13.92, $p = 0.001$) and FO$^+$ (OR 4.73, 95% CI 2.29–9.76, $p = 0.001$). In conclusion, alteplase seems to improve functional outcome in patients with "mild stroke". However, in our experience, this beneficial effect is strongly influenced by FD at admission.

Keywords: intravenous thrombolysis; NIHSS; Barthel index; functional dependence

1. Introduction

Many patients with acute ischemic strokes (AIS) have a low National Institutes of Health Stroke Scale (NIHSS) score at presentation [1,2]. Although the presence of these mild symptoms represents the most common reason for renouncing intravenous thrombolysis (IVT) [3], only 68% of these patients can be discharged home without a residual disability [4]. Thus, there is increasing interest in the use of IVT in AIS patients with a low NIHSS score at admission. Results coming from clinical studies on this topic are conflicting, since functional outcome results, as assessed by the modified Rankin scale (mRS) sometimes improve, and at other times, are not modified by IVT treatment [5–10].

Previous American Heart Association/American Stroke Association guidelines suggested to use IVT treatment in persons with a *wide spectrum* of neurological deficits (1996) and with *measurable* neurological deficits (2007) [11,12]. This concept has been updated in the most version of the guidelines, recommending that IVT should also be used in patients with mild, but nevertheless disabling symptoms [13]. However, the NIHSS is not able to assess severity of disability. For instance, it cannot be used to accurately assess posterior circulation disease, which may cause very disabling symptoms. In fact, already in 2013, Wendt et al. reported that language impairment, distal paresis, and gait disorder were common disabling deficits in patients with low NIHSS scores. The authors suggest that the judgment of whether a stroke is disabling should not be based on the NIHSS score, but on the assessment of individual neurologic deficits and their impact on functional impairment [14].

To date, only a trial has been performed to compare the efficacy of alteplase versus aspirin for AIS patients with minor and non-disabling neurological deficits (the PRISMS trial). The authors observed that alteplase did not increase the likelihood of favorable outcome compared to aspirin [15,16]. Although the PRISMS was a prospective, double-blind, and placebo-controlled trial, it suffered from two significant limitations. In fact, the study was terminated early because patient recruitment was below target and it adopted a definition of "not clearly disabling" that was subjective and required interpretation by individual clinicians. Thus, conclusions of the PRISMS trial cannot be generalized.

A possible reason for the uncertain effectiveness of alteplase in minor strokes is that patients with a low NIHSS score at admission may respond to IVT treatment in different ways, depending on their level of functional dependence (FD) at admission. In addition, we suggest that the severity of FD should be assessed by a standard measure, such as the Barthel index (BI), instead of using a subjective selection based on the judgment of each physician. The aims of our study were: (1) to investigate the effects of IVT in patients with "mild stroke", defined as a NIHSS score of 0–5 at presentation; (2) to explore the role of FD in influencing response to IVT in AIS patients with "mild stroke".

2. Materials and Methods

2.1. Patients

This study was based on a retrospective analysis of a prospectively-collected database of consecutive patients admitted to the Udine University Hospital for AIS from January 2015 to December 2018. Inclusion criteria were: age 18 years or older and NIHSS score of 0 to 5. Exclusion criteria were: presence of a pre-stroke mRS score > 1, large vessel occlusion on cranial CT-angiography, and time interval > 4.5 h from symptoms onset. Out of 1636 patients admitted for AIS, 389 were considered suitable for the study after considering inclusion and exclusion criteria. The study sample was stratified into 2 groups: AIS patients who received IVT (IVT$^+$) and patients to whom IVT was denied because of mild symptoms (IVT$^-$).

2.2. Data Collection

The following variables were collected: age, sex, vascular risk factors such as previous transient ischemic attack or previous stroke, ischemic heart disease, peripheral artery disease, obesity defined as a BMI $\geq$ 30, atrial fibrillation, hypertension, diabetes mellitus, hypercholesterolemia, current smoking status, and pharmacological treatment. Stroke severity was determined with the NIHSS at admission. Presence of intracranial hemorrhage (ICH) was detected. Definition of symptomatic ICH (sICH) was based on the European Cooperative Acute Stroke Study (ECASS) III protocol [17]. Functional outcome was assessed by means of the mRS score 3 months after the stroke, and of the BI score, calculated at admission and recalculated at 3-months. The mRS and the BI scores after discharge were recorded at the patients' routine clinical visit during a face-to-face examination.

2.3. Outcome Measures

Our efficacy endpoints were: (1) rate of positive disability outcome (DO$^+$), defined as a 3-month mRS score of 0 or 1; (2) rate of positive functional outcome (FO$^+$), defined as an mRS score of 0 or 1 *plus* a BI score of 95 or 100 at 3 months. The safety endpoints were: (1) rate of mortality at 3 months; (2) presence of sICH.

2.4. Statistical Analysis

Baseline characteristics and outcomes of the two patient groups (IVT$^+$ versus IVT$^-$) were compared by means of the chi-square test (Fisher's exact test) for categorical variables and the Student's *t*-test for independent samples when the continuous variables had a normal distribution.

The Mann–Whitney U test was used when the continuous variables had an abnormal distribution and for ordinal variables. Binary logistic regression was used to explore variables associated with outcome measures.

In order to explore whether there was a significant interaction between the types of presenting symptoms (according to the Barthel index) and the efficacy of thrombolysis, both patients treated and not treated with IVT were differentiated as: (1) patients without FD; (2) patients with FD predominantly due to weakness; (3) patients with FD predominantly due to imbalance; (4) patients with FD predominantly due to neglect and/or hemianopsia; (5) patients with FD predominantly due to other neurological symptoms, e.g., aphasia and confusion.

With the aim to verify if the level of FD at admission might influence response to IVT in AIS patients with "mild stroke", we divided our sample into subjects with a BI score < 80 (FD$^+$) and those with a BI score ≥ 80 (FD$^-$). We tested this hypothesis comparing the efficacy endpoints between FD$^+$ and FD$^-$ patients, treated and not treated with IVT.

Data are displayed in tables as means and standard deviations (SD), if not otherwise specified. All probability values are two-tailed. A *p* value of < 0.05 was considered to be statistically significant. Statistical analysis was carried out using the SPSS Statistics, Version 20.0 for Windows (Chicago, IL, USA).

3. Results

Our sample of 389 patients was composed of 235 males (60.4%) with a mean age of 68.5 ± 13.6 years, a median NIHSS score of 2 (IQR 1–3), and a median BI score of 75 (IQR 60-90). Almost one-half (51.7%) of our patients with "mild stroke" had a BI score < 80 at admission (FD$^+$ patients). Figure 1 shows the distribution of the BI score at admission in our sample.

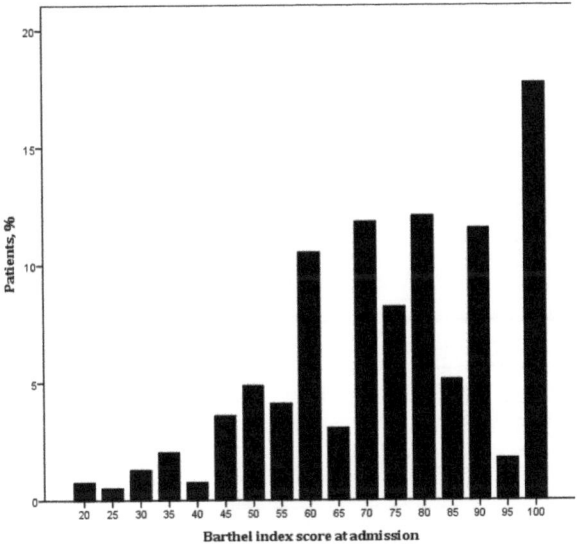

Figure 1. Barthel index score distribution in our sample.

Of the 389 enrolled patients with "mild stroke", 113 (29%) were treated with IVT (IVT$^+$), whereas in 276 (71%), IVT was denied because of mild symptoms (IVT$^-$). Baseline characteristics in IVT$^+$ and IVT$^-$ patients are summarized in Table 1. The two groups differed only in median NIHSS score and use of anticoagulants.

Table 1. Baseline characteristics.

	IVT$^+$ (n = 113)	IVT$^-$ (n = 276)	p
Demographic data and baseline clinical characteristics			
Age, years	68.2 ± 12.0	68.7 ± 14.2	0.7
Males, n (%)	67 (59.3)	168 (60.9)	0.8
NIHSS score at admission, median (IQR)	3 (2–4)	2 (1–3)	0.001
BI score at admission, median (IQR)	60 (75–90)	60 (75–90)	0.5
Medications prior to onset, n (%)			
Antiplatelet agents	39 (34.5)	79 (28.6)	0.2
Anticoagulant agents	1 (0.9)	25 (9.1)	0.003
Glucose level, mg/dl	126.4 ± 35.3	134.2 ± 64.7	0.3
Vascular risk factors			
Previous transient ischemic attack/stroke, n (%)	15 (13.3)	45 (16.3)	0.4
Ischemic heart disease, n (%)	19 (18.3)	27 (10.8)	0.06
Peripheral artery disease, n (%)	2 (1.9)	2 (0.8)	0.6
Obesity, n (%)	9 (8.7)	22 (8.8)	0.9
Atrial fibrillation, n (%)	19 (16.8)	67 (24.3)	0.1
Hypertension, n (%)	68 (60.2)	184 (66.7)	0.2
Diabetes mellitus, n (%)	17 (15.0)	63 (22.8)	0.08
Hypercholesterolemia, n (%)	43 (38.1)	102 (37.0)	0.8
Current smoking, n (%)	29 (26.1)	53 (21.1)	0.3

IVT = intravenous thrombolysis; NIHSS = National Institute of Health Stroke scale; BI = Barthel index.

At 3-months, IVT treatment improved both measures of outcome (DO$^+$ and FO$^+$). Although IVT$^+$ patients showed higher rates of sICH than those IVT$^-$, the prevalence of 3-month mortality did not differ between the two groups (see Table 2).

Table 2. Efficacy and safety endpoints in patients treated and not treated with IVT.

	IVT$^+$ (n = 113)	IVT$^-$ (n = 276)	p
Efficacy endpoints			
DO$^+$, n (%)	98 (86.7)	195 (70.7)	0.001
FO$^+$, n (%)	94 (83.9)	179 (65.6)	0.001
Safety endpoints			
Mortality at 3-months, n (%)	1 (0.9)	3 (1.1)	0.8
sICH, n (%)	5 (4.4)	3 (1.1)	0.03

IVT = intravenous thrombolysis; DO$^+$ (3-month mRS score of 0 or 1) = positive disability outcome; FO$^+$ (mRS score of 0 or 1, *plus* BI score of 95 or 100 at 3-months) = positive functional outcome; sICH = symptomatic intracranial hemorrhage.

By univariate analysis, apart from IVT treatment, a positive disability outcome (DO+) was also associated with younger age (OR for 1-year increment in age 0.98, 95% CI 0.96–0.99, p = 0.02), lower NIHSS score at admission (OR 0.72 for 1-point increase in the scale, 95% CI 0.60–0.85, p = 0.001), higher BI score at admission (OR 1.06, 95% CI 1.05–1.08, p = 0.001), lower serum glucose at admission (OR 0.98 for each mg/dl increase in glucose, 95% CI 0.97–0.99, p = 0.01), a history of previous transient ischemic attack/stroke (OR 0.42, 95% CI 0.24–0.75, p = 0.003), obesity (OR 0.41, 95% CI 0.19–0.91, p = 0.02), and of diabetes mellitus (OR 0.45, 95% CI 0.27–0.77, p = 0.003). Regarding instead positive functional outcome (FO+), younger age (OR for 1-year increment in age 0.98, 95% CI 0.96–0.99, p = 0.008), lower NIHSS score at admission (OR 0.72 for 1-point increase in the scale, 95% CI 0.61–0.85, p = 0.001), higher BI score at admission (OR 1.06, 95% CI 1.04–1.07, p = 0.001), a history of previous transient ischemic attack/stroke (OR 0.45, 95% CI 0.26–0.80, p = 0.005), hypertension (OR 0.61, 95% CI 0.38–0.98, p = 0.04), and diabetes mellitus (OR 0.52, 95% CI 0.31–0.87, p = 0.01) were related to FO+ at 3 months.

By multivariate analysis, after controlling for variables significantly associated with the two efficacy endpoints at the univariate analysis, IVT treatment remained an independent predictor of DO+ and FO+ in patients with "mild stroke" (see Table 3).

Table 3. Multivariable analyses showing independent predictors of positive disability outcome and positive functional outcome.

DO+	OR	95% CI	p
IVT treatment			
No	1.00		
Yes	3.12	1.34–7.27	0.008
Age	0.95	0.92–0.98	0.003
BI score at admission	1.06	1.04–1.09	0.001
FO+	**OR**	**95% CI**	**p**
IVT treatment			
No	1.00		
Yes	4.70	2.38–9.26	0.001
Age	0.98	0.96–0.99	0.02
NIHSS score at admission	0.77	0.61–0.97	0.03
BI score at admission	1.06	1.04–1.07	0.001
Diabetes mellitus			
No	1.00		
Yes	0.53	0.29–0.98	0.04

DO+ (3-month mRS score of 0 or 1) = positive disability outcome; FO+ (mRS score of 0 or 1 plus BI score of 95 or 100 at 3-months) = positive functional outcome; IVT = intravenous thrombolysis; NIHSS = National Institute of Health Stroke scale; BI = Barthel index.

A beneficial effect of IVT was observed only in patients with FD predominantly due to weakness who significantly improved after treatment (DO+: OR 4.88, 95% CI 2.01–11.83, p = 0.001; FO+: OR 5.03, 95% CI 2.23–11.32, p = 0.001), different from patients without FD, or with other types of presenting symptoms (data not shown).

As shown in Figure 2, the prevalence of DO+ was significantly higher in FD+ IVT+ patients than in those FD+ IVT− (FD+ IVT+: 83.9% vs. FD+ IVT−: 52.5%, p = 0.001); differently, IVT treatment did not influence DO+ in FD− patients (FD− IVT+: 90.2% vs. FD− IVT−: 89.1%, p = 0.8). Similarly, for functional outcome, FO+ was significantly more common in FD+ IVT+ patients than in those FD+ IVT− (FD+ IVT+: 77.4% vs. FD+ IVT−: 44.6%, p = 0.001), whereas rates of FO+ were similar in FD− IVT+ and FD− IVT− patients (90.2% vs. 85.4%, p = 0.4) (see Figure 3).

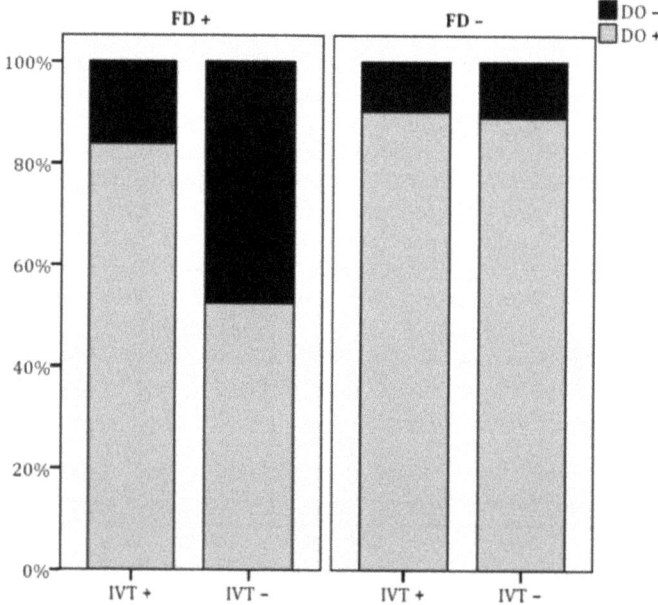

Figure 2. Effect of IVT on disability outcome rates in groups of patients with different levels of functional dependence at admission. DO = disability outcome; FD = functional dependence; IVT = intravenous thrombolysis.

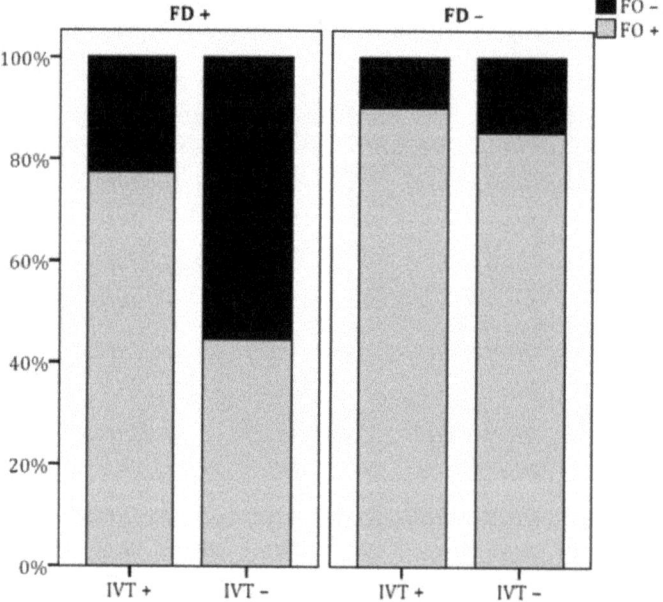

Figure 3. Effect of IVT on functional outcome rates in groups of patients with different levels of functional dependence at admission. FO= functional outcome; FD = functional dependence; IVT = intravenous thrombolysis.

In FD$^+$ patients, the following variables were independent predictors of outcome: IVT treatment (OR 6.01, 95% CI 2.59–13.92, $p = 0.001$), BI score at admission (OR 1.07, 95% CI 1.04–1.10, $p = 0.001$), a history of previous transient ischemic attack/stroke (OR 0.41, 95% CI 0.18–0.92, $p = 0.03$), and diabetes mellitus (OR 0.42, 95% CI 0.18–0.94, $p = 0.04$) for DO$^+$; IVT treatment (OR 4.73, 95% CI 2.29–9.76, $p = 0.001$), BI score at admission (OR 1.04, 95% CI 1.02–1.07, $p = 0.001$), and a history of previous transient ischemic attack/stroke (OR 0.44, 95% CI 0.20–0.96, $p = 0.04$) for FO$^+$. In contrast, IVT treatment did not affect functional outcome in FD$^-$ patients; in fact, BI score at admission was the only independent predictor of DO$^+$ (OR 1.22, 95% CI 1.07–1.39, $p = 0.002$), and FO$^+$ (OR 1.13, 95% CI 1.05–1.21, $p = 0.001$).

4. Discussion

For the first time we demonstrated that patients with "mild stroke", as defined as a NIHSS score of 0–5, should be selected for IVT on the basis of their level of FD at admission. In particular, subjects with moderate or severe FD, as assessed by the BI score, should be treated with IVT as soon as possible. In contrast, treatment with alteplase seems to be ineffective on patients who are functionally independent or with slight FD at admission. Thus, our study gives support to the latest American Heart Association/American Stroke Association guidelines recommending that IVT should be used for patients with mild but also disabling symptoms [13].

There is ongoing debate concerning what is a "mild stroke". In 2010, Fisher et al. explored the relationship of 6 different "minor stroke" definitions and outcomes. Since patients with a NIHSS score ≤ 3 had the best short- and medium-term outcome, the authors suggested to use this easily-applicable definition [18]. Although this definition has been used in some studies [19,20], a recent review of this topic reported that the NIHSS—with a score ranging from 0 to 5—is the most commonly used tool to define a "mild stroke" [21]. Similarly, we utilized an NIHSS score of 0 to 5 for identifying patients with supposed "mild" symptoms; our patients had a median NIHSS score of 2. However, despite their low NIHSS, several of them were affected by severe FD at admission; in fact, we observed a median BI score of 75, and 51.7% of the sample had a BI score < 80. This discrepancy may be due to the fact that the NIHSS is not able to detect symptoms of posterior circulation stroke, such as postural instability, gait disturbance, and dysphagia that can cause very severe disability. Thus, we think that patients with a low NIHSS score at presentation should be carefully evaluated regarding the presence of possible disabling symptoms before being labeled as affected by "mild stroke".

Originally published in 1965, the BI was developed to give physicians a suitable standard tool to assess and measure FD [22]. In fact, the BI covers all activities considered part of any assessment of activities of daily living, has an excellent reliability and validity, is easy to use, and only takes a few minutes [23]. Thus, we suggest adopting this tool in patients with "mild stroke", in order to correctly recognize patients with non-disabling symptoms.

Obviously, the exact distinction between stroke with disabling or non-disabling symptoms becomes extremely important when patients are affected by AIS and are suitable for IVT treatment. In our sample, more than 70% of AIS patients were not treated with IVT because they were deemed too good to be treated. This rate is perfectly in line with previous studies on this topic [6,9,10]. As shown in Table 1, the decision to treat or not to treat with IVT was merely based on the NIHSS score, whereas the level of FD was absolutely neglected. Use of anticoagulant agents was, as expected, significantly higher in AIS patients with "mild stroke" who were not treated, than in those who received IVT.

Previous studies on IVT treatment in AIS patients with mild symptoms report conflicting results [5–10]. In 2012 Huisa et al. investigated 133 patients with minor ischemic strokes, defined as an admission NIHSS score ≤ 5, and observed similar outcomes between patients treated and not treated with alteplase [5]. An Italian study of 128 patients with mild ischemic stroke confirmed that alteplase did not improve functional outcome [6]. Of 276 patients with mild ischemic stroke symptoms that were analyzed by Spokoyny et al., 83 were IVT treated. Treated and untreated patients had similar baseline characteristics except that the treated group had higher baseline NIHSS. Prevalence of mRS 2–6 at 90 days was 37.4% in the treated group and 31.1% in the untreated group ($p = 0.44$) [9]. In contrast, Urra et al. reported that IVT was associated with a greater proportion of patients with mild stroke who shifted down on the mRS score at 3 months (OR 2.66; 95% CI 1.49–4.74, $p = 0.001$) [7]. In a case-control study of 890 Austrian patients with a NIHSS score 0–5 at admission, IVT was associated with a better outcome after 3 months (OR 1.49, 95% CI 1.17–1.89, $p < 0.001$) [8]. More recently, Haeberlin et al. compared 3-month functional outcomes in 370 consecutive AIS patients with a NIHSS score ≤ 6. Although patients with mild AIS had a high chance of favorable outcomes irrespective of treatment type, subjects receiving IVT more often achieved complete remission of symptoms (mRS score = 0) (OR 3.33, $p < 0.0001$) [10]. Similarly to Urra et al. [7] and Haeberlin et al. [10], we observed a major beneficial effect of IVT on the outcome measures. Interestingly, it would seem that IVT efficacy is more pronounced in AIS patients affected by "mild stroke" than in those enrolled in regulatory randomized controlled trials, in which patients with minor symptoms were largely underrepresented [24]. We think that this discrepancy may be due to different study design between observational studies and randomized controlled trials. In fact, more often, non-interventional studies tend to overestimate the effects of the treatment and show more variability in estimates of the effects because of residual confounding, errors, and bias.

Discording results of IVT efficacy in "mild strokes" may be explained by differences in clinical characteristics among patients with minor symptoms. In particular, our patients who underwent IVT had a better 3-month functional outcome than those IVT$^-$, but presence of neurological symptoms due to weakness and level of FD at admission played a major role in influencing this association. If patients with "mild stroke" *plus* disabling symptoms (FD$^+$) were treated with alteplase, there was a significant improvement in functional outcome compared to those which were not treated. Indeed, more than 50% of patients with a BI score < 80 for whom IVT was denied did not achieve functional independence 3 months after stroke. In patients with "mild stroke" *plus* disabling symptoms, IVT represented the strongest predictor of DO$^+$ (OR: 6.01) and FO$^+$ (OR: 4.73). On the other hand, rates of favorable outcomes were very high in patients without disability, regardless of treatment type. In these patients, BI score at admission was the only independent predictor of DO$^+$ and FO$^+$, while IVT treatment did not influence functional outcomes. In contrast, Urra et al. report that IVT was associated with a greater proportion of patients with non-disabling minor strokes who shifted down on the mRS score at 3-months [7].

To date, only the PRISMS trial has been designed to assess the efficacy of IVT for the treatment of AIS with NIHSS 0–5, and without clearly disabling deficits. The authors designed a multicenter, randomized, double-blind, placebo-controlled trial with a sample size of 948 subjects [15]. Unfortunately, the study was terminated early because of low patient recruitment. Results of the 313 patients enrolled failed to demonstrate more favorable functional outcomes in patients treated with alteplase, as compared to those receiving only aspirin. However, the trial's early termination precludes any definitive conclusions on this topic. Moreover, definition of "not clearly disabling" was left to the subjective interpretation of individual clinicians [16].

Regarding safety endpoints, in our sample, alteplase treatment significantly increased the risk of sICH, even if rates of mortality were similar in patients IVT$^+$ and IVT$^-$. Bearing in mind that higher NIHSS scores predict a higher rate of sICH, it could be argued that our sICH rate in patients with "mild stroke" was high. However, a previous study performed in patients with minor stroke reported a sICH rate as high as 5% when IVT was administered [5].

Several limitations of this study need to be acknowledged. First, the retrospective design of our study was certainly a limit; however, all data were prospectively collected. Second, measures of outcome were obtained by physicians that were not blinded to IVT treatment, which may have influenced their rating. Third, information on intervals between stroke onset and IVT was not collected, thus we cannot exclude that elapsed time from symptoms onset may have influenced physicians' decisions to perform or not perform IVT treatment. Finally, since this was a hypothesis-generating study, further surveys are needed to test our preliminary hypotheses. In particular, interventional trials should be performed in order to exclude the presence of a bias by indication that could have affected our observational study.

In conclusion, alteplase seems to improve functional outcome in patients with a low NIHSS score. However, in our experience, this beneficial effect is strongly influenced by FD at admission. In patients with "mild stroke" *plus* disabling symptoms, IVT treatment should be administered as soon as possible; on the contrary, alteplase may not be used if minor and non-disabling deficits are diagnosed. In order to distinguish mild ischemic stroke patients with disabling or non-disabling symptoms, we suggest to use the BI. Our observational study brings further evidence to the results coming from a few other non-interventional studies and from one randomized trial interrupted before completion. Thus, further large interventional studies are needed to confirm our preliminary findings.

Author Contributions: Conceptualization, G.M. and C.S.; methodology, G.M. and C.S.; software, G.M. and C.S.; validation, S.L., G.L.G. and M.V.; formal analysis, G.M.; investigation, C.S., S.L. and A.S.; resources, C.S., S.L. and A.S.; data curation, G.M.; writing—original draft preparation, G.M.; writing—review and editing, G.M.; visualization, G.L.G; supervision, M.V. All authors have read and agreed to the published version of the manuscript.

Funding: This research received no external funding.

Conflicts of Interest: The authors declare no conflict of interest.

References

1. Reeves, M.; Khoury, J.; Alwell, K.; Moomaw, C.; Flaherty, M.; Woo, D.; Khatri, P.; Adeoye, O.; Ferioli, S.; Kissela, N.; et al. Distribution of national institutes of health stroke scale in the Cincinnati/Northern Kentucky stroke study. *Stroke* **2013**, *44*, 3211–3213. [CrossRef]
2. Dhamoon, M.S.; Moon, Y.P.; Paik, M.C.; Boden-Albala, B.; Rundek, T.; Sacco, R.L.; Elkind, M.S. Long-term functional recovery after first ischemic stroke. *Stroke* **2009**, *40*, 2805–2811. [CrossRef]
3. Messé, S.R.; Khatri, P.; Reeves, M.J.; Smith, E.E.; Saver, J.L.; Bhatt, D.L.; Grau-Sepulveda, M.V.; Cox, M.; Peterson, E.D.; Fonarow, G.C.; et al. Why are acute ischemic stroke patients not receiving IV tPA? Results from a national registry. *Neurology* **2016**, *87*, 1565–1574. [CrossRef]
4. Barber, P.A.; Zhang, J.; Demchuk, A.M.; Hill, M.D.; Buchan, A.M. Why are stroke patients excluded from TPA therapy? An analysis of patient eligibility. *Neurology* **2001**, *56*, 1015–1020. [CrossRef] [PubMed]
5. Huisa, B.N.; Raman, R.; Neil, W.; Ernstrom, K.; Hemmen, T. Intravenous tissue plasminogen activator for patients with minor ischemic stroke. *J. Stroke Cerebrovasc. Dis.* **2012**, *21*, 732–736. [CrossRef] [PubMed]
6. Nesi, M.; Lucente, G.; Nencini, P.; Fancellu, L.; Inzitari, D. Aphasia predicts unfavorable outcome in mild ischemic stroke patients and prompts thrombolytic treatment. *J. Stroke Cerebrovasc. Dis.* **2014**, *23*, 204–208. [CrossRef] [PubMed]
7. Urra, X.; Ariño, H.; Llull, L.; Amaro, S.; Obach, V.; Cervera, A.; Chamorro, A. The outcome of patients with mild stroke improves after treatment with systemic thrombolysis. *PLoS ONE* **2013**, *8*, e59420. [CrossRef] [PubMed]
8. Greisenegger, S.; Seyfang, L.; Kiechl, S.; Lang, W.; Ferrari, J. Austrian Stroke Unit Registry Collaborators. Thrombolysis in patients with mild stroke: Results from the Austrian Stroke Unit Registry. *Stroke* **2014**, *45*, 765–769. [CrossRef]
9. Spokoyny, I.; Raman, R.; Ernstrom, K.; Khatri, P.; Meyer, D.M.; Hemmen, T.M.; Meyer, B.C. Defining mild stroke: Outcomes analysis of treated and untreated mild stroke patients. *J. Stroke Cerebrovasc. Dis.* **2015**, *24*, 1276–1281. [CrossRef]
10. Haeberlin, M.I.; Held, U.; Baumgartner, R.W.; Georgiadis, D.; Valko, P.O. Impact of intravenous thrombolysis on functional outcome in patients with mild ischemic stroke without large vessel occlusion or rapidly improving symptoms. *Int. J. Stroke* **2019**. [CrossRef]
11. Adams, H.P., Jr.; Brott, T.G.; Furlan, A.J.; Gomez, C.R.; Grotta, J.; Helgason, C.M.; Kwiatkowski, T.; Lyden, P.D.; Marler, J.R.; Torner, J.; et al. Guidelines for thrombolytic therapy for acute stroke: A supplement to the guidelines for the management of patients with acute ischemic stroke. A statement for healthcare professionals from a special writing group of the Stroke Council, American Heart Association. *Stroke* **1996**, *27*, 1711–1718. [PubMed]

12. Adams, H.O., Jr.; del Zoppo, G.; Alberts, M.J.; Bhatt, D.L.; Brass, L.; Furlan, A.; Grubb, R.L.; Higashida, R.T.; Jauch, E.C.; Kidwell, C.; et al. American Heart Association, American Stroke Association Stroke Council, Clinical Cardiology Council, Cardiovascular Radiology and Intervention Council, Atherosclerotic Peripheral Vascular Disease and Quality of Care Outcomes in Research Interdisciplinary Working Groups. Guidelines for the early management of adults with ischemic stroke: A guideline from the American Heart Association/American Stroke Association Stroke Council, Clinical Cardiology Council, Cardiovascular Radiology and Intervention Council, and the Atherosclerotic Peripheral Vascular Disease and Quality of Care Outcomes in Research Interdisciplinary Working Groups: The American Academy of Neurology Affirms the Value of This Guideline as an Educational Tool for Neurologists. *Stroke* **2007**, *38*, 1655–1711. [PubMed]
13. Powers, W.J.; Rabinstein, A.A.; Ackerson, T.; Adeoye, O.M.; Bambakidis, N.C.; Becker, K.; Biller, J.; Brown, M.; Demaerschalk, B.M.; David, L.; et al. American Heart Association Stroke Council. 2018 guidelines for the early management of patients with acute ischemic stroke: A guideline for healthcare professionals from the American Heart Association/American Stroke Association. *Stroke* **2018**, *49*, e46–e110. [CrossRef] [PubMed]
14. Wendt, M.; Tutuncu, S.; Fiebach, J.B.; Scheitz, J.F.; Audebert, H.J.; Nolte, C.H. Preclusion of ischemic stroke patients from intravenous tissue plasminogen activator treatment for mild symptoms should not be based on low National Institutes of Health Stroke Scale scores. *J. Stroke Cerebrovasc. Dis.* **2013**, *22*, 550–553. [CrossRef] [PubMed]
15. Yeatts, S.D.; Broderick, J.P.; Chatterjee, A.; Jauch, E.C.; Levine, S.R.; Romano, J.G.; Saver, J.L.; Vagal, A.; Purdon, B.; Devenport, J.; et al. Alteplase for the treatment of acute ischemic stroke in patients with low National Institutes of Health Stroke Scale and not clearly disabling deficits (Potential of rtPA for Ischemic Strokes with Mild Symptoms PRISMS): Rationale and design. *Int. J. Stroke* **2018**, *13*, 654–661. [CrossRef] [PubMed]
16. Khatri, P.; Kleindorfer, D.O.; Devlin, T.; Sawyer, R.N.; Starr, M.; Mejilla, J.; Broderick, J.; Chatterjee, A.; Jauch, E.C.; Levine, S.R.; et al. Effect of alteplase vs. aspirin on functional outcome for patients with acute ischemic stroke and minor nondisabling neurlogic deficits: The PRISMS randomized clinical trial. *JAMA* **2018**, *320*, 156–166. [CrossRef]
17. Hacke, W.; Kaste, M.; Bluhmki, E.; Brozman, M.; Davalos, A.; Guidetti, D.; Larrue, V.; Lees, K.R.; Medeghri, Z.; Machnig, T.; et al. Thrombolysis with alteplase 3 to 4.5 h after acute ischemic stroke. *N. Engl. J. Med.* **2008**, *359*, 1317–1329. [CrossRef]
18. Fischer, U.; Baumgartner, A.; Arnold, M.; Nedeltchev, K.; Gralla, J.; Marco De Marchis, G.; Kappeler, L.; Mono, M.-L.; Brekenfeld, C.; Schroth, G.; et al. What is a minor stroke? *Stroke* **2010**, *41*, 661–666. [CrossRef]
19. Luengo-Fernandez, R.; Gray, A.M.; Rothwell, P.M. Effect of urgent treatment for transient ischaemic attack and minor stroke on disability and hospital costs (EXPRESS study): A prospective population-based sequential comparison. *Lancet Neurol.* **2009**, *8*, 218–219. [CrossRef]
20. Coutts, S.B.; Hill, M.D.; Campos, C.R.; Choi, Y.B.; Subramaniam, S.; Kosior, J.C.; Demchuk, A.M. Recurrent events in transient ischemic attack and minor stroke. *Stroke* **2008**, *39*, 2461–2466. [CrossRef]
21. Schwartz, J.K.; Capo-Lugo, C.E.; Akinwuntan, A.E.; Roberts, P.; Krishnan, S.; Belagaje, S.R.; Lovic, M.; Burns, S.P.; Hu, X.; Danzl, M.; et al. Classification of mild stroke: A mapping review. *Pm&r* **2019**, *11*, 996–1003.
22. Mahoney, F.I.; Barthel, D.W. Functional evaluation: The Barthel index. *Md. State Med. J.* **1965**, *14*, 61–65. [PubMed]
23. Barak, S.; Duncan, P.W. Issues in selecting outcome measures to assess functional recovery after stroke. *NeuroRx* **2006**, *3*, 505–524. [CrossRef] [PubMed]
24. Wardlaw Wardlaw, J.M.; Murray, V.; Berge, E.; del Zoppo, G.J. Thrombolysis for acute ischemic stroke. *Cochrane Database Syst. Rev.* **2014**, *7*, CD000213.

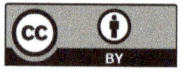

© 2020 by the authors. Licensee MDPI, Basel, Switzerland. This article is an open access article distributed under the terms and conditions of the Creative Commons Attribution (CC BY) license (http://creativecommons.org/licenses/by/4.0/).

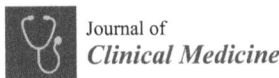

Article

Improving the Clinical Outcome in Stroke Patients Receiving Thrombolytic or Endovascular Treatment in Korea: from the SECRET Study

Young Dae Kim [1], Ji Hoe Heo [1], Joonsang Yoo [1,2], Hyungjong Park [1,2], Byung Moon Kim [3], Oh Young Bang [4], Hyeon Chang Kim [5], Euna Han [6], Dong Joon Kim [3], JoonNyung Heo [1], Minyoung Kim [1], Jin Kyo Choi [1], Kyung-Yul Lee [7], Hye Sun Lee [8], Dong Hoon Shin [9], Hye-Yeon Choi [10], Sung-Il Sohn [2], Jeong-Ho Hong [2], Jang-Hyun Baek [11,12], Gyu Sik Kim [13], Woo-Keun Seo [4], Jong-Won Chung [4], Seo Hyun Kim [14], Tae-Jin Song [15], Sang Won Han [16], Joong Hyun Park [16], Jinkwon Kim [7,17], Yo Han Jung [18], Han-Jin Cho [19], Seong Hwan Ahn [20], Sung Ik Lee [21], Kwon-Duk Seo [13,21] and Hyo Suk Nam [1,*]

1. Department of Neurology, Yonsei University College of Medicine, Seoul 03722, Korea; neuro05@yuhs.ac (Y.D.K.); jhheo@yuhs.ac (J.H.H.); JSYOO@yuhs.ac (J.Y.); hjpark209042@gmail.com (H.P.); jnheo@jnheo.com (J.H.); bestmykim@gmail.com (M.K.); JKSNAIL85@yuhs.ac (J.K.C.)
2. Department of Neurology, Brain Research Institute, Keimyung University School of Medicine, Daegu 41931, Korea; sungil.sohn@gmail.com (S.-I.S.); neurohong79@gmail.com (J.-H.H.)
3. Department of Radiology, Yonsei University College of Medicine, Seoul 03722, Korea; BMOON21@yuhs.ac (B.M.K.); DJKIMMD@yuhs.ac (D.J.K.)
4. Department of Neurology, Samsung Medical Center, Sungkyunkwan University School of Medicine, Seoul 06351, Korea; ohyoung.bang@samsung.com (O.Y.B.); mcastenosis@gmail.com (W.-K.S.); neurocjw@gmail.com (J.-W.C.)
5. Department of Preventive Medicine, Yonsei University College of Medicine, Seoul 03722, Korea; hckim@yuhs.ac
6. College of Pharmacy, Yonsei Institute for Pharmaceutical Research, Yonsei University, Incheon 21983, Korea; eunahan@yonsei.ac.kr
7. Department of Neurology, Gangnam Severance Hospital, Severance Institute for Vascular and Metabolic Research, Yonsei University College of Medicine, Seoul 06273, Korea; KYLEE@yuhs.ac (K.-Y.L.); antithrombus@gmail.com (J.K.)
8. Department of Research Affairs, Biostatistics Collaboration Unit, Yonsei University College of Medicine, Seoul 06273, Korea; HSLEE1@yuhs.ac
9. Department of Neurology, Gachon University Gil Medical Center, Incheon 21565, Korea; sphincter@naver.com
10. Department of Neurology, Kyung Hee University Hospital at Gangdong, Kyung Hee University School of Medicine, Seoul 05278, Korea; hyechoi@gmail.com
11. Department of Neurology, National Medical Center, Seoul 04564, Korea; janghyun.baek@gmail.com
12. Department of Neurology, Kangbuk Samsung Hospital, Sungkyunkwan University School of Medicine, Seoul 03181, Korea
13. Department of Neurology, National Health Insurance Service Ilsan Hospital, Ilsan 10444, Korea; gskim@nhimc.or.kr (G.S.K.); seobin7@naver.com (K.-D.S.)
14. Department of Neurology, Yonsei University Wonju College of Medicine, Wonju 26426, Korea; s-hkim@yonsei.ac.kr
15. Department of Neurology, Seoul Hospital, Ewha Womans University College of Medicine, Seoul 07804, Korea; knstar@hanmail.net
16. Department of Neurology, Sanggye Paik Hospital, Inje University College of Medicine, Seoul 01757, Korea; sah1puyo@gmail.com (S.W.H.); truelove1@hanmail.net (J.H.P.)
17. Department of Neurology, CHA Bundang Medical Center, CHA University, Seongnam 13496, Korea
18. Department of Neurology, Changwon Fatima Hospital, Changwon 51394, Korea; eyasyohan@gmail.com
19. Department of Neurology, Pusan National University School of Medicine, Busan 49241, Korea; chohj75@gmail.com
20. Department of Neurology, Chosun University School of Medicine, Gwangju 61453, Korea; shahn@Chosun.ac.kr

21 Department of Neurology, Sanbon Hospital, Wonkwang University School of Medicine, Sanbon 15865, Korea; neurologist@hanmail.net
* Correspondence: hsnam@yuhs.ac; Tel.: +82-2-2228-1617; Fax: +82-2-393-0705

Received: 23 January 2020; Accepted: 2 March 2020; Published: 6 March 2020

Abstract: We investigated whether there was an annual change in outcomes in patients who received the thrombolytic therapy or endovascular treatment (EVT) in Korea. This analysis was performed using data from a nationwide multicenter registry for exploring the selection criteria of patients who would benefit from reperfusion therapies in Korea. We compared the annual changes in the modified Rankin scale (mRS) at discharge and after 90 days and the achievement of successful recanalization from 2012 to 2017. We also investigated the determinants of favorable functional outcomes. Among 1230 included patients, the improvement of functional outcome at discharge after reperfusion therapy was noted as the calendar year increased ($p < 0.001$). The proportion of patients who were discharged to home significantly increased (from 45.6% in 2012 to 58.5% in 2017) ($p < 0.001$). The successful recanalization rate increased over time from 78.6% in 2012 to 85.1% in 2017 ($p = 0.006$). Time from door to initiation of reperfusion therapy decreased over the years ($p < 0.05$). These secular trends of improvements were also observed in 1203 patients with available mRS data at 90 days ($p < 0.05$). Functional outcome was associated with the calendar year, age, initial stroke severity, diabetes, preadmission disability, intervals from door to reperfusion therapy, and achievement of successful recanalization. This study demonstrated the secular trends of improvement in functional outcome and successful recanalization rate in patients who received reperfusion therapy in Korea.

Keywords: reperfusion; therapy; ischemic stroke; outcome

1. Introduction

Stroke is one of the diseases with the highest burden worldwide. Although the age-standardized risk of stroke or case fatality has been improving, there is still an increase in the absolute number of stroke or stroke-related death [1]. The Global Burden of Disease Study demonstrated that the burden of cerebrovascular disease increased over several decades and ranked second in the highest burden of diseases in 2015 [2].

Intravenous tissue plasminogen activator (IV t-PA) therapy and endovascular treatment (EVT) are established treatments for eligible patients with acute ischemic stroke [3,4]. Although these modalities can lead to successful recanalization, which is a strong determinant of a good outcome [5], many patients who received reperfusion therapy did not achieve a favorable outcome [6]. Over the past decades, there has been an improvement in the stroke care program, imaging techniques, treatment devices, and experience in EVT. As a result, overall outcome of reperfusion therapy for acute ischemic stroke could be improved at a national level [7]. In Korea, there have been improvements in the care system for acute stroke patients, including easy and rapid accessibility to medical services, establishment of stroke units or centers, and acute stroke codes for reperfusion therapy [8–10]. Considering these secular trends in the stroke care system, clinical and radiologic outcomes after reperfusion therapy might have changed in Korea.

We investigated whether there was an annual change in outcomes in patients who received IV t-PA therapy or EVT in Korea. We also determined which factors had played a role in these changes using the nationwide thrombolytic and EVT registry.

2. Materials and Methods

2.1. Patients Inclusion

The study population was derived from the Selection Criteria in Endovascular Thrombectomy and thrombolytic therapy (SECRET) registry (Clinicaltrials.gov NCT02964052, https://clinicaltrials.gov/ct2/show/NCT02964052?term=NCT02964052&rank=1). The SECRET registry is a nationwide multicenter registry for exploring the selection criteria of patients who would benefit from reperfusion therapies. The SECRET registry was started on May 2016. This registry consisted of four parts: (1) clinical information, (2) information on reperfusion therapy, (3) comorbidities, and (4) imaging data.

The clinical information section includes the demographics, vascular risk factors, previous medication status, laboratory findings, and neurologic status or premorbidity before stroke. In the reperfusion therapy section, the information on time parameters, angiographic findings before and after treatment, devices used during the procedure, periprocedural complications, and concomitant thrombolytic agents used was collected. The modified Rankin scale (mRS) at discharge and after 90 days, along with mortality within 6 months, was determined in each patient during the follow-up. If a patient died, we also assessed the cause of death.

For the comorbidities section, we determined the presence of the component of the Charlson comorbidity index (CCI) for each patient. In the stroke population, we used a modified version of the CCI, which consisted of 19 diseases, including myocardial infarction, congestive heart failure, peripheral vascular disease, previous stroke, atrial fibrillation, dementia, depression, chronic pulmonary disease, ulcer disease, mild liver disease, moderate or severe renal disease, connective tissue disease or rheumatic disease, anemia, diabetes, acquired immune deficiency syndrome, cancer, leukemia, lymphoma, and metastatic cancer [11].

The imaging data section included the occlusion site, infarction core, collateral status, and thrombus characteristics on thin-section computed tomography (CT). The imaging findings were ascertained by the imaging adjudication committee (6 stroke neurologists and 4 neuroradiologists). The audit was conducted every two weeks, and the data management center verified the completeness and accuracy of the data. For this study, we used the demographics, vascular risk factors, underlying vascular diseases, time parameters, occlusion site, angiographic findings before and after treatment, and functional outcome variables.

This registry included 1026 patients who had been registered retrospectively from 15 hospitals between January 2012 and December 2015 and 333 patients who had been registered prospectively from 13 hospitals between November 2016 and December 2017. For prospectively-enrolled patients, written informed consent was obtained from patients or the next of kin. This registry was approved by the institutional review board in each participating hospital.

2.2. Reperfusion Therapy

IV t-PA and EVT was used in patients who met the criteria based on current guidelines. IV t-PA (Actilyse; Boehringer-Ingelheim, Ingelheim, Germany) was used in patients who had a stroke within 4.5 h from symptom onset and met the criteria based on current guidelines with a standard dose (0.9 mg/kg) [12,13]. If patients had large vessel occlusion on initial angiographic studies and could be treated within 8 h from symptom onset, EVT was considered. The EVT was performed primarily using mechanical devices rather than chemical agents. Among the mechanical devices, Solitaire stent retriever (Medtronic Neurovascular, Iirvine, CA, USA), Trevo retriever (Stryker Neurovascular, Fremont, CA, USA), or Penumbra reperfusion catheter (Penumbra, Alameda, CA, USA) was available in Korea and used based on target vessel site, tortuosity, or neurointerventionalist's preference. Intra-arterial thrombolysis with urokinase (Green Cross, Seoul, Korea) or glycoprotein IIb/IIIa antagonists was used as an adjuvant therapy in certain cases including those with re-occlusion or distal embolization.

If the onset of symptom was unclear, EVT was performed based on imaging findings and physician's discretion. Brain magnetic resonance imaging and magnetic resonance angiography were performed 24 h after reperfusion therapy. When brain MRI could not be performed, brain CT and/or CT angiography was performed. During hospitalization, each patient was treated on the basis of current stroke guidelines [14,15].

2.3. Outcome Measures

In this study, functional outcome was assessed with mRS at discharge and after 90 days. Favorable functional was defined as having mRS score of 0–2 and excellent functional outcomes was defined as mRS score of 0–1. In terms of radiologic outcomes, successful recanalization was determined using digital subtraction angiography (DSA), CT angiography (CTA), or magnetic resonance angiography (MRA). In this study, successful recanalization was defined as thrombolysis in cerebral infarction grade of 2b or 3 on final DSA among patients with EVT [16]. In patients who received IV t-PA only, successful recanalization was defined as arterial occlusive lesion (AOL) scoring of 3 on CTA or MRA performed within 24 h. Symptomatic intracerebral hemorrhage was defined as having any type of hemorrhage causing neurologic deterioration with National Institutes of Health Stroke Scale (NIHSS) score ≥ 4 or leading to death or surgery within 7 days of stroke onset based on the criteria in the European Cooperative Acute Stroke Study (ECASS) III trial [12].

2.4. Statistical Analysis

When we compared the baseline characteristics according to the calendar year, Student's independent t-test was used to compare age, time interval, and laboratory findings, and Pearson's χ^2 test or Fisher's exact test was used in the analysis of categorical data. Wilcoxon rank sum test was used to compare baseline NIHSS scores. Because the number of patients who received reperfusion therapy in December 2016 and registered in the SECRET registry was small, these patients were merged into the patient group treated in 2017 for this analysis. When we investigated the trends of outcomes by year, linear-by-linear or Jonckheere-Terpstra test was used for the analysis. To determine the independent predictors of outcomes, logistic regression or ordinal regression analysis was used. A multivariable analysis was performed using all variables with a p-value < 0.1 in the univariable analysis. All p-values were two-sided, and a p-value < 0.05 was considered statistically significant. All statistical analysis was performed using Windows SPSS package (version 23.0, IBM Corp., Armonk, NY, USA) and R version 3.2.1 (R Foundation for Statistical Computing, Vienna, Austria, http://www.R-project.org).

3. Results

3.1. Baseline Characteristics

Between January 2012 and December 2017, a total of 1359 patients who received reperfusion therapy with either IV t-PA therapy or EVT were registered. First, we excluded 38 patients who received intra-arterial chemical thrombolytic treatment as primary therapeutic modality. Then, we also excluded 86 patients who had in-hospital ischemic stroke, and nine patients who were transferred to the study hospital from other local hospitals ("drip-and-ship" case) because there were insufficient data on time parameters such as the intervals from stroke onset to first hospital arrival, CT, or IV t-PA. Finally, 1226 patients were included in this analysis (Figure 1).

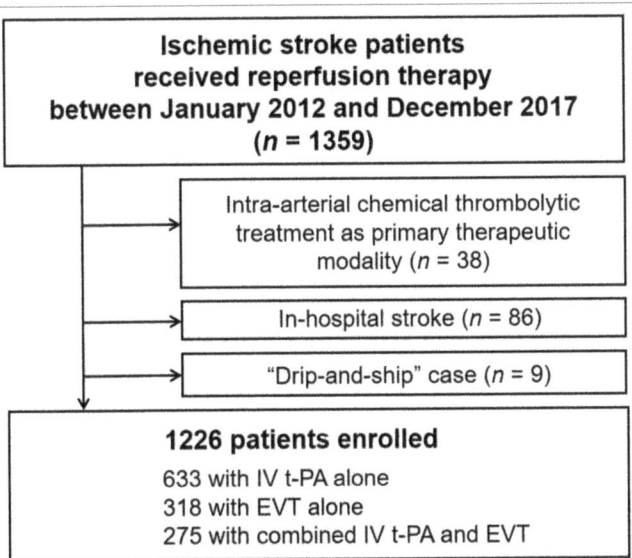

Figure 1. Flow diagram for the selection of patients in this study. IV, intravenous; t-PA, tissue plasminogen activator; EVT, endovascular.

Baseline characteristics of patients are presented in Table 1. The mean age was 68.9 ± 11.6 years, and 724 patients (58.9%) were male. The most common risk factor was hypertension (70.9%), followed by atrial fibrillation or atrial flutter (48.3%). The median NIHSS score was 12 (interquartile range [IQR], 7–17). Six-hundred and thirty-three (51.6%) patients received IV t-PA treatment alone, 318 (25.9%) patients received EVT alone, and the remaining 275 (22.4%) received combined IV t-PA and EVT. The number of patients who received IV t-PA and registered in SECRET registry was larger than those registered after EVT with/without IV t-PA, except in 2017. We could determine the location of large artery occlusion in 851 of 1021 patients who underwent angiographic studies before reperfusion therapy. The most common occlusion site was the middle cerebral artery (MCA) (56.1%, n = 477), followed by the internal carotid artery (ICA) (27.1%, n = 231), vertebrobasilar (VBA) artery (12.1%, n = 103), and others (4.7%, n = 40). During study period, thrombectomy devices including Solitaire, Trevo, and Penumbra system were available in Korea. Among 593 patients treated with EVT, Solitaire was most frequently selected in 433 (73%), followed by Penumbra system (n = 69, 11.6%), and Trevo (n = 69, 11.6%).

Table 1. Baseline characteristics of the included patients by year.

	Total	Calendar Year					p-Value for Trends
		2012 (n = 103)	2013 (n = 231)	2014 (n = 284)	2015 (n = 302)	2017 (n = 306)	
Age	68.9 ± 11.6	68.7 ± 10.3	68.8 ± 11.2	68.8 ± 11.7	70.0 ± 11.3	67.9 ± 12.6	0.941
Male sex	723 (59.0)	58 (56.3)	142 (61.5)	162 (57.0)	168 (55.6)	193 (63.1)	0.328
Hypertension	869 (70.9)	79 (76.7)	168 (72.7)	193 (68.0)	213 (70.5)	216 (70.6)	0.437
Diabetes	499 (40.7)	53 (51.5)	101 (43.7)	110 (38.7)	108 (35.8)	127 (41.5)	0.187
Hyperlipidemia	408 (33.3)	33 (32.0)	60 (26.0)	98 (34.5)	87 (28.8)	130 (42.5)	0.001
Current smoking	273 (22.3)	22 (21.4)	52 (22.5)	70 (24.6)	64 (21.2)	65 (21.2)	0.630
Coronary disease	212 (17.3)	21 (20.4)	31 (13.4)	55 (19.4)	52 (17.2)	53 (17.3)	0.903
Valvular heart disease	47 (3.8)	4 (3.9)	3 (1.3)	10 (3.5)	20 (6.6)	10 (3.3)	0.408
Mechanical valvular disease	18 (1.5)	4 (3.9)	2 (0.9)	3 (1.1)	4 (1.3)	5 (1.6)	0.714
Mitral stenosis	29 (2.4)	0 (0.0)	1 (0.4)	7 (2.5)	16 (5.3)	5 (1.6)	0.182
Atrial fibrillation or atrial flutter	592 (48.3)	55 (53.4)	112 (48.5)	144 (50.7)	159 (52.6)	122 (39.9)	0.008
Congestive heart failure	68 (5.5)	5 (4.9)	16 (6.9)	18 (6.3)	16 (5.3)	13 (4.2)	0.265
Peripheral arterial occlusive diseases	22 (1.8)	3 (2.9)	8 (3.5)	4 (1.4)	2 (2.2)	5 (1.6)	0.141
Previous stroke	246 (20.1)	26 (25.2)	42 (18.2)	60 (21.1)	55 (18.2)	63 (20.3)	0.754
Preadmission disability	50 (4.1)	8 (7.8)	10 (4.3)	16 (5.6)	8 (2.6)	8 (2.6)	0.020
Location site (n = 1021)							0.170
ICA	231 (22.6)	26 (34.7)	35 (19.7)	53 (24.5)	54 (21.7)	63 (20.8)	
MCA	477 (46.7)	24 (32.0)	81 (45.5)	110 (50.9)	125 (50.2)	137 (45.2)	
VBA	103 (10.1)	11 (14.7)	20 (11.2)	23 (10.6)	18 (7.2)	31 (10.2)	
Others	40 (3.9)	2 (2.7)	10 (5.6)	7 (3.2)	7 (2.8)	14 (4.6)	
No Occlusion	170 (16.7)	12 (16.0)	32 (18.0)	23 (10.6)	45 (18.1)	58 (19.1)	
Systolic blood pressure	149.9 ± 28.8	153.3 ± 33.6	152.5 ± 30.1	148.3 ± 27.6	149.2 ± 28.8	148.8 ± 27.3	0.078
Diastolic blood pressure	85 ± 16.6	87.4 ± 21.1	86.3 ± 15.9	86.3 ± 16.6	84.1 ± 16.4	82.8 ± 15.3	0.018
Last normal to ED	144.3 ± 180.4	117.6 ± 159.2	131.7 ± 146.6	139.4 ± 178.3	148.9 ± 174.5	162.8 ± 213.8	0.015

Table 1. Cont.

	Total	Calendar Year				p-Value for Trends
		2012 (n = 103)	2013 (n = 231)	2014 (n = 284)	2015 (n = 302)	2017 (n = 306)	
ED to CT (n = 1212)	18.5 ± 21.7	21.5 ± 16.1	18.4 ± 42.3	16.5 ± 12.5	17.8 ± 11.6	20.1 ± 14.1	0.450
ED to t-PA infusion (n = 908)	47.1 ± 23.1	56.5 ± 24.9	47.8 ± 22	47.1 ± 21.8	48.7 ± 25.5	41.1 ± 20.6	<0.001
ED to groin puncture (n = 593)	124.1 ± 57.7	137.2 ± 63.7	133.7 ± 66.5	131.6 ± 50.8	123.1 ± 60.3	112.8 ± 53.1	0.009
ED to final recanalization (n = 497)	192.3 ± 76.8	240.1 ± 99.1	206.6 ± 89.1	208.8 ± 69.2	181.8 ± 78.4	172.9 ± 62.6	<0.001
Last normal to final recanalization (n = 497)	389.9 ± 244.2	401.3 ± 184.8	402.1 ± 206.9	395.0 ± 249.0	395.7 ± 257.0	367.8 ± 256.6	0.127
NIHSS score at stroke onset	12 (7–17)	13 (7–18)	13 (7–17)	13 (7–18)	12 (6–17)	12 (5–16)	0.004
Treatment modality							<0.001
IV t-PA alone	633 (51.6)	58 (56.3)	144 (62.3)	154 (54.2)	172 (57.0)	105 (34.3)	
EVT alone	318 (25.9)	25 (24.3)	49 (21.2)	71 (25.0)	73 (24.2)	100 (32.7)	
EVT + IV t-PA	275 (22.4)	20 (19.4)	38 (16.5)	59 (20.8)	57 (18.9)	101 (33.0)	
Use of stentriever *	499 (48.1)	31 (68.9)	60 (69.0)	107 (82.3)	115 (88.5)	186 (92.5)	<0.001

Values are presented as n (%), unless otherwise indicated. ICA, internal carotid artery; MCA, middle cerebral artery; VBA, vertebrobasilar artery; ED, emergency department; NIHSS, National Institutes of Health Stroke Scale; IV, intravenous; EVT, endovascular; t-PA, tissue plasminogen activator. * Among 499 patients who received EVT with/without IV t-PA.

3.2. Secular Trends of Functional and Radiologic Outcomes

There was an increase in the number of patients who received the reperfusion therapy and the number of patients was 103 in 2012, 231 in 2013, 284 in 2014, 302 in 2015, and 306 in 2017. When we compared the baseline characteristics annually, initial diastolic blood pressure, NIHSS score at admission, and frequency of atrial fibrillation or atrial flutter decreased, while frequency of dyslipidemia or preadmission disability (mRS score of >2 before stroke) increased (Table 1). However, there were no differences in demographics or other vascular risk factors between calendar years. In time parameters, the intervals from stroke onset to arrival to emergency department (ED) increased, while those from door to initiation of IV t-PA (in 908 patients who received IV t-PA) or groin puncture (in 593 patients who received EVT) decreased over the years (all $p < 0.05$, Table 1). Especially, in 497 patients who had achieved final recanalization using EVT, the intervals from door to final recanalization [decreased from 240.1 ± 99.1 min in 2012 to 172.9 ± 62.6 min in 2017 ($p < 0.001$). During the study period, total number of stroke neurologist of study hospitals slightly increased (34 in 2012, 37 in 2013, 38 in 2014, 40 in 2015, 41 in 2017), while the number of neurointerventionalists or neurosurgeons involving EVT was similar (35 in 2012, 37 in 2013, 36 in 2014, 35 in 2015, 37 in 2017).

During the study period, patients achieved favorable functional outcome (mRS score of 0–2) in 48.6% and excellent functional outcome (mRS score of 0–1) in 31.3% at discharge. Among 1203 patients with available mRS data at 90 days, 501 (41.8%) patients achieved favorable functional outcome and 703 (58.6%) patients did excellent functional outcome at 90 days. The improvement in functional outcome at discharge after reperfusion therapy was noted as calendar year increased (Figure 2). The proportion of patients who were discharged home significantly increased (from 45.6% in 2012 to 58.5% in 2017) ($p < 0.001$). Likewise, functional outcome at 90 days was also different between calendar years ($p < 0.05$). There was an increase in favorable functional outcome (mRS score of 0–2) or excellent outcome (mRS score of 0–1) at discharge or after 90 days (all $p < 0.05$) (Table 2). In addition, the mortality rate at discharge or after 90 days significantly decreased with an increase in calendar year (all $p < 0.05$). These secular trends were consistently observed regardless of treatment modalities (Figure 2).

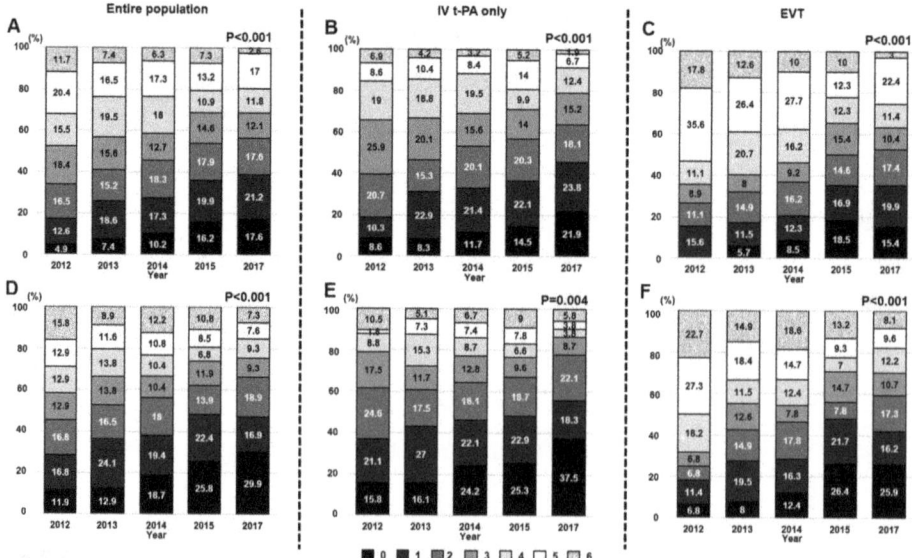

Figure 2. Secular trends in functional outcome at discharge (**A**–**C**) and after 90 days (**D**–**F**). Distribution of mRS scores of the entire population (**A** and **D**), those who received IV t-PA alone (**B**,**E**), and those who received EVT with/without IV t-PA (**C**,**F**).

Table 2. Clinical and radiologic outcome.

	Total	Calendar Year					p-Value for Trends
		2012	2013	2014	2015	2017	
mRS score of 0–1 at discharge	384 (31.3)	18 (17.5)	60 (26.0)	78 (27.5)	109 (36.1)	119 (38.9)	<0.001
mRS score of 0–2 at discharge	596 (48.6)	35 (34.0)	95 (41.1)	130 (45.8)	163 (54.0)	173 (56.5)	<0.001
Discharge route							<0.001
Transfer to rehabilitation	168 (13.7)	18 (17.5)	25 (10.8)	42 (14.8)	27 (8.9)	56 (18.3)	
Home	662 (54.0)	47 (45.6)	114 (49.4)	140 (49.3)	182 (60.3)	179 (58.5)	
Transfer to other hospitals or departments	318 (25.9)	26 (25.2)	76 (32.9)	82 (28.9)	71 (23.5)	63 (20.6)	
Death	78 (6.4)	12 (11.7)	16 (6.9)	20 (7.0)	22 (7.3)	8 (2.6)	
mRS score of 0–1 at 90 days	501 (41.8)	29 (28.7)	83 (37.1)	106 (38.1)	142 (48.1)	141 (46.8)	<0.001
mRS score of 0–2 at 90 days	703 (58.6)	46 (45.5)	120 (53.6)	156 (56.1)	183 (62.0)	198 (65.8)	<0.001
Successful recanalization immediately after EVT	478 (80.6)	37 (82.2)	66 (75.9)	99 (76.2)	101 (77.7)	175 (87.1)	0.02
Successful recanalization within 24 h	628 (78.1)	47 (78.3)	95 (71.4)	135 (75.8)	143 (75.7)	208 (85.2)	0.004
Symptomatic intracranial hemorrhage	46 (3.8)	4 (3.9)	13 (5.6)	12 (4.2)	13 (4.3)	4 (1.3)	0.018

Values are presented as n (%), unless otherwise indicated. mRS, modified Rankin score; EVT, endovascular treatment.

Successful recanalization rate could be evaluated in 804 patients who had undergone follow-up angiographic studies within 24 h after IV t-PA therapy or EVT. The successful recanalization rate increased over time from 78.3% in 2012 to 85.2% in 2017 ($p = 0.004$) (Table 2). On the contrary, the development of symptomatic intracerebral hemorrhage has declined over time ($p = 0.018$).

3.3. Determinants of Functional Outcomes

We investigated the determinants associated with functional outcomes. The univariable analysis demonstrated that favorable outcome (mRS score of 0–2) at discharge was associated with age, male sex, diabetes, current smoking, atrial fibrillation or atrial flutter, previous stroke, preadmission disability, initial stroke severity, and intervals from stroke onset to ED or from ED to reperfusion therapy, along with the calendar year (all $p < 0.05$). Among 804 patients who had large vessel occlusion and underwent angiographic studies before and after reperfusion therapy, favorable outcome was associated with occlusion site or achievement of successful recanalization. After adjusting these significant variables ($p < 0.05$) in the univariable analysis, the independent and significant predictors for favorable functional outcome at discharge were age, diabetes, preadmission disability, initial stroke severity, intervals from door to reperfusion therapy, achievement of successful recanalization, and calendar year (Supplementary Table S1). When we investigated the independent factor for functional outcome at 90 days. the same variables were independently associated with favorable outcome at 90 days (Table 3).

Further, we performed the univariable and multivariable ordinal regression analysis to obtain a significant factor for a shift in mRS at discharge and 90 days. The independent determinants of mRS at discharge and 90 days included age, diabetes, previous stroke, preadmission disability, initial stroke severity, intervals from door to reperfusion therapy, and achievement of successful recanalization, along with the calendar year (Supplementary Table S1 and Table 3).

Table 3. Independent determinants for functional outcome at 90 days.

	Ordinal Logistic Regression (Increase in mRS)				Binary Logistic Regression (mRS ≤ 2 vs. mRS > 2)			
	OR (95% CI)	p-Value *	OR (95% CI)	p-Value †	OR (95% CI)	p-Value *	OR (95% CI)	p-Value †
Calendar year								
2012	1		1		1		1	
2013	0.882 (0.579–1.343)	0.559	0.686 (0.391–1.203)	0.188	1.209 (0.701–2.088)	0.495	1.776 (0.813–3.882)	0.15
2014	0.796 (0.529–1.198)	0.274	0.579 (0.339–0.991)	0.046	1.464 (0.857–2.501)	0.163	2.650 (1.241–5.661)	0.012
2015	0.626 (0.417–0.942)	0.025	0.525 (0.306–0.900)	0.019	1.706 (1.000–2.909)	0.05	2.014 (0.950–4.273)	0.068
2017	0.507 (0.337–0.762)	0.001	0.467 (0.276–0.791)	0.005	2.131 (1.246–3.645)	0.006	2.395 (1.142–5.023)	0.021
Age	1.03 (1.019–1.04)	<0.001	1.027 (1.014–1.039)	<0.001	0.966 (0.953–0.980)	<0.001	0.968 (0.951–0.985)	<0.001
Male sex	0.936 (0.746–1.173)	0.565	0.85 (0.642–1.125)	0.255	1.083 (0.802–1.461)	0.604	1.262 (0.857–1.859)	0.239
Diabetes	2.421 (1.955–2.997)	<0.001	2.791 (2.139–3.643)	<0.001	0.382 (0.290–0.503)	<0.001	0.329 (0.230–0.469)	<0.001
Current smoking	1.037 (0.785–1.369)	0.799	0.912 (0.634–1.313)	0.621	0.976 (0.673–1.417)	0.9	1.112 (0.672–1.842)	0.679
Atrial fibrillation or atrial flutter	0.721 (0.579–0.897)	0.003	0.8 (0.613–1.046)	0.103	1.468 (1.100–1.959)	0.009	1.216 (0.843–1.753)	0.296
Congestive heart failure	1.294 (0.823–2.035)	0.265	1.333 (0.801–2.219)	0.269	0.742 (0.530–1.039)	0.082	0.793 (0.526–1.195)	0.267
Previous stroke	1.359 (1.05–1.759)	0.02	1.418 (1.05–1.914)	0.023	0.094 (0.035–0.251)	<0.001	0.178 (0.062–0.510)	0.001
Preadmission disability	3.888 (2.268–6.673)	<0.001	2.855 (1.565–5.202)	0.001	0.999 (0.999–1.000)	0.104	0.999 (0.999–1.000)	0.126
Last normal to ED	1.001 (1.000–1.001)	0.08	1.001 (1.000–1.001)	0.095	0.996 (0.994–0.999)	0.002	0.995 (0.992–0.998)	0.001
ED to treatment	1.003 (1.001–1.005)	0.002	1.003 (1.001–1.005)	0.002	0.878 (0.857–0.900)	<0.001	0.860 (0.832–0.890)	<0.001
NIHSS at stroke onset	1.119 (1.099–1.139)	<0.001	1.126 (1.100–1.152)	<0.001				
Location site								
ICA	1		1		1		1	
MCA			0.871 (0.647–1.174)	0.365			0.834 (0.554–1.257)	0.386
VBA			1.215 (0.787–1.878)	0.379			0.723 (0.391–1.338)	0.302
Others			1.212 (0.608–2.414)	0.584			0.544 (0.211–1.403)	0.208
Successful recanalization within 24 h			0.221 (0.159–0.307)	<0.001			6.477 (4.056–10.345)	<0.001

ED, emergency department; NIHSS, National Institutes of Health Stroke Scale; ICA, internal carotid artery; MCA, middle cerebral artery; VBA, vertebrobasilar artery. * Adjusted for significant variables in the univariable analysis among the entire study population (n = 1199). † Adjusted for significant variables in the univariable analysis among patients who had arterial occlusion at initial angiographic studies and could determine whether a successful recanalization was achieved at follow-up angiographic studies (n = 783).

4. Discussion

We investigated whether clinical or radiologic outcomes after reperfusion therapy changed over time using nationwide, multicenter data covering real clinical practice between 2012 and 2017 in Korea. We demonstrated that there was an increase in the number of patients who received reperfusion therapy, especially EVT, and the clinical outcomes of patients who received reperfusion therapy significantly improved over the past five years. The favorable trend in functional outcomes may be partly ascribed to the increases in successful recanalization rate and decreases in the door-to-treatment intervals and hemorrhagic complications. Of note, the calendar year was a significant factor for functional outcome even after adjusting for significant determinants.

The rate of favorable outcome in this study was comparable to or even better than those of the previous randomized controlled trials. For example, in previous trials investigating the usefulness of IV t-PA, the proportions of patients with mRS score of 0–1 at 90 days were 39% in the National Institute of Neurological Disorders and Stroke study [13], 52.4% in ECASS III [12], and 39% in Safe Implementation of Thrombolysis in Stroke-Monitoring Study [17]. A previous study using the data of Get with the Guidelines-Stroke hospitals showed that in-hospital mortality and discharge-to-home rates were 8.25% and 42.7%, respectively, among patients received IV t-PA therapy [18].

In this analysis, 45.3% of patients had a mRS score of 0–1 at 90 days, and 62.4% of patients could be discharged to home among patients with IV t-PA alone.

The meta-analysis of pooled patient data from five randomized trials after 2015 showed that 46% of patients achieved mRS score of 0–2 at 90 days [4]. In our patients who received EVT with/without IV t-PA, 50.7% of patients had an mRS score of 0–2 at 90 days. In addition, successful recanalization rate in our study population was 83%–87%, which was similar to those in recent EVT trials [19]. Although comparison of clinical outcomes between studies might be difficult because of different patient characteristics, feasibilities of procedures, types of devices, or treatment modalities between studies, our data suggested the benefits of current reperfusion therapy can be reproduced in the real clinical practice.

Our study also demonstrated that some characteristics of patients who received the reperfusion therapy have changed. Although age, vascular risk factors other than dyslipidemia, and occlusion site did not change over time, stroke severity slightly decreased. This may be ascribed to the increase in reperfusion therapy for minor stroke and decrease in the prevalence of atrial fibrillation- or atrial flutter-related stroke [20,21]. Furthermore, time from stroke onset to ED was longer than those in previous studies because patient eligibility for EVT might be based more on imaging parameters recently, instead of the time window paradigm [22]. Increase in the intervals from stroke onset to arrival to ED over years might be partly because more patients with delayed presentation to ED might have been treated with the reperfusion therapy over the years, thanks to advances in selection of patients by multimodal neuroimaging.

In this study, we reaffirm the importance of earlier treatment and achieving successful recanalization to improve patient outcome. Reducing the time from stroke onset to treatment is beneficial to not only reduce the ischemic core but also to remove thrombus [23–25]. Earlier treatment would also reduce the risk of symptomatic intracranial hemorrhage. [26,27] In Korea, there have been continuing efforts on reducing the time delay for patients with stroke using the stroke code system based on the computerized physician order entry system [9,27]. Actually, our data showed that mean time from door to initiation of treatment was continuously decreasing (up to 41.1 min for IV t-PA or 113 min for groin puncture).

Moreover, completely reopening the occluded artery is known as one of the essential components in reperfusion therapy [5]. Currently, the stentriever is the most commonly preferred device in approximately 90% of hospitals in Korea [8]. Stentriever use had some advantages such as easy handling, faster and complete reperfusion, temporal opening, and lesser bleeding complications [28,29]. There were increasing trends in successful recanalization (up to 87% in 2017) and rapid recanalization (mean intervals from door to final recanalization from 240.1 min in 2014 to 173 min in 2017) and decreasing trends in symptomatic intracranial hemorrhage, which might be related with growing use of stentriever over time in Korea.

The calendar year was one of significant factors for favorable outcome even after adjusting for significant variables including age, initial stroke severity, comorbidities, and time from door to needle or achievement of successful recanalization. This implied that the advances in certain factors over time could also play a role for these trends. First, optimal medical treatment before and after reperfusion therapy would prevent complications or early neurologic deterioration and favorably affect the outcome. In this context, the role of the stroke team is important even in the era of EVT for acute stroke. Over the past decades, there has been an improvement in stroke care in Korea: Increase in stroke unit-based centers, multidisciplinary stroke team, guideline-based clinical practice, certification of stroke center, use of antithrombotics or statin in preventing stroke, development of networks among regional comprehensive and primary stroke centers, and provision of nationwide quality care for stroke [10,30–32]. Additionally, there was a possibility of advancement in the selection of eligible candidates who would benefit from reperfusion therapy. Many stroke centers in Korea use imaging parameters, such as collateral status, diffusion/perfusion mismatch, clot characteristics, or ASPECTS score, for identifying patients who are more suitable for reperfusion therapy [8,33].

There are some limitations to this study. First, the decision regarding the method of reperfusion therapy was based on discretion of the stroke neurologist or neurointerventionalist at each study center. The selection of EVT device, number of EVT passes, and use of balloon-guided catheter was not standardized. However, most stroke centers are collaborative in terms of sharing experience and protocols. Second, there were some unmeasured variables, such as socioeconomic status, educational level, and medication adherence before/after stroke, that could affect the functional outcome after stroke.

5. Conclusions

Our analysis demonstrated the increase in favorable outcomes among patients who received reperfusion therapy in Korea. There were a changing patterns, such as an improvement in time parameters, increase in successful recanalization rate, and decrease in bleeding complication rate, leading to the improvement in stroke metrics. However, there is still room for additional efforts, such as rapid notification or communication, for reduction in time delay before arrival to the hospital. Our data also suggest the need for support of personnel or infrastructure to continue the optimum treatment.

Supplementary Materials: The following are available online at http://www.mdpi.com/2077-0383/9/3/717/s1, Table S1: Independent determinants for functional outcome at discharge.

Author Contributions: Conceptualization: Y.D.K., H.S.N.; methodology: Y.D.K., J.H.H., H.S.L., H.S.N.; formal analysis: Y.D.K., H.S.L.; investigation: Y.D.K., J.H.H., J.Y., H.P., B.M.K., O.Y.B., H.C.K., E.H., D.J.K., J.H., M.K., J.K.C., K.-Y.L., H.S.L., D.H.S., H.-Y.C., S.-I.S., J.-H.H., J.-H.B., G.S.K., W.-K.S., J.-W.C., S.H.K., T.-J.S., S.W.H., J.H.P., J.K., Y.H.J., H.-J.C., S.H.A., S.I.L., K.-D.S., H.S.N.; data curation: Y.D.K., J.H.H., J.Y., H.P., B.M.K., O.Y.B., H.C.K., E.H., D.J.K., J.H., M.K., J.K.C., K.-Y.L., H.S.L., D.H.S., H.-Y.C., S.-I.S., J.-H.H., J.-H.B., G.S.K., W.-K.S., J.-W.C., S.H.K., T.-J.S., S.W.H., J.H.P., J.K., Y.H.J., H.-J.C., S.H.A., S.I.L., K.-D.S., H.S.N.; writing—original draft preparation: Y.D.K., H.S.N.; writing—review and editing: Y.D.K., J.H.H., J.Y., H.P., B.M.K., O.Y.B., H.C.K., E.H., D.J.K., J.H., M.K., J.K.C., K.-Y.L., H.S.L., D.H.S., H.-Y.C., S.-I.S., J.-H.H., J.-H.B., G.S.K., W.-K.S., J.-W.C., S.H.K., T.-J.S., S.W.H., J.H.P., J.K., Y.H.J., H.-J.C., S.H.A., S.I.L., K.-D.S., H.S.N.; supervision: H.J.J., H.S.N.; funding acquisition: H.S.N. All authors have read and agreed to the published version of the manuscript.

Funding: This work was supported by the National Research Foundation of Korea (NRF) grant funded by the Korea government (MSIT) (2019R1H1A1079907) and a faculty research grant of Yonsei University College of Medicine (6-2019-0065).

Conflicts of Interest: The authors declare no conflicts of interest.

References

1. Wang, H.; Naghavi, M.; Allen, C.; Barber, R.M.; Bhutta, Z.A. Global, regional, and national life expectancy, all-cause mortality, and cause-specific mortality for 249 causes of death, 1980–2015: A systematic analysis for the global burden of disease study 2015. *Lancet (Lond. Engl.)* **2016**, *388*, 1459–1544. [CrossRef]

2. Kassebaum, N.J.; Arora, M.; Barber, R.M.; Bhutta, Z.A.; Brown, J.; Carter, A.; Casey, D.C.; Charlson, F.J.; Coates, M.M.; Coggeshall, M.; et al. Global, regional, and national disability-adjusted life-years (dalys) for 315 diseases and injuries and healthy life expectancy (hale), 1990–2015: A systematic analysis for the global burden of disease study 2015. *Lancet* **2016**, *388*, 1603–1658. [CrossRef]
3. Donnan, G.A.; Fisher, M.; Macleod, M.; Davis, S.M. Stroke. *Lancet (Lond. Engl.)* **2008**, *371*, 1612–1623. [CrossRef]
4. Goyal, M.; Menon, B.K.; van Zwam, W.H.; Dippel, D.W.; Mitchell, P.J.; Demchuk, A.M.; Davalos, A.; Majoie, C.B.; van der Lugt, A.; de Miquel, M.A.; et al. Endovascular thrombectomy after large-vessel ischaemic stroke: A meta-analysis of individual patient data from five randomised trials. *Lancet (Lond. Engl.)* **2016**, *387*, 1723–1731. [CrossRef]
5. Rha, J.H.; Saver, J.L. The impact of recanalization on ischemic stroke outcome: A meta-analysis. *Stroke* **2007**, *38*, 967–973. [CrossRef] [PubMed]
6. Fargen, K.M.; Meyers, P.M.; Khatri, P.; Mocco, J. Improvements in recanalization with modern stroke therapy: A review of prospective ischemic stroke trials during the last two decades. *J. Neurointerv. Surg.* **2013**, *5*, 506–511. [CrossRef]
7. Jansen, I.G.H.; Mulder, M.; Goldhoorn, R.B.; investigators, M.C.R. Endovascular treatment for acute ischaemic stroke in routine clinical practice: Prospective, observational cohort study (mr clean registry). *BMJ* **2018**, *360*, k949. [CrossRef]
8. Seo, K.-D.; Suh, S.H. Endovascular treatment in acute ischemic stroke: A nationwide survey in korea. *Neurointervention* **2018**, *13*, 84–89. [CrossRef]
9. Heo, J.H.; Kim, Y.D.; Nam, H.S.; Hong, K.S.; Ahn, S.H.; Cho, H.J.; Choi, H.Y.; Han, S.W.; Cha, M.J.; Hong, J.M.; et al. A computerized in-hospital alert system for thrombolysis in acute stroke. *Stroke* **2010**, *41*, 1978–1983. [CrossRef]
10. Kim, J.Y.; Kang, K.; Kang, J.; Koo, J.; Kim, D.H.; Kim, B.J.; Kim, W.J.; Kim, E.G.; Kim, J.G.; Kim, J.M.; et al. Executive summary of stroke statistics in korea 2018: A report from the epidemiology research council of the korean stroke society. *J. Stroke* **2019**, *21*, 42–59. [CrossRef]
11. Goldstein, L.B.; Samsa, G.P.; Matchar, D.B.; Horner, R.D. Charlson index comorbidity adjustment for ischemic stroke outcome studies. *Stroke* **2004**, *35*, 1941–1945. [CrossRef]
12. Hacke, W.; Kaste, M.; Bluhmki, E.; Brozman, M.; Dávalos, A.; Guidetti, D.; Larrue, V.; Lees, K.R.; Medeghri, Z.; Machnig, T.; et al. Thrombolysis with alteplase 3 to 4.5 h after acute ischemic stroke. *N. Engl. J. Med.* **2008**, *359*, 1317–1329. [CrossRef] [PubMed]
13. Tissue Plasminogen Activator for Acute Ischemic Stroke. The national institute of neurological disorders and stroke rt-pa stroke study group. *N. Engl. J. Med.* **1995**, *333*, 1581–1587.
14. Jauch, E.C.; Saver, J.L.; Adams, H.P.; Bruno, A.; Connors, J.J.; Demaerschalk, B.M.; Khatri, P.; McMullan, P.W.; Qureshi, A.I.; Rosenfield, K.; et al. Guidelines for the early management of patients with acute ischemic stroke: A guideline for healthcare professionals from the american heart association/american stroke association. *Stroke* **2013**, *44*, 870–947. [CrossRef] [PubMed]
15. Kernan, W.N.; Ovbiagele, B.; Black, H.R.; Bravata, D.M.; Chimowitz, M.I.; Ezekowitz, M.D.; Fang, M.C.; Fisher, M.; Furie, K.L.; Heck, D.V.; et al. Guidelines for the prevention of stroke in patients with stroke and transient ischemic attack: A guideline for healthcare professionals from the american heart association/american stroke association. *Stroke* **2014**, *45*, 2160–2236. [CrossRef] [PubMed]
16. Higashida, R.T.; Furlan, A.J. Trial design and reporting standards for intra-arterial cerebral thrombolysis for acute ischemic stroke. *Stroke* **2003**, *34*, e109–e137. [CrossRef] [PubMed]
17. Wahlgren, N.; Ahmed, N.; Davalos, A.; Ford, G.A.; Grond, M.; Hacke, W.; Hennerici, M.G.; Kaste, M.; Kuelkens, S.; Larrue, V.; et al. Thrombolysis with alteplase for acute ischaemic stroke in the safe implementation of thrombolysis in stroke-monitoring study (sits-most): An observational study. *Lancet* **2007**, *369*, 275–282. [CrossRef]
18. Fonarow, G.C.; Zhao, X.; Smith, E.E.; Saver, J.L.; Reeves, M.J.; Bhatt, D.L.; Xian, Y.; Hernandez, A.F.; Peterson, E.D.; Schwamm, L.H. Door-to-needle times for tissue plasminogen activator administration and clinical outcomes in acute ischemic stroke before and after a quality improvement initiative. *JAMA* **2014**, *311*, 1632–1640. [CrossRef]
19. Hong, K.S.; Ko, S.B.; Lee, J.S.; Yu, K.H.; Rha, J.H. Endovascular recanalization therapy in acute ischemic stroke: Updated meta-analysis of randomized controlled trials. *J. Stroke* **2015**, *17*, 268–281. [CrossRef]

20. Baek, J.H.; Kim, B.M. Angiographical identification of intracranial, atherosclerosis-related, large vessel occlusion in endovascular treatment. *Front. Neurol.* **2019**, *10*, 298. [CrossRef]
21. Yoo, J.; Sohn, S.I.; Kim, J.; Ahn, S.H.; Lee, K.; Baek, J.H.; Kim, K.; Hong, J.H.; Koo, J.; Kim, Y.D.; et al. Delayed intravenous thrombolysis in patients with minor stroke. *Cerebrovasc. Dis.* **2018**, *46*, 52–58. [CrossRef] [PubMed]
22. Kim, J.T.; Cho, B.H.; Choi, K.H.; Park, M.S.; Kim, B.J.; Park, J.M.; Kang, K.; Lee, S.J.; Kim, J.G.; Cha, J.K.; et al. Magnetic resonance imaging versus computed tomography angiography based selection for endovascular therapy in patients with acute ischemic stroke. *Stroke* **2019**, *50*, 365–372. [CrossRef] [PubMed]
23. Meretoja, A.; Keshtkaran, M.; Saver, J.L.; Tatlisumak, T.; Parsons, M.W.; Kaste, M.; Davis, S.M.; Donnan, G.A.; Churilov, L. Stroke thrombolysis: Save a minute, save a day. *Stroke* **2014**, *45*, 1053–1058. [CrossRef] [PubMed]
24. Kim, Y.D.; Nam, H.S.; Kim, S.H.; Kim, E.Y.; Song, D.; Kwon, I.; Yang, S.H.; Lee, K.; Yoo, J.; Lee, H.S.; et al. Time-dependent thrombus resolution after tissue-type plasminogen activator in patients with stroke and mice. *Stroke* **2015**, *46*, 1877–1882. [CrossRef]
25. Bourcier, R.; Goyal, M.; Liebeskind, D.S.; Muir, K.W.; Desal, H.; Siddiqui, A.H.; Dippel, D.W.J.; Majoie, C.B.; van Zwam, W.H.; Jovin, T.G.; et al. Association of time from stroke onset to groin puncture with quality of reperfusion after mechanical thrombectomy: A meta-analysis of individual patient data from 7 randomized clinical trials. *JAMA Neurol.* **2019**, *76*, 405–411. [CrossRef] [PubMed]
26. Fonarow, G.C.; Smith, E.E.; Saver, J.L.; Reeves, M.J.; Bhatt, D.L.; Grau-Sepulveda, M.V.; Olson, D.M.; Hernandez, A.F.; Peterson, E.D.; Schwamm, L.H. Timeliness of tissue-type plasminogen activator therapy in acute ischemic stroke: Patient characteristics, hospital factors, and outcomes associated with door-to-needle times within 60 min. *Circulation* **2011**, *123*, 750–758. [CrossRef] [PubMed]
27. Jeon, S.B.; Ryoo, S.M.; Lee, D.H.; Kwon, S.U.; Jang, S.; Lee, E.J.; Lee, S.H.; Han, J.H.; Yoon, M.J.; Jeong, S.; et al. Multidisciplinary approach to decrease in-hospital delay for stroke thrombolysis. *J. Stroke* **2017**, *19*, 196–204. [CrossRef]
28. Song, D.; Heo, J.H.; Kim, D.I.; Kim, D.J.; Kim, B.M.; Lee, K.; Yoo, J.; Lee, H.S.; Nam, H.S.; Kim, Y.D. Impact of temporary opening using a stent retriever on clinical outcome in acute ischemic stroke. *PLoS ONE* **2015**, *10*, e0124551. [CrossRef]
29. Touma, L.; Filion, K.B.; Sterling, L.H.; Atallah, R.; Windle, S.B.; Eisenberg, M.J. Stent retrievers for the treatment of acute ischemic stroke: A systematic review and meta-analysis of randomized clinical trials. *JAMA Neurol.* **2016**, *73*, 275–281. [CrossRef]
30. Choi, H.Y.; Cha, M.J.; Nam, H.S.; Kim, Y.D.; Hong, K.S.; Heo, J.H.; Korean Stroke Unit Study, C. Stroke units and stroke care services in korea. *Int. J. Stroke* **2012**, *7*, 336–340. [CrossRef]
31. Kim, Y.D.; Jung, Y.H.; Saposnik, G. Traditional risk factors for stroke in east asia. *J. Stroke* **2016**, *18*, 273–285. [CrossRef] [PubMed]
32. Kim, J.; Hwang, Y.H.; Kim, J.T.; Choi, N.C.; Kang, S.Y.; Cha, J.K.; Ha, Y.S.; Shin, D.I.; Kim, S.; Lim, B.H. Establishment of government-initiated comprehensive stroke centers for acute ischemic stroke management in south korea. *Stroke* **2014**, *45*, 2391–2396. [CrossRef] [PubMed]
33. Yoo, J.; Baek, J.H.; Park, H.; Song, D.; Kim, K.; Hwang, I.G.; Kim, Y.D.; Kim, S.H.; Lee, H.S.; Ahn, S.H.; et al. Thrombus volume as a predictor of nonrecanalization after intravenous thrombolysis in acute stroke. *Stroke* **2018**, *49*, 2108–2115. [CrossRef] [PubMed]

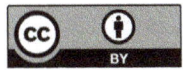 © 2020 by the authors. Licensee MDPI, Basel, Switzerland. This article is an open access article distributed under the terms and conditions of the Creative Commons Attribution (CC BY) license (http://creativecommons.org/licenses/by/4.0/).

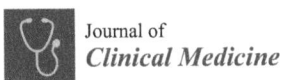

Article

High On-Treatment Platelet Reactivity Affects the Extent of Ischemic Lesions in Stroke Patients Due to Large-Vessel Disease

Adam Wiśniewski [1,*], Joanna Sikora [2], Agata Sławińska [3], Karolina Filipska [4], Aleksandra Karczmarska-Wódzka [2], Zbigniew Serafin [3] and Grzegorz Kozera [5]

1. Department of Neurology, Faculty of Medicine, Nicolaus Copernicus University in Toruń, Collegium Medicum in Bydgoszcz, 85-094 Bydgoszcz, Poland
2. Experimental Biotechnology Research and Teaching Team, Department of Transplantology and General Surgery, Faculty of Medicine, Nicolaus Copernicus University in Toruń, Collegium Medicum in Bydgoszcz, 85-094 Bydgoszcz, Poland; joanna.sikora@cm.umk.pl (J.S.); akar@cm.umk.pl (A.K.-W.)
3. Department of Radiology and Diagnostic Imaging, Faculty of Medicine, Nicolaus Copernicus University in Toruń, Collegium Medicum in Bydgoszcz, 85-094 Bydgoszcz, Poland; agataslawinska@cm.umk.pl (A.S.); serafin@cm.umk.pl (Z.S.)
4. Department of Neurological and Neurosurgical Nursing, Faculty of Health Sciences, Nicolaus Copernicus University in Toruń, Collegium Medicum in Bydgoszcz, 85-821 Bydgoszcz, Poland; karolinafilipskakf@gmail.com
5. Medical Simulation Centre, Faculty of Medicine, Medical University of Gdańsk, 80-210 Gdańsk, Poland; gkozera1@wp.pl
* Correspondence: adam.lek@wp.pl; Tel.: +48-790-813-513; Fax: +48-52-5854032

Received: 13 December 2019; Accepted: 15 January 2020; Published: 17 January 2020

Abstract: Background: Excessive platelet activation and aggregation plays an important role in the pathogenesis of ischemic stroke. Correlation between platelet reactivity and ischemic lesions in the brain shows contradictory results and there are not enough data about the potential role of stroke etiology and its relationships with chronic lesions. The aim of this study is to assess the relationship between platelet reactivity and the extent of ischemic lesions with the particular role of etiopathogenesis. Methods: The study involved 69 patients with ischemic stroke, including 20 patients with large-vessel disease and 49 patients with small-vessel disease. Evaluation of platelet reactivity was performed within 24 h after the onset of stroke using two aggregometric methods (impedance and optical), while ischemic volume measurement in the brain was performed using magnetic resonance imaging (in diffusion-weighted imaging (DWI) and fluid-attenuated inversion recovery (FLAIR) sequences) at day 2–5 after the onset of stroke. Results: In the large-vessel disease subgroup, a correlation was found between platelet reactivity and acute ischemic focus volume (correlation coefficient (R) = 0.6858 and p = 0.0068 for DWI; R = 0.6064 and p = 0.0215 for FLAIR). Aspirin-resistant subjects were significantly more likely to have a large ischemic focus (Odds Ratio (OR) = 45.00, 95% Confidence Interval (CI) = 1.49–135.36, p = 0.0285 for DWI; OR = 28.00, 95% CI = 1.35–58.59, p = 0.0312 for FLAIR) than aspirin-sensitive subjects with large-vessel disease. Conclusion: In patients with ischemic stroke due to large-vessel disease, high on-treatment platelet reactivity affects the extent of acute and chronic ischemic lesions.

Keywords: platelet reactivity; ischemic stroke; aspirin resistance; infarction volume; multiplate

1. Introduction

Stroke is one of the main causes of morbidity and long-term disability, and the second most frequent cause of death globally [1]. The updated definition of ischemic stroke by the American Heart

Association/American Stroke Association (AHA/ASA) recognizes stroke as when clinical symptoms last less than 24 h and neuroimaging studies have demonstrated acute ischemic infarctions [2].

Currently, magnetic resonance (MR) imaging of the head is the gold standard in neuroimaging of the acute phase of ischemic stroke and aggregometry is the most popular methodology for the evaluation of platelet reactivity in the acute stage of stroke. In magnetic resonance (MR) imaging of the head, ischemic changes in the T2 and fluid-attenuated inversion recovery (FLAIR) sequences are described as hyper-intensive (i.e., with higher density than cerebral tissue). Additionally, imaging by means of the diffusion-weighted imaging (DWI) sequence, which is currently the most sensitive and the most specific method for imaging ischemic changes, shows the ischemic change just a few minutes after the onset of symptoms [3]. The ischemic focus in the DWI sequence is described as the area undergoing diffusion restriction. In order to assess the extent of an ischemic focus, its volume measurement via MR volumetry is used. Measurement of the volume of the area of interest is the most frequently performed technique, which consists of marking out the contours of the studied area in MR images, with further creation of a spatial structure and volume measures using dedicated software [4].

Platelet reactivity plays a role in the pathology of ischemic stroke, especially in nonembolic mechanisms (i.e., in patients with large and small vessels). Antiplatelet agents are the current standard in the secondary prevention of ischemic stroke, and European and American guidelines recommend acetylsalicylic acid (ASA) as the drug of first choice [5]. The efficacy of ASA can be decreased by a phenomenon called aspirin resistance [6]. Various platelet reactivity tests have been used to assess platelet activation and aggregation capacity, which allow for the assessment of platelet reactivity in response to the antiplatelet drug. High levels of platelet reactivity indicate a weak antiplatelet effect of the drug, which is estimated as laboratory resistance [7].

Previous studies reporting on the impact of aspirin resistance for ischemic lesion volumes in patients with stroke are scarce and have contradictory results. Some authors showed significant correlations between high platelet reactivity and large ischemic volumes in the brain [8,9], but there is still a lack of data about the potential roles of the etiology of strokes and relationships with the level of advancement of chronic vascular lesions in the brain. The aim of this study is to assess the platelet reactivity in patients in the acute phase of ischemic stroke and to investigate the relationships between platelet reactivity (estimated by impedance and optical aggregometry) and the volume of acute ischemic focus (volumetry in MR; DWI and FLAIR sequences) and chronic vascular changes (estimated using the Fazekas scale) in the brain with the particular role of cerebral ischemia etiopathogenesis.

2. Material and Methods

2.1. Research Subjects

The study was conducted in the Department of Neurology from February 2016 to December 2017 at the University Hospital No. 1 in Bydgoszcz. The prospective study included 69 subjects with diagnosis of ischemic stroke according to the updated definition of AHA/ASA. At the time of admission, all patients had been treated with ASA at a dose of 150 mg. Considering the etiopathogenesis of cerebral ischemia, patients were divided into groups with large-vessel disease (large artery atherosclerosis, LAA; $n = 20$ subjects) and small-vessel disease (SVD; $n = 49$ subjects). In the LAA group, significant atherosclerotic changes in the internal carotid artery was the cause of stroke; in the SVD group, lacunar changes in deep structures of the brain tissue were responsible for stroke symptoms. The LAA group included patients with a carotid artery stenosis >50% on the side, corresponding to the symptoms of stroke conforming to a Doppler ultrasound examination of the carotid arteries. The SVD group included patients with no significant hemodynamic stenoses of large precranial vessels or cardiogenic embolic backgrounds, in which neuroimaging confirmed the presence of a lacunar focus and revealed chronic vascular changes with a typical location and morphology for small-vessel disease (i.e., subcortical lesions, periventricular lesions, and leukoaraiosis features) [10]. The following exclusion criteria were used: lack of informed consent for the patient to participate in the study (quantitative disturbances of consciousness or aphasia), cardioembolic etiology of stroke (documented atrial fibrillation, dilated cardiomyopathy, thrombus in the heart cavities), chronic inflammatory processes (chronic lower limb ischemia or chronic venous thrombosis of the lower limbs), stroke or transient ischemic attack (TIA) in the previous 2 years, documented neoplasms, taking acetylsalicylic acid before admission to the clinic, past significant bleeding in the previous 2 years (e.g., gastrointestinal bleeding), level of hemoglobin < 9 g/dL, thrombocytopenia < 100 thousands/uL, or value of hematocrit <35%. The general characteristics of the studied population and a comparison of the groups of patients with large-vessel disease and small-vessel disease are shown in Table 1.

Table 1. Comparison of the selected risk factors and biochemical parameters obtained in subjects with stroke in both etiological subgroups of cerebral ischemia.

Parameter	LAA N = 20	SVD N = 49	p Values
Age median (range) *	67 (45–85)	68 (40–89)	0.7761
Sex, male, N (%) **	14 (70%)	21 (42.9%)	**0.0408**
Hypertension, N (%) **	17 (85%)	44 (89.7%)	0.6822
Diabetes, N (%) **	8 (40%)	17 (34.7%)	0.7842
Hyperlipidemia, N (%) **	10 (50%)	18 (36.7%)	0.4185
Smoking, N (%) **	11 (55%)	13 (26.5%)	**0.0299**
Ischemic heart disease, N (%) **	3 (15.0%)	6 (12.2%)	0.7120
CRP (mg/L) median (range) *	4.90 (0.43–30.45)	4,79 (0.36–29.15)	0.7660
HbA1c (%) median (range) *	5.9 (5.2–10.04)	5.6 (5.0–9.8)	0.2313
Homocystein (µmolµ/L) median (range) *	10.67 (5.1–30.92)	10.87 (3.52–48.6)	0.6153
Fibrinogen (mg/dL) median (range) *	312.5 (234–590)	300 (369–540)	0.2992
Obesity, N (%) **	12 (60%)	36 (73.47%)	0.2699
The volume of ischemic focus DWI (cm^3) median (range) *	2.23 (0.12–10.3)	0.89 (0.09–1.5)	0.0694
The volume of ischemic focus FLAIR (cm^3) Median (range) *	3.46 (0.35–31.8)	0.99 (0.18–1.71)	0.0846
Platelet reactivity: optical aggregometry (AUC) median (range) *	17.1 (0–208.6)	20.4 (0–154.2)	0.7147
Platelet reactivity: impedance aggregometry (AUC) median (range) *	42 (9–101)	27.5 (6–108)	0.0622
Resistance to ASA (multiplate), % **	52.3%	22.9%	**0.0286**

* U Mann-Whitney test; ** chi square test. Note: FLAIR = fluid-attenuated inversion recovery; ASA = acetylsalicylic acid; AUC = area under the curve; DWI- diffusion-weighted imaging; CRP = C-reactive protein; HbA1c- glycated hemoglobin; LAA = large artery atherosclerosis; SVD = small-vessel disease; N = number of subjects, bold font = statistically significant p Values.

All subjects signed an informed consent form to participate in the study and read the protocol. The study protocol received a positive opinion from the Bioethics Committee of the Nicolaus Copernicus University in Torun at Collegium Medicum of Ludwik Rydygier in Bydgoszcz (KB number 73/2016).

2.2. Platelet Reactivity Research Methodology

The platelet reactivity assessment was performed by optical aggregometry and impedance aggregometry in the Laboratory of Biotechnology at Collegium Medicum in Bydgoszcz. Blood tests were performed at a similar time of day (10:00–12:00) in the first 24 h of onset of stroke symptoms. The optical aggregometry test was performed using a Chrono-Log aggregometer with the Agrolink software for Windows (Havertown, PA, USA). Using the apparatus, the ability of platelet aggregation in platelet-rich plasma was evaluated in vitro by measuring the change in transmission of light passing through the platelet suspension in response to the addition of a platelet agonist. After the activation of platelets by the agonist, the plasma suspension cleared before the formation of platelet aggregates; thus, the amount of light absorbed by the photometer increased. Arachidonic acid was used as the agonist, which activated the cyclo-oxygenase No 1 (COX-1) enzyme, the point of action of acetylsalicylic acid. The aggregometer analyzed changes in transmitted light in percentage and automatically converted this to a graphical curve that reflected changes in light transmission as a result of platelet aggregation. The most important element visually was the area under the curve (AUC), which depicted the amount of light absorbed over time. An average increase in absorbance above 20% (or AUC units > 115) was considered as ASA resistance, equivalent to a high on-treatment platelet reactivity induced by arachidonic acid. Approximately 9.4 mL of blood was collected in the morning on an empty stomach from the veins of the forearm into tubes with an admixture of 3.2% sodium citrate at a ratio of 1:9. Tests were performed up to 2 h after blood collection. Samples were centrifuged at 100 g for 10 min at room temperature to obtain platelet-rich plasma (PRP), and at 2400 g for 20 min at a temperature of 40 °C to obtain platelet-poor plasma (PPP). The number of platelets was calculated before the activation was assessed and the number was corrected to 250,000/μL. The percentage of aggregation induced with arachidonic acid in the final concentration of 0.5 μM was assessed [11]. The evaluation of optical aggregometry was performed in 43 out of 69 subjects due to aggregometer failure.

The Multiplate–Dynabyte multichannel platelet function analyzer (Roche Diagnostics, France) was used to perform impedance aggregometry. The Multiplate system, based on the impedance aggregation method in whole blood, used the so-called multiple electrode aggregation (i.e., a double marking was performed during each measurement). In this study, the acetylsalicylic acid platelet inhibitor (ASPI) test (measuring aggregation dependent on cyclo-oxygenase) was applied with arachidonic acid as a platelet activator. Two electrodes were immersed in a blood sample with a stirrer and the blood platelets aggregated after the addition of the agonist, causing them to accumulate onto the electrodes, resulting in a change in electrical resistance (impedance) between them. Impedance changes were then converted into a graphical model depicting the change in platelet aggregation over time. The AUC parameter was reported as the final result of the determination. The results above 40 AUC units were considered to be high on-treatment platelet reactivity induced by arachidonic acid, similar to ASA resistance (see Figure 1). Subjects with AUC values under 30 were treated as sensitive to ASA, while from 30–40 was considered as mild sensitivity to ASA. From each patient, approximately 2.6 mL of blood was collected in the morning from the forearm veins into a Sarstedt r-hirudin-type tube. After collection, the blood was kept for at least 30 min but for no more than 2 h. At first, 300 μL of sodium chloride was prepared and heated up to 37 degrees C, then 300 μL of whole blood was prepared in a special Dynabyte disposable test chamber with a magnetic stirrer, placed into four consecutive measuring stations, and connected to the device. Then, after 3 min of incubation, 20 μL of the reagent (arachidonic acid) was added. The aggregation test was assessed for 6 min, and the final result (in the form of AUC units) was the mean of the two measurements in the form of a curve [12]. The evaluation of impedance aggregometry with the use of the Multiplate system was performed in all 69 subjects.

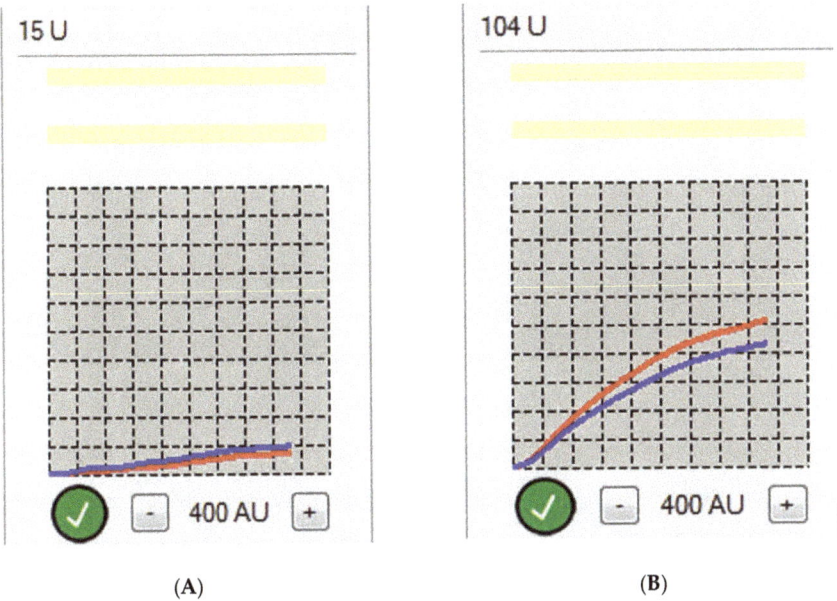

Figure 1. Curves of platelet reactivity assessed by impedance aggregometry: (**A**) Aspirin (ASA)-sensitive subject with 15 area under the curve (AUC) (**B**) ASA-resistant subject with 104 AUC. First measurement- blue line, second measurement- red line.

2.3. Doppler Examination of the Carotid Arteries

Doppler examination of the carotid arteries was performed in all subjects within 5 days after the onset of symptoms of cerebral ischemia using a MyLab C Class (ESAOTE, Genoa, Italy) in the Doppler Laboratory of the Neurological Department of Dr A. Jurasz University Hospital No. 1 in Bydgoszcz. The study was performed based on the guidelines of the American Neurological Society [13].

2.4. Magnetic Resonance Imaging of the Head with Volumetric Evaluation

Magnetic resonance imaging was performed during hospitalization in the Department of Neurology within 2–5 days from the onset of symptoms of cerebral ischemia in the Magnetic Resonance Laboratory of the Department of Radiology, Dr A. Jurasz University Hospital No. 1, Bydgoszcz, with a 1,5 T Signa HDX apparatus (G.E. Healthcare, Chicago, IL, USA). The study was performed without a contrast agent following the so-called "stroke protocol", evaluating brain images in T1, T2, FLAIR, and DWI sequences. The volumetric evaluation (shown in Figure 2) in the FLAIR and DWI sequences was estimated on a "layer-by-layer" basis, using the G.E. Advanced Workstation 4.6 by an experienced radiologist and given in millimeters (1 mL = 1 cm^3) [4]. Based on the volumetry method of the subjects with stroke, they were divided into patients with a large ischemic focus (> 2.5 mL in DWI and > 3.5 mL in FLAIR) and a small ischemic focus in the brain.

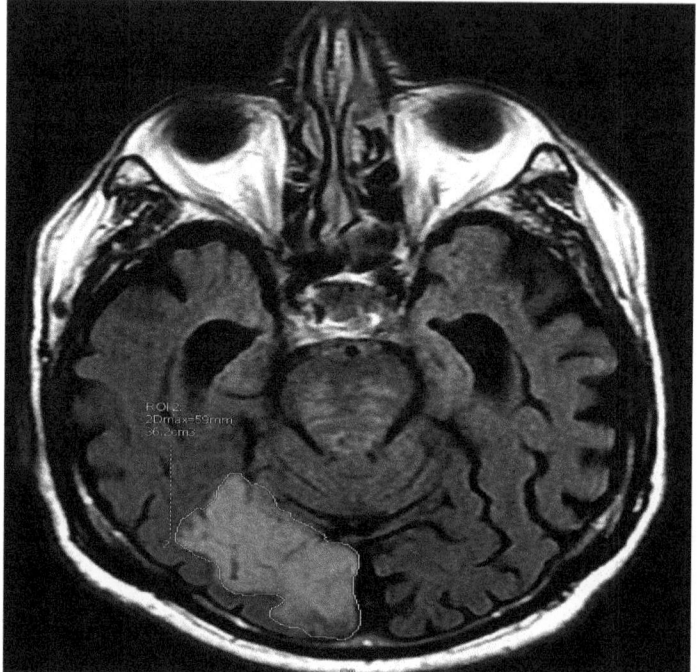

Figure 2. Volumetric evaluation of ischemic focus size in magnetic resonance (MR) in fluid-attenuated inversion recovery (FLAIR) sequence.

The extent and the degree of chronic ischemic changes in periventricular white matter was estimated by the periventricular white matter (PVWM) Fazekas scale, and in deep white matter by the deep white matter (DWM) Fazekas scale. A total of 14 subjects with LAA and 43 with SVD underwent MRI examination.

2.5. Statistical Evaluation Methods

Nonparametric tests due to the incompatibility of the distribution of features with the normal distribution were used: the chi-square test (relations between categorized variables), Spearman's rank correlation test (relations between variables), and the Mann–Whitney U test (relations between binary and continuous variables). Logistic regression analysis was performed to estimate the probability of a large ischemic outbreak, comparing ASA-sensitive and -resistant subjects. The significance level of $p < 0.05$ was considered to be statistically significant. Statistical evaluation was performed with STATISTICA software (version 13.1, Dell Inc., Round Rock, TX, USA).

3. Results

3.1. All Subjects

The median of ischemic focus volume was 1.81 mL (minimum 0.09 mL, maximum 10.1 mL) in the DWI sequence and 2.41 mL (minimum 0.18 mL, maximum 31.8 mL) in the FLAIR sequence. In patients with stroke, there were no statistically significant correlations between platelet reactivity and the size of the ischemic lesion, as assessed both in the DWI (with the Multiplate method, $R = 0.0700$ and $p = 0.6243$; with optical aggregometry, $R = -0.0670$ and $p = 0.7064$), and FLAIR (with the Multiplate method, $R = 0.083$ and $p = 0.5648$; with optical aggregometry, $R = -0.0500$ and $p = 0.7783$) sequences.

In ASA-resistant patients (by Multiplate), the median ischemic focal size did not differ significantly from the median ischemic focus size in ASA-sensitive patients in both DWI and FLAIR sequences (DWI median: 3.94 versus 1.305 mL, $p = 0.4755$; FLAIR median: 4.88 versus 2.09 mL, $p = 0.5241$). There were also no significant differences in platelet reactivity between the groups of patients with large and small ischemic focuses (DWI sequence median: 31.5 AUC versus 23 AUC, $p = 0.3226$; FLAIR sequence median: 33.5 AUC versus 23 AUC, $p = 0.3559$). No significant correlations between platelet reactivity and the extent and degree of chronic ischemic lesions in periventricular or deep white matter were found either (PVWM Fazekas $R = 0.0067$, $p = 0.9667$; DWM Fazekas $R = 0.00547$, $p = 0.9742$).

3.2. Subgroups of LAA and SVD Subjects

In the subgroup of patients with LAA, there was a significant positive correlation between the platelet reactivity in the impedance aggregometry method and the ischemic focal size, as assessed both in the DWI (Figure 3A) and FLAIR sequences ($R = 0.6858$ and $p = 0.0068$ for DWI; $R = 0.6064$ and $p = 0.0215$ for FLAIR). There was no correlation between platelet reactivity and ischemic focus size in the SVD subgroup ($R = -0.1107$ and $p = 0.5139$ for DWI; $R = -0.1055$ and $p = 0.5342$ for FLAIR).

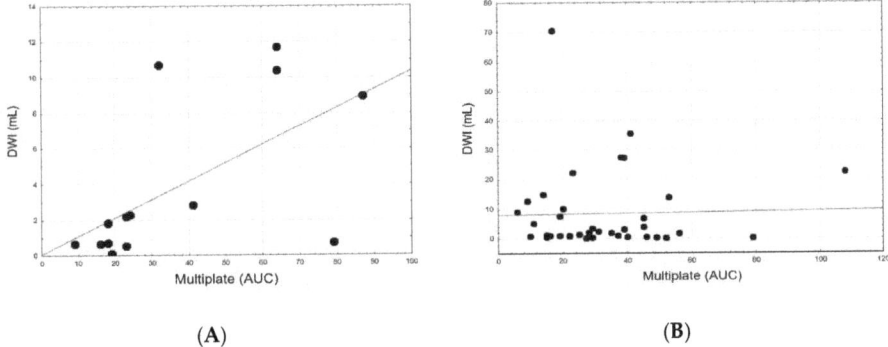

(A)   (B)

Figure 3. Correlation between platelet reactivity as assessed by Multiplate method (in area under the curve (AUC) units) with the ischemic focus size assessed in diffusion-weighted imaging (DWI) (in mL) sequence in the large-artery atherosclerosis subgroup (**A**) and small-vessel disease subgroup (**B**).

There were no significant correlations between platelet reactivity and the ischemic volume in either subgroups based on the optical aggregometry method. In the subgroup with LAA, ASA-resistant patients (assessed by Multiplate) had a significantly larger median volume of ischemic focus, both in DWI (Figure 4A) and FLAIR, as compared to patients sensitive to ASA (DWI median: 8.93 versus 0.68 mL, $p = 0.0157$; FLAIR median: 11.0 versus 1.21 mL, $p = 0.0338$). In the SVD subgroup, no similar significant relationships were found ($p = 0.8259$ for DWI; $p = 0.7084$ for FLAIR). In the subgroup of subjects with LAA, the median platelet reactivity assessed by the Multiplate method was higher in the subgroup of patients with a large ischemic focus in the DWI sequence than in the group with small ischemic focus (median: 41 versus 18 AUC, $p = 0.0253$) (Figure 5A). There were no significant relationships in the FLAIR sequence (median: 41 versus 19 AUC, $p = 0.0639$) in the LAA subgroup and in SVD subjects, either with the impedance or optical aggregometry methods.

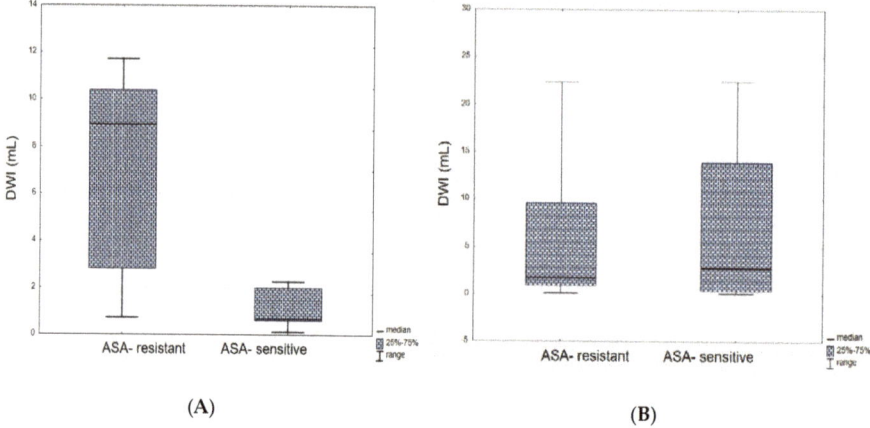

Figure 4. Comparison of ischemic focus size (in mL) in the diffusion-weighted imaging (DWI) sequence in the group of patients resistant and sensitive to Aspirin (ASA) in the large artery atherosclerosis subgroup (**A**) and the small-vessel disease subgroup (**B**).

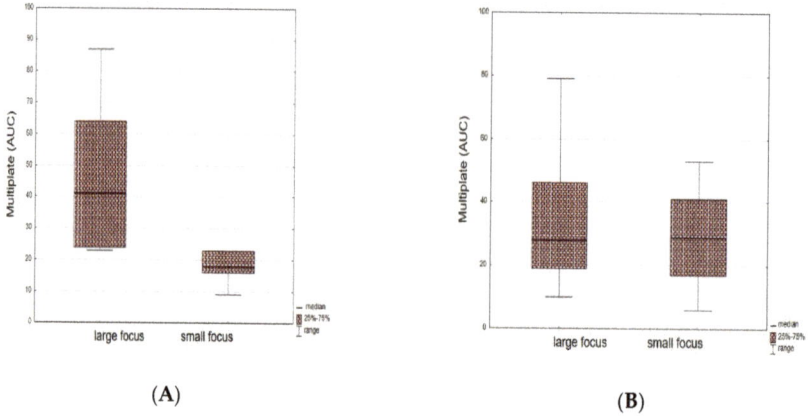

Figure 5. Comparison of the platelet reactivity (in area under the curve (AUC) units) assessed by the Multiplate method in subjects with a large and small ischemic focus in the diffusion-weighted imaging (DWI) sequence, in both the large-artery atherosclerosis subgroup (**A**) and the small-vessel disease subgroup (**B**).

In the LAA subgroup, a significant correlation between platelet reactivity in the Multiplate method and the extent and degree of chronic ischemic lesions was demonstrated, both in periventricular and deep white matter (PVWM Fazekas R = 0.5569, p = 0.0386; DWM Fazekas R = 0.5590, p = 0.0377). In the SVD subgroup, no significant relationships in this subject were found (PVWM Fazekas R = −0.1613, p = 0.3403; DWM Fazekas R = −0.2479, p = 0.1356).

Logistic regression analysis showed that in the subgroup of patients with LAA, ASA-resistant patients (by Multiplate) had a significantly higher probability of a large ischemic focus than patients who were sensitive to ASA (OR = 45.00, 95% CI 1.49–135.36; p = 0.0285 for DWI and OR = 28.00, 95% CI 1.35–58.59; p = 0.0312 for FLAIR). There were no similar significant relationships in the subgroup of patients with SVD (OR = 1.0, 95% CI 0.22–4.56, p = 1.0 for DWI and FLAIR) and in the whole group of patients with stroke (OR = 2.55, 95% CI 0.70–9.31, $p = 0.1566$ for DWI; OR = 2.70, 95% CI 0.74–9.81, $p = 0.1313$ for FLAIR).

4. Discussion

It has been proven that ASA-resistant subjects are at significantly higher risk of stroke recurrence, heart attack, and death due to vascular disease. Furthermore, resistance to ASA has been associated with the male gender and smoking [14,15]. The spread of aspirin resistance in subjects with stroke has been estimated at 5–65% [16]. In our own research, based on the method of impedance aggregometry, ASA resistance was estimated among patients with stroke at 31.8% and at 7% in the method of optical aggregometry, which coincides with the data from the literature. Considering the increasing incidence of stroke (20% increase predicted by 2030 as a result of population aging) [17], it is necessary to study the impact of ASA resistance on the size of the ischemic focus.

Our study demonstrated the significant effect of etiopathogenesis of ischemic stroke on the relationship between platelet reactivity and the size of an ischemic focus. There was a highly positive correlation observed between platelet reactivity and size of the acute ischemic focus in the subgroup of patients with large artery atherosclerosis. Moreover, it was noted that aspirin-resistant patients with carotid artery pathology had a larger stroke volume than patients who were sensitive to ASA, and at the same time, that the large ischemic focus in DWI was related to higher platelet reactivity. Additionally, there was a highly positive correlation observed with the extent and the degree of chronic ischemic changes in white matter in large artery atherosclerosis subgroup. This should be treated as novelty in this field, because the literature does not address the impact of stroke etiopathogenesis on the correlation of platelet reactivity and the size of the acute ischemic focus. To the best of our knowledge, we are first to underline the role of high on-treatment platelet reactivity for the extent of chronic vascular lesions in the brain.

However, the results presented in this study did not lead to finding any significant relationship between platelet reactivity and the size of an ischemic focus in the whole group of patients with stroke. Oh et al. [8] documented that patients with ASA resistance had a statistically significantly larger ischemic focus size, as assessed in MR-DWI (median 5.4 mL versus 1.7 mL), than the group of patients sensitive to ASA. Similar results were presented by Cheng et al. [9], whose differences between the ASA-resistant and -sensitive groups were even more significant (13.21 mL versus 4.26 mL). In addition, they showed a significant correlation between the reactivity of the platelets and the size of the ischemic focus (R = 0.63). In turn, Agayeva et al. [18] and El-Mitwalli et al. [19] did not show the influence of platelet reactivity on the ischemic focus size, as assessed by MR-DWI in the brain. Discrepancies with the results of Oh et al. [8] and Cheng et al. [9] may have resulted from several important elements. First of all, the methodology was as follows: all of the above tests were performed based on turbidimetry aggregometry, which as demonstrated by Larsen et al. [20] and Ko et al. [21], poorly correlates with the Multiplate method. Secondly, other publications have studied patients with all types of strokes (including embolic). Due to other mechanisms of activation of the coagulation cascade, the limited therapeutic effect of ASA, and the possible use of low molecular weight heparin therapy in a treatment dose from day 1 of the stroke, patients with embolic stroke were excluded from this study. The aim of this procedure was also to unify the group of subjects to only those in which the pathology of platelet function is of the greatest importance in the etiopathogenesis of stroke (thrombotic mechanism) and in which the benefits of ASA therapy are the greatest. Thirdly, in all of the above studies, the patients took acetylsalicylic acid at least 7 days before the onset of the stroke. It is worth mentioning that the population of patients studied in this study included only those who had not taken acetylsalicylic acid before the onset of stroke. The aim of this procedure was not only to unify the study group, but also to maintain the right proportions in relation to the epidemiology of stroke, as the data from the literature showed that the vast majority of patients, at the same time of developing stroke, did not previously take ASA [22]. Data from the literature provides information that the fact of taking ASA before stroke is relevant to the results obtained. Rosafio et al. [23] and Sabra et al. [24] showed significant differences in platelet reactivity between a group that took ASA for the first time in the acute phase of stroke and a group that had received ASA prior to stroke. In addition, some authors have shown that taking ASA before has a potential effect on the size of an ischemic focus [25]. It is worth mentioning that Cheng et al. [9] always evaluated the size of the ischemic focus size in DWI within the first day of stroke, and Oh et al. [8] within 48 h. In this study, the MR examination was performed up to 5 days after, usually on the 3rd or 4th day, but never within the first 24 h. It cannot be excluded that these time discrepancies, which have no effect on the size of the ischemic focus, may have contributed to the contradictory results. During the first few hours of stroke, the area of ischemia in DWI may include—aside from the area of irreversibly damaged tissue—the penumbra area (i.e., the area at risk of infarction progression), which after several hours (sometimes even after 24 h) may be remitted due to reperfusion [26,27].

Theoretically, greater activation and aggregation of platelets in the presence of the platelet inhibitory effect by ASA should create microaggregates from platelets and platelet–thrombin complexes, and the release of pro-spasmodic factors, leading to a larger vascular plug formation, occlusion of the larger vessel, and finally leading to a larger area of cerebral ischemia [28]. However, the authors of this study believe that this mechanism may be important, but only at the level of arteries of a larger caliber. In patients with small-vessel disease, small arterioles and capillaries, which are initially narrowed by advanced atherosclerotic processes, ultimately close when the thrombus is formed, leading to a relatively small ischemic outbreak. In this case, excessive activation of platelets, which may lead to the closure of several additional fine arterioles in the areas, does not significantly affect the size of the ischemic focus. Nevertheless, in the case of patients with large-vessel disease, excessive activation and platelet aggregation may significantly affect the closure of the larger vessel, which will lead to a globally larger ischemic area from the larger vascularization basin. This relationship was demonstrated in this analysis, finding a high correlation between the platelet reactivity and the size of the ischemic focus—the higher the activity of platelets in patients with a larger vessel closure, the larger the ischemic focus in the brain. However, it is worth noting that this study was dominated by patients with small-vessel disease and globally small ischemic foci, in which no correlation with platelet reactivity was demonstrated. This can be used to explain the fact that in this study, patients with ASA resistance and higher platelet reactivity obtained larger median sizes of ischemic focal size in all analyses; however, these values were not significant for the entire stroke group, even at the level of statistical tendency.

The obtained results of this study suggest that large artery atherosclerosis appears to be an important factor in activating platelets. Independent authors have demonstrated, by means of various methods of assessing platelet reactivity, higher platelet activation in patients with the large extracranial vessel disease [29–32]. Moreover, the beneficial role of surgical interventions on the carotid artery in improving platelet function has also been emphasized. Kinsella et al. [33] showed that high platelet reactivity was observed in patients after stroke in the course of carotid artery stenting after carotid stenting decreased below the level found in asymptomatic patients, who were treated only with the antiplatelet drug. The above results undoubtedly prove the important role of platelets in the pathogenesis of stroke in patients with carotid artery stenosis, which additionally, in the light of the results of this analysis, puts the group of patients with large artery atherosclerosis as special beneficiaries of optimal antiplatelet therapy. The authors of this study also believe that the effects of etiopathogenesis of ischemic stroke may also result from a pathomorphic basis. In patients with LAA, the classic atherosclerotic process dominates, in which the role of platelet activation is indisputable and primary; in patients with small-vessel disease (especially in small arteries under 200 μm), fibrosis, glazing, calcification, and lypohialinose processes prevail, which pathomorphologically different than the classical atherosclerotic process and in which the role of platelets is limited and marginal [34]. These pathomorphological differences can undoubtedly result in the relationship between excessive activation of platelets and a larger area of cerebral ischemia.

However, the current study has its limitations: The size of the studied population was moderate, but seemed sufficient to make conclusions. Additional studies on larger populations of subjects are needed to confirm our theories. Due to the failure of the optical aggregometer, most conclusions were based only on the results of impedance aggregometry (Multiplate analyzer), which similar to other platelet reactivity tests, is poorly standardized with agreed resistance criteria [35]. The main limitation of our study is that it is a one-time, single measurement of platelet activation at different times after the onset of stroke symptoms and after the dose of acetylsalicylic acid, which may be insufficient to properly assess the relationships between ASA resistance and the size of an ischemic focus. An optimal approach seems to be the sequential determination of platelet reactivity on successive days [36–38]. Another limitation is poor correlation between biochemical (laboratory) and clinical ASA resistance [39]. Thus, the results of the ex vivo platelet reactivity tests do not always translate to the therapeutic effect of the antiplatelet drug. Agayeva et al. [40] suggested that the reason for this may be the heterogeneity of the pathophysiological basis of ischemic brain stroke. One should also remember the anti-inflammatory and neuroprotective activities of ASA, which take place by mechanisms independent of the platelets [41]. Another limitation seems to be the lack of assessment of the potential impacts of other drugs used by stroke patients (such as statins, which are routinely recommended in the secondary prevention of stroke) and the ASA dose itself on platelet reactivity. Due to the low detectability of atrial fibrillation as a cause of stroke, the authors of the study are also uncertain whether there was a small percentage of patients in the study population with embolic cerebral ischemia. In turn, for formal reasons (i.e., conscious consent for the study given to the Bioethics Committee), the analysis did not include patients with a severe neurological deficit (e.g., patients with impaired consciousness); hence, the study does not include a full cross-section of patients with stroke, but only patients with milder clinical conditions.

5. Conclusions

In stroke patients with large-vessel disease, high on-treatment platelet reactivity is associated with a larger extent of acute ischemic focus and chronic ischemic lesions in the brain. The important roles of etiopathogenesis of stroke in the occurrence of significant relationships between platelet reactivity and the extent of both acute and chronic brain lesions have been highlighted. Further research is needed to determine the optimal therapeutic strategies in stroke due to large-vessel disease coexisting with high on-treatment platelet reactivity.

Author Contributions: Conceptualization, A.W. and G.K.; methodology, A.W., G.K., J.S., and A.K.-W.; software, J.S.; validation, G.K.; formal Analysis, A.W., K.F., and G.K.; investigation, A.W.; resources, J.S.; data curation, J.S., A.K.-W., and A.S.; writing—original draft preparation, A.W. and K.F.; writing—review and editing, G.K.; visualization, A.W.; supervision, G.K. and Z.S.; project administration, A.W. and G.K. All authors have read and agreed to the published version of the manuscript.

Funding: This research received no external funding.

Conflicts of Interest: The authors declare no conflict of interest.

References

1. Naghavi, M.; Wang, H.; Lozano, R.; Davis, A.; Liang, X.; Zhou, M.; Vollset, S.E.; Ozgoren, A.A.; Abdalla, S.; Abd-Allah, F.; et al. Global, regional, and national age-sex specific all-cause and cause-specific mortality for 240 causes of death, 1990–2013: A systematic analysis for the Global Burden of Disease Study 2013. *Lancet* **2015**, *385*, 117–171.
2. Sacco, R.L.; Kasner, S.E.; Broderick, J.P.; Caplan, L.R.; Connors, J.J.; Culebras, A.; Elkind, M.S.; George, M.G.; Hamdan, A.D.; Higashida, R.T.; et al. An updated definition of stroke for the 21st century: A statement for healthcare professionals from the American Heart Association/American Stroke Association. *Stroke* **2013**, *44*, 2064–2089. [CrossRef]
3. Okrój-Lubecka, J.; Szurowska, E.; Kozera, G. Neuroimaging of acute phase of ischemic stroke in clinical practice. *For. Med. Rodz.* **2015**, *9*, 391–401.

4. Keller, S.S.; Roberts, N. Measurement of brain volume using MRI: Software, techniques, choices and prerequisites. *J. Anthropol. Sci.* **2009**, *87*, 127–151. [PubMed]
5. Ahmed, N.; Steiner, T.; Caso, V.; Wahlgren, N. Recommendations from the ESO- Karolinska Stroke Update Conference, Stockholm 13–15 November 2016. *Eur. Stroke J.* **2017**, *2*, 95–102. [CrossRef] [PubMed]
6. Ozben, S.; Ozben, B.; Tanrikulu, A.M.; Ozer, F.; Ozben, T. Aspirin resistance in patients with acute ischemic stroke. *J. Neurol.* **2011**, *258*, 1979–1986. [CrossRef]
7. Paniccia, R.; Priora, R.; Liotta, A.A.; Agatina, A. Platelet function tests: A comparative review. *Vasc. Health Risk Manag.* **2015**, *11*, 133–148. [CrossRef] [PubMed]
8. Oh, M.S.; Yu, K.H.; Lee, J.H.; Jung, S.; Kim, C.; Jang, M.U.; Lee, J.; Lee, B.C. Aspirin resistance is associated with increased stroke severity and infarct volume. *Neurology* **2016**, *86*, 1808–1817. [CrossRef] [PubMed]
9. Cheng, X.; Xie, N.C.; Hu, H.L.; Chen, C.; Lian, Y.J. Biochemical aspirin resistance is associated with increased stroke severity and infarct volumes in ischemic stroke patients. *Oncotarget* **2017**, *8*, 77086–77095. [CrossRef]
10. Wardlaw, J.M.; Smith, E.E.; Biessels, G.J.; Cordonnier, C.; Fazekas, F.; Frayne, R.; Lindley, R.I.; O'Brien, J.T.; Barkhof, F.; Benavente, O.R.; et al. Neuroimaging standards for research into small vessel disease and its contribution to ageing and neurodegeneration. *Lancet Neurol.* **2013**, *12*, 822–838. [CrossRef]
11. Sibbing, D.; Braun, S.; Jawansky, S.; Vogt, W.; Mehilli, J.; Schömig, A.; Kastrati, A.; von Beckerath, N. Assessment of ADP-induced platelet aggregation with light transmission aggregometry and multiplate electrode platelet aggregometry before and after clopidogrel treatment. *Thromb. Haemost.* **2008**, *99*, 121–126. [PubMed]
12. Tóth, O.; Calatzis, A.; Penz, S.; Losonczy, H.; Siess, W. Multiple electrode aggregometry: A new device to measure platelet aggregation in whole blood. *Thromb. Haemost.* **2006**, *96*, 781–788. [PubMed]
13. Wojczal, J.; Tomczyk, T.; Luchowski, P. Standards in neurosonology. *J. Ultrason.* **2016**, *16*, 44–45. [CrossRef] [PubMed]
14. Wiśniewski, A.; Sikora, J.; Filipska, K.; Kozera, G. Assessment of the relationship between platelet reactivity, vascular risk factors and gender in cerebral ischaemia patients. *Neurol. Neurochir. Pol.* **2019**, *53*, 258–264. [CrossRef] [PubMed]
15. Gremmel, T.; Steiner, S.; Seidinger, D.; Koppensteiner, R.; Panzer, S.; Kopp, C.W. Comparison of methods to evaluate aspirin- mediated platelet inhibition after percutaneous intervention with stent implantation. *Platelets* **2011**, *22*, 188–195. [CrossRef] [PubMed]
16. Crescente, M.; Di Castelnuovo, A.; Iacoviello, L.; Vermylen, J.; Cerletti, C.; de Gaetano, G. Response variability to aspirin as assessed by the platelet function analyzer (PFA)-100. *Thromb. Haemost.* **2008**, *99*, 14–26. [CrossRef]
17. Go, A.S.; Mozaffarian, D.; Roger, V.L.; Benjamin, E.J.; Berry, J.D.; Blaha, M.J.; Dai, S.; Ford, E.S.; Fox, C.S.; Franco, S.; et al. Heart disease and stroke statistics—2014 update: A report from the American Heart Association. *Circulation* **2014**, *129*, e28–e292. [CrossRef]
18. Agayeva, N.; Topcuoglu, M.A.; Arsava, E.M. The Interplay between Stroke Severity, Antiplatelet Use, and Aspirin Resistance in Ischemic Stroke. *J. Stroke Cerebrovasc. Dis.* **2016**, *25*, 397–403. [CrossRef]
19. El-Mitwalli, A.; Azzam, H.; Abu-Hegazy, M.; Gomma, M.; Wasel, Y. Clinical and biochemical aspirin resistance in patients with recurrent cerebral ischemia. *Clin. Neurol. Neurosurg.* **2013**, *115*, 944–947. [CrossRef] [PubMed]
20. Larsen, P.D.; Holley, A.S.; Sasse, A.; Al-Sinan, A.; Fairley, S.; Harding, S.A. Comparison of Multiplate and VerifyNow platelet function tests in predicting clinical outcome in patients with acute coronary syndromes. *Thromb. Res.* **2017**, *152*, 14–19. [CrossRef] [PubMed]
21. Ko, Y.G.; Suh, J.W.; Kim, B.H.; Lee, C.J.; Kim, J.S.; Choi, D.; Hong, M.K.; Seo, M.K.; Youn, T.J.; Chae, I.H.; et al. Comparison of 2 point-of-care platelet function tests, VerifyNow Assay and Multiple Electrode Platelet Aggregometry, for predicting early clinical outcomes in patients undergoing percutaneous coronary intervention. *Am. Heart J.* **2011**, *161*, 383–390. [CrossRef] [PubMed]
22. Greisenegger, S.; Tentschert, S.; Weber, M.; Ferrari, J.; Lang, W.; Lalouschek, W. Prior therapy with antiplatelet agents is not associated with outcome in patients with acute ischemic stroke/TIA. *J. Neurol.* **2006**, *253*, 648–652. [CrossRef] [PubMed]
23. Rosafio, F.; Lelli, N.; Mimmi, S.; Vandelli, L.; Bigliardi, G.; Dell'Acqua, M.L.; Picchetto, L.; Pentore, R.; Ferraro, D.; Trenti, T.; et al. Platelet Function Testing in Patients with Acute Ischemic Stroke: An Observational Study. *J. Stroke Cerebrovasc. Dis.* **2017**, *26*, 1864–1873. [CrossRef] [PubMed]

24. Sabra, A.; Stanford, S.N.; Storton, S.; Lawrence, M.; D'Silva, L.; Morris, R.H.; Evans, V.; Wani, M.; Potter, J.F.; Evans, P.A. Assessment of platelet function in patients with stroke using multiple electrode platelet aggregometry: A prospective observational study. *BMC Neurol.* **2016**, *16*, 254. [CrossRef] [PubMed]
25. Sobol, A.B.; Mochecka, A.; Selmaj, K.; Loba, J. Is there a relationship between aspirin responsiveness and clinical aspects of ischemic stroke? *Adv. Clin. Exp. Med.* **2009**, *18*, 473–479.
26. Warach, S. Use of diffusion and perfusion magnetic resonance imaging as a stroke clinical trials. *Curr. Control. Trials Cardiovasc. Med.* **2001**, *2*, 38–44. [CrossRef]
27. Guadagno, J.V.; Warburton, E.A.; Aigbirhio, F.I.; Smielewski, P.; Fryer, T.D.; Harding, S.; Price, C.J.; Gillard, J.H.; Carpenter, T.A.; Baron, J.C. Does the acute diffusion-weighted imaging lesion represent penumbra as well as core? A combined quantitative PET/MRI voxel-based study. *J. Cereb. Blood Flow Metabol.* **2004**, *24*, 1249–1254. [CrossRef]
28. Jastrzębska, M.; Siennicka, A.; Chełstowski, K.; Ciechanowicz, A.; Nowacki, P.; Wódecka, A. Laboratory evaluation of response for treatment with acetylsalicilic acid (ASA) in patients with acute phase of ischemic stroke—Appication of flow aggregometry (PFA-100) and impedance (Multiplate) aggregometry. *J. Lab. Diagn.* **2011**, *47*, 155–163.
29. Tsai, N.W.; Chang, W.N.; Shaw, C.F.; Jan, C.R.; Chang, H.W.; Huang, C.R.; Chen, S.D.; Chuang, Y.C.; Lee, L.H.; Wang, H.C.; et al. Levels and value of platelet activation markers in different subtypes of acute non-cardio-embolic ischemic stroke. *Thromb. Res.* **2009**, *124*, 213–218. [CrossRef]
30. Zheng, A.S.; Churilov, L.; Colley, R.E.; Goh, C.; Davis, S.M.; Yan, B. Association of aspirin resistance with increased stroke severity and infarct size. *JAMA Neurol.* **2013**, *70*, 208–213. [CrossRef]
31. Kinsella, J.A.; Tobin, W.O.; Hamilton, G.; McCabe, D.J. Platelet activation, function, and reactivity in atherosclerotic carotid artery stenosis: A systematic review of the literature. *Int. J. Stroke* **2013**, *8*, 451–464. [CrossRef] [PubMed]
32. Dawson, J.; Quinn, T.; Lees, K.R.; Walters, M.R. Microembolic signals and aspirin resistance in patients with carotid stenosis. *Cardiovasc. Ther.* **2012**, *30*, 234–239. [CrossRef] [PubMed]
33. Kinsella, J.A.; Tobin, W.A.; Tierney, S. Assessment of 'on-treatment platelet reactivity' and relationship with cerebral micro-embolic signals in asymptomatic and symptomatic carotid stenosis. *J. Neurol. Sci.* **2017**, *376*, 133–139. [CrossRef] [PubMed]
34. Dymecki, J.; Kulczycki, J. *Clinical Neuropathology*, 1rd ed.; Institute of Psychiatrics and Neurology: Warsaw, Poland, 1997; pp. 98–99.
35. Paniccia, R.; Antonucci, E.; Maggini, N.; Romano, E.; Gori, A.M.; Marcucci, R.; Prisco, D.; Abbate, R. Assessment of platelet function on whole blood by multiplate electrode platelet aggregometry in high-risk patients with coronary artery disease receiving antiplatelet therapy. *Am. J. Clin. Pathol.* **2009**, *131*, 834–842. [CrossRef]
36. McCabe, D.J.; Harrison, P.; Mackie, I.J.; Sidhu, P.S.; Lawrie, A.S.; Purdy, G.; Machin, S.J.; Brown, M.M. Assessment of the antiplatelet effects of low to medium dose aspirin in the early and late phases after ischaemic stroke and TIA. *Platelets* **2005**, *16*, 269–280. [CrossRef]
37. Kim, J.T.; Heo, S.H.; Choi, K.H.; Nam, T.S.; Choi, S.M.; Lee, S.H.; Park, M.S.; Kim, B.C.; Kim, M.K.; Saver, J.L.; et al. Clinical Implications of Changes in Individual Platelet Reactivity to Aspirin Over Time in Acute Ischemic Stroke. *Stroke* **2015**, *46*, 2534–2540. [CrossRef]
38. Kim, J.T.; Heo, S.H.; Lee, J.S.; Choi, M.J.; Choi, K.H.; Nam, T.S.; Lee, S.H.; Park, M.S.; Kim, B.C.; Kim, M.K.; et al. Aspirin resistance in the acute stages of acute ischemic stroke is associated with the development of new ischemic lesions. *PLoS ONE* **2015**, *10*, e0120743. [CrossRef]
39. Kour, D.; Tandon, V.R.; Kapoor, B.; Mahajan, A.; Parihar, A.; Somtra, S. Aspirin Resistance. *New Horiz.* **2006**, *8*, 116–117.
40. Agayeva, N.; Gungor, L.; Topcuoglu, M.A.; Arsava, E.M. Pathophysiologic, rather than laboratory-defined resistance drives aspirin failure in isch-emic stroke. *J. Stroke Cerebrovasc. Dis.* **2015**, *24*, 745–750. [CrossRef]
41. Alberts, M.J.; Bergman, D.L.; Molner, E.; Jovanovic, B.D.; Ushiwata, I.; Teruya, J. Antiplatelet effect of aspirin in patients with cerebrovascular disease. *Stroke* **2004**, *35*, 175–178. [CrossRef]

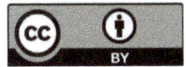

© 2020 by the authors. Licensee MDPI, Basel, Switzerland. This article is an open access article distributed under the terms and conditions of the Creative Commons Attribution (CC BY) license (http://creativecommons.org/licenses/by/4.0/).

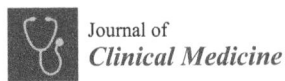

Article

One-Stop Management of 230 Consecutive Acute Stroke Patients: Report of Procedural Times and Clinical Outcome

Marios-Nikos Psychogios [1,2,*], Ilko L. Maier [3], Ioannis Tsogkas [1], Amélie Carolina Hesse [1], Alex Brehm [1,2], Daniel Behme [1], Marlena Schnieder [3], Katharina Schregel [1], Ismini Papageorgiou [4], David S. Liebeskind [5], Mayank Goyal [6], Mathias Bähr [3], Michael Knauth [1] and Jan Liman [3]

[1] Department of Neuroradiology, University Medical Center Goettingen, 37075 Goettingen, Germany; ioannis.tsogkas@usb.ch (I.T.); amelie.hesse@med.uni-goettingen.de (A.C.H.); alex.brehm@usb.ch (A.B.); daniel.behme@med.uni-goettingen.de (D.B.); katharina.schregel@med.uni-goettingen.de (K.S.); michael.knauth@med.uni-goettingen.de (M.K.)
[2] Department of Neuroradiology, Clinic for Radiology & Nuclear Medicine, University Hospital Basel, 4031 Basel, Switzerland
[3] Department of Neurology, University Medical Center Goettingen, 37075 Goettingen, Germany; ilko.maier@med.uni-goettingen.de (I.L.M.); marlena.schnieder@med.uni-goettingen.de (M.S.); mbaehr@gwdg.de (M.B.); jliman@gwdg.de (J.L.)
[4] Department of Neuroradiology, Südharz Klinikum, 99734 Nordhausen, Germany; ismini.e.papageorgiou@gmail.com
[5] Neurovascular Imaging Research Core and Stroke Center, Department of Neurology, University of California Los Angeles, Los Angeles, CA 90095, USA; davidliebeskind@yahoo.com
[6] Calgary Stroke Program, Department of Clinical Neurosciences, University of Calgary, Calgary, AB 2500, Canada; mgoyal@ucalgary.ca
* Correspondence: marios.psychogios@usb.ch; Tel.: +41-613-28-6370

Received: 20 November 2019; Accepted: 6 December 2019; Published: 11 December 2019

Abstract: Background and purpose: Rapid thrombectomy for acute ischemic stroke caused by large vessel occlusion leads to improved outcome. Optimizing intrahospital management might diminish treatment delays. To examine if one-stop management reduces intrahospital treatment delays and improves functional outcome of acute stroke patients with large vessel occlusion. Methods: We performed a single center, observational study from June 2016 to November 2018. Imaging was acquired with the latest generation angiography suite at a comprehensive stroke center. Two-hundred-thirty consecutive adults with suspected acute stroke presenting within 6 h after symptom onset with a moderate to severe National Institutes of Health Stroke Scale (≥10 in 2016; ≥7 since January 2017) were directly transported to the angiography suite by bypassing multidetector CT. Noncontrast flat-detector CT and biphasic flat-detector CT angiography were acquired with an angiography system. In case of a large vessel occlusion patients remained in the angiography suite, received intravenous rtPA therapy and underwent thrombectomy. As primary endpoints, door-to-reperfusion times and functional outcome at 90 days were recorded and compared in a case-control analysis with matched prior patients receiving standard management. Results: A total of 230 patients (123 women, median age of 78 years (Interquartile Range (IQR) 69–84)) were included. Median symptom-to-door time was 130 min (IQR 70–195). Large vessel occlusion was diagnosed in 166/230 (72%) patients; 64/230 (28%) had conditions not suitable for thrombectomy. Median door-to-reperfusion time for M1 occlusions was 64 min (IQR 56–87). Compared to 43 case-matched patients triaged with multidetector CT, median door-to-reperfusion time was reduced from 102 (IQR 85–117) to 68 min (IQR 53–89; $p < 0.001$). Rate of good functional outcome was significantly better in the one-stop management group ($p = 0.029$). Safety parameters (mortality, sICH, any hemorrhage) did not differ significantly between groups. Conclusions: One-stop management for stroke triage reduces intrahospital time delays in our specific hospital setting.

Keywords: stroke; hemorrhage; thrombectomy; cone-beam computed tomography; cerebral angiography

1. Introduction

Swift and complete reperfusion of the occluded vessel territory is the key of every revascularization therapy in stroke patients with large vessel occlusion (LVO) [1,2]. Thrombectomy became the new standard of LVO-therapy after publication of multiple trials showing higher reperfusion rates and improved functional outcomes in patients receiving the combination of thrombectomy and medical therapy as opposed to medical therapy alone [3–7]. However, door-to-groin times have been consistently longer than one hour, even in trials focusing on rapid treatment of stroke patients [2,6]. The primary limitation leading to time-delays in the treatment of LVO-patients is the lack of a fast, reliable and affordable prehospital screening tool in stroke treatment akin to e.g., the electrocardiogram in patients with an acute coronary syndrome. While STEMI-patients with a positive electrocardiogram are directly transported to the angiography-suite, stroke patients are usually first triaged with a noninvasive imaging method in one room, or even hospital, and then transported to a different room, or even different hospital, for thrombectomy.

In order to minimize intrahospital times at the treating hospital, we recently proposed a method of noninvasive triage with a flat-detector computed tomography (FDCT) capable angiography-suite, IV lysis and thrombectomy in the same room (one-stop management) with the potential of significant reduction of door-to-groin and door-to-reperfusion times [8]. We demonstrated in prior work, that a rather simple, fast and commercially available non-enhanced FDCT protocol can be used to detect intracranial hemorrhage (ICH) with a very high sensitivity, which is comparable to multi-detector CT (MDCT) [9]. Furthermore, biphasic FDCT angiography enabled us to reliable detect LVOs and grade collaterals [10]. These advancements made the aforementioned paradigm feasible for the triage of mothership, who are eligible for IV lysis, as well as transfer patients.

In this study, we report the first 230 consecutive stroke patients diagnosed and treated with a one-stop management and analyze the 90 days functional outcomes, compared to patients managed with an optimized stroke workflow previously published [11].

2. Materials and Methods

2.1. Patient Selection

This observational study includes all 230 consecutive adult patients treated with one-stop management in our hospital from June 2016 to November 2018. All patients presented with clinical signs of an ischemic stroke within 6 h after symptom onset and a National Institutes of Health Stroke Scale (NIHSS) (≥10 in 2016; ≥7 since January 2017) were included in our study. Unknown symptom onset, prolonged time from symptom onset, a low NIHSS (<10 in 2016; <7 since January 2017) or occupation of the FDCT-capable angiography-suite during admission were exclusion criteria. Data were prospectively collected and documented in an Institutional Review Board-approved database. A neurological assessment was performed (i) at hospital admission, (ii) hospital discharge and (iii) 90 days after stroke by a certified stroke neurologist. The imaging data were documented by the treating physician and re-evaluated by a core-team, consisting of an experienced neurointerventionalist (>10 years of experience) and a neuroradiology resident. A patient's consent for treatment was obtained according to the institutional guidelines. The local ethics committee waived the need for a formal application or a separate consent concerning the inclusion in our observational database.

2.2. Image Acquisition and Processing

Images were acquired using an Artis Q angiography system (Siemens Healthcare GmbH, Forchheim, Germany) as described before [8,12]. First, an FDCT was acquired to exclude intracranial hemorrhage. A commercially available 20 s rotational acquisition was used (20 s DCT Head, 109 kV, 1.8 µGy/frame, 200° angle, 0.4°/frame angulation step; effective dose ~2.5 mSv; Siemens Healthineers AG, Erlangen, Germany) and raw data were instantly and automatically reconstructed in 5 mm multiplanar reconstructions on a commercially available workstation (syngo × Workplace; Siemens Healthineers AG, Erlangen, Germany). Next, a commercially available biphasic FDCT-angiography (biFDCTA) was acquired for detection of arterial occlusion and evaluation of intracranial collaterals (2 × 10 s DSA, 70kV, 1.2 µGy/frame, 200° angle, 0.8°/frame angulation step; effective dose ~ 2.5 mSv; Siemens Healthineers AG, Erlangen, Germany) after intravenous injection of 60 mL contrast media (Imeron 400; Bracco Imaging Inc, Konstanz, Germany) at a flow rate of 5 mL/s followed by 60 mL saline chaser at 5 mL/s. Both FDCTA datasets were instantly and automatically reconstructed on the aforementioned workstation and 24 mm transversal maximal intensity projections of the first and second phase were simultaneously viewable on the workstation. Timing for the start of the first (arterial) phase acquisition was determined using a bolus-tracking acquisition. The second (venous) phase was acquired automatically with a delay of 5 s from the end of the first rotation. The acquisition, reconstruction and evaluation of all datasets do not require more than 2 min.

2.3. Management After Imaging

Patients with no hemorrhage and with an LVO were treated, if eligible, with intravenous recombinant tissue plasminogen activator (IV rtPA) and with thrombectomy. As per institutional guidelines, a low Alberta Stroke Program Early CT Scale (ASPECTS) or low collateral score was not an exclusion criterion for thrombectomy in the first 6 h after symptom onset. Patients with no hemorrhage and with a small vessel occlusion (SVO) were treated with IV rtPA only, if eligible. Patients with no hemorrhage and with no arterial occlusion were started on IV rtPA, if eligible, and received an additional stroke MRI to decide on further treatment. Patients with an intracranial hemorrhage and no occlusion were treated as per institutional standards. Lastly, patients with an intracranial hemorrhage (ICH) and LVO were treated with thrombectomy after an individualized case discussion between the neurologist, interventional neuroradiologist and patient or his/her next of kin.

2.4. Statistical Analysis

Characteristics and time-metrics of the one-stop database are reported by descriptive statistics. Time-intervals are documented with median, interquartile range (IQR) and 90th percentile, as recently proposed [13]. A case-matched analysis is performed between the one-stop database and the standard workflow (multidetector CT (MDCT)-triaged patients) database with the following criteria: patient's age, admission NIHSS, ASPECTS and symptom-to-door time. Only standard-workflow-patients that arrived in our hospital with an NIHSS ≥7 while the angiography-suite was not occupied were included in the case-matched analysis in order to simulate a similar scenario for matching purposes. The maximum allowed difference for case-matching was chosen arbitrarily and was 10 years for age, six points for NIHSS, 3 points for ASPECTS and 45 min for symptom-to-door time. Continuous variables were compared between one-stop management and optimized workflow patients either by t-test, in the case of normal distribution, or by the Wilcoxon test, in the case of non-normal or ordinal distribution. Categorical variables were compared between the 2 groups by the Fisher's exact test. The probability of favorable outcome (modified Rankin scale (mRS) ≤ 2) between the two groups at 90 days was further assessed by logistic regression using selected variables. Statistical analyses were performed with the MedCalc Statistical Software version 18 (MedCalc Software bv, Ostend, Belgium; http://www.medcalc.org; 2018).

3. Results

Two-hundred-thirty one-stop managed patients were included in our study (123 women; median age of 78 years (IQR 69–84)). The overall admission NIHSS was 15 (IQR 12–19) and 166/230 (72%) patients were diagnosed with an LVO, 25/230 (11%) with an SVO, 24/230 (10%) with an ICH, 11/230 (5%) with a Todd's paresis and 4/230 (2%) with a recanalized LVO after transfer, respectively (Table 1). One-hundred-twenty-seven out of 230 (55%) cases were direct admissions, while 103/230 (45%) were transfer patients from a peripheral stroke center with a confirmed LVO. Of the 127 direct admission patients 74/127 (58%) were LVOs, 19/127 (15%) were SVOs, 23/127 (18%) were ICHs and 11/127 (9%) were Todd's paresis. Of the 103 transfer patients, 61/103 (59%) received IV rtPA at the peripheral stroke center ("drip and ship"), 1/103 (1%) was diagnosed with a new subdural hematoma on FDCT that was not present on the initial external MDCT and 4/103 (4%) showed complete revascularization on baseline FDCTA at our center. The median time required between the external MDCT and the FDCT was 124 min (110–155; 90th percentile 218).

The overall door-to-FDCT time was 15 min (IQR 10–20; 90th percentile 26) and door-to-IVrtPA was 22 min (IQR 20–30; 90th percentile 41). The median door-to-groin time for LVO patients was 29 min (IQR 22–39; 90th percentile 50) with a median door-to-reperfusion time of 72 min (IQR 58–91; 90th percentile 117; Table 2). Patients with an M1 occlusion had a median door-to-reperfusion time of 64 min (IQR 56–87; 90th percentile 102). Any hemorrhage was depicted in 25/166 (15%), a parenchymal hematoma type-2 in 2/166 (1%) and a symptomatic intracranial hemorrhage (sICH) in 6/166 (4%) of the LVOs on follow-up imaging. Overall mortality was 22%. A favorable outcome was documented in 65/166 (39%) of the LVO patients at discharge. Nineteen LVO patients were lost to follow-up; favorable outcome and mortality for mothership patients with a pre-stroke mRS less than three were 57% and 31% while overall favorable outcome and mortality of mothership LVO patients were 51% and 32% respectively at 90 days after stroke onset.

The case-control analysis revealed 43 LVO matches for each group (one-stop vs. traditional management). Matching variables were not significantly different between one-stop and traditional workflow patients; other baseline and imaging characteristics (e.g., collaterals) were also balanced between the two groups (Table 3). We observed a significant reduction of door-to-groin and door-to-reperfusion times, both during working and off-duty hours, for direct admission and transfer patients. Safety variables, such as sICH, any hemorrhage on follow-up imaging or mortality were comparable between the two groups. Median discharge and 90 d mRS in the one-stop group was three (IQR 1–5) and two (IQR 1–5), respectively. The rate of good functional outcome at 90 days was significantly higher in the one-stop management group with 58% (25/43) as compared to 33% (14/43) in the normal workflow group ($p = 0.029$). In the logistic regression model comparing predictors of favorable clinical outcome in the matched population, the one-stop management (odds ratio (OR) 3.75; 95% confidence interval (CI) 1.13–12.44; $p = 0.031$) and successful reperfusion (OR 2.58; 95% CI 1.19–5.55; $p = 0.015$) were significant contributors to the prediction of a favorable outcome (Figure 1).

Table 1. Clinical, angiographic, and procedural details of the 100 one-stop-management patients.

	All, n = 230	LVO, n = 166	SVO, n = 25	ICH, n = 24	Todd's, n = 11	RLVO, n = 4
Age, median (IQR)	78 (69–84)	77 (68–84)	79 (71–87)	78 (75–83)	79 (73–82)	81 (77–86)
Admission NIHSS	15 (12–19)	16 (13–19)	13 (11–15)	15 (10–17)	12 (11–15)	13 (11–13)
Female	123 (54%)	90 (54%)	12 (48%)	12 (50%)	5 (46%)	4 (100%)
IV-rtPA	144 (63%)	112 (68%)	23 (92%)	1	4 (36%)	4 (100%)
Hemorrhage on initial FDCT	25 (11%)	1 (1%)	0 (0%)	24 (100%)	0 (0%)	0 (0%)
Occlusion site						
ICA-T		41 (25%)				
M1		88 (53%)				
M2		15 (9%)				
Other		22 (13%)				
Tandem occlusion		34 (21%)				
Times, min (IQR; 90th Percentile)						
Symptom to door	130 (70–195; 253)	154 (67–205; 264)	82 (66–134; 205)	105 (69–129; 204)	131 (95–146; 186)	229 (181–259)
Door to FDCT	15 (10–20; 26)	14 (9–19; 25)	16 (12–24; 32)	17 (14–22; 30)	21 (13–23; 31)	16 (14–16)
Door to IV-rtPA	22 (20–30; 41)	22 (20–29; 38)	26 (20–45; 53)			
Door to treatment start[α]				21 (18–33; 34)	27 (19–32; 37)	
Door to groin		29 (22–39; 50)				
Groin to reperfusion		40 (28–60; 80)				
FDCT to reperfusion		59 (45–82; 101)				
Door to reperfusion		72 (58–91; 117)				
Door to reperfusion M1		64 (56–87; 102)				
extCT to FDCT		124 (110–155; 218)				

Table 1. Cont.

	All, n = 230	LVO, n = 166	SVO, n = 25	ICH, n = 24	Todd's, n = 11	RLVO, n = 4
Direct admission	127 (55%)	74 (45%)	19 (76%)	23 (96%)	11 (100%)	0 (0%)
Working hours$^\beta$	95 (41%)	68 (41%)	13 (52%)	11 (46%)	2 (18%)	1 (25%)
Reperfusion, mTICI2b-3		142 (86%)				
Any hemorrhage on FU	49 (21%)	25 (15%)	0 (0%)	24 (100%)	0 (0%)	
PH-2 hematoma on FU		2 (1%)				
sICH		6 (4%)				
Discharge NIHSS	5 (2–10)	5 (2–12)	7 (4–10)	5 (1–9)	4 (1–6)	6 (4–7)
Discharge mRS	4 (1–5)	4 (1–5)	4 (2–5)	2 (2–6)	3 (1–4)	3 (3–4)
Mortality	45/230 (20%)	36 (22%)	2 (8%)	5 (30%)	2 (18%)	0 (0%)
90 d mRS		4 (1–6)				
90 d favorable outcome	54/147 (37%)					

LVO, large vessel occlusion; SVO, small vessel occlusion; ICH, intracranial hemorrhage; RLVO, recanalized LVO during transfer; IQR, interquartile range, NIHSS, National Institutes of Health Stroke Scale; IV-rtPA, intravenous recombinant tissue plasminogen activator; FDCT, flat-detector CT; extCT, external CT in primary stroke center; mTICI, modified thrombolysis in cerebral infarction score; FU, follow-up; mRS, modified Rankin scale; α, intravenous injection of antihypertensive drugs in case of ICB or sedative drugs in case of seizures; β, weekdays 08:00 to 17:00.

Table 2. Procedural details of one-stop-management patients with large vessel occlusion.

Direct Admission n = 74	Min (IQR; 90th Percentile)
Door to FDCT	15 (12–20; 24)
Door to IV–rtPA	22 (20–29; 38)
Door to groin	34 (28–45; 51)
Groin to reperfusion	41 (26–55; 73)
FDCT to reperfusion	61 (47–81; 93)
Door to reperfusion	76 (61–92; 116)
Door to reperfusion of M1	68 (58–89; 101)
Occluded vessel	ICA-T 13 (18%), M1 42 (58%), M2 9 (12%)
Tandem occlusions	15 (20%)
Transfer patients n = 92	
extCT to FDCT	124 (110–155; 218)
Door to FDCT	10 (8–17; 25)
Door to groin	25 (19–33; 41)
Groin to reperfusion	38 (29–65; 87)
FDCT to reperfusion	56 (44–86; 110)
Door to reperfusion	68 (53–90; 126)
Door to reperfusion of M1	59 (52–84; 118)
Occluded vessel	ICA-T 28 (30%), M1 46 (50%), M2 6 (7%)
Tandem occlusions	19 (20%)
Working hours n = 68	
Door to FDCT	12 (7–16; 21)
Door to IV–rtPA	22 (20–26; 34)
Door to groin	25 (19–33; 41)
Groin to reperfusion	38 (25–53; 85)
FDCT to reperfusion	61 (42–69; 101)
Door to reperfusion	66 (52–85; 105)
Off-hours n = 98	
Door to FDCT	15 (10–21; 27)
Door to IV–rtPA	23 (19–29; 38)
Door to groin	33 (25–42; 60)
Groin to reperfusion	38 (25–53; 86)
FDCT to reperfusion	52 (42–69; 101)
Door to reperfusion	66 (52–85; 105)

Table 3. Case-control study of FDCT vs. MDCT patients, n =86.

	MDCT, n = 43	FDCT, n = 43	p-Value
Age median (IQR) *	77 (69–81)	77 (69–82)	0.962
Admission NIHSS *	17 (14–20)	16 (13–20)	0.796
CT ASPECTS *	8 (7–9)	9 (7–10)	0.138
Onset to door, min (IQR; 90th) *	129 (76–200; 244)	160 (74–202; 221)	0.511
Female	26 (61%)	26 (61%)	1.000
IV-rtPA	36 (84%)	30 (70%)	0.201
Hypertension	35 (81%)	33 (77%)	0.791
Hyperlipidemia	14 (33%)	20 (47%)	0.266
PAD	2 (5%)	5 (12%)	0.433
DM	11 (26%)	17 (40%)	0.249
Collateral grading	7 (5–8)	7 (4–8)	0.699
Direct admissions	30 (70%)	18 (42%)	**0.016**
Working hours	22 (51%)	19 (44%)	0.666
Door to CT, min (IQR; 90th)	15 (11–20; 24)	9 (6–14; 16)	**<0.001**
Door to IV-rtPA	27 (22–34; 35)	19 (12–22; 34)	**0.016**
Door to groin	60 (48–68; 79)	25 (19–30; 38)	**<0.001**
Working hours	60 (42–65; 85)	21 (17–25; 41)	**<0.001**
Off-hours	62 (53–69; 75)	25 (21–32; 38)	**<0.001**
Direct admissions	61 (54–67; 83)	26 (25–38; 44)	**<0.001**
Transfer patients	40 (30–69; 75)	21 (19–26; 35)	**<0.001**
Groin to reperfusion	42 (27–62; 94)	43 (33–60; 78)	0.866
CT to reperfusion	84 (71–99; 144)	59 (44–75; 96)	**<0.001**
Door to reperfusion	102 (85–117; 166)	68 (53–89; 104)	**<0.001**
Working hours	102 (79–145; 191)	62 (52–81; 104)	**0.006**
Off-hours	103 (93–116; 126)	74 (55–90; 109)	**<0.001**
Direct admissions	103 (85–121; 184)	72 (58–87; 103)	**0.001**
Transfer patients	102 (68–109; 120)	64 (51–88; 108)	**0.05**
ICA-T	7 (16%)	13 (30%)	0.179
M1	26 (61%)	25 (58%)	0.888
M2	9 (21%)	3 (7%)	0.117
Tandem occlusion	6 (14%)	7 (16%)	1
Successful reperfusion (mTICI2b-3)	31 (72%)	38 (88%)	0.102
sICH	3 (7%)	2 (5%)	1
Any hemorrhage	11 (26%)	7 (16%)	0.427
PH–2 hemorrhage	1 (2%)	1 (2%)	1
Discharge mRS	4 (2–5)	3 (1–5)	0.374
90d mRS	4 (1–5)	2 (1–5)	0.153
90d mRS of 0–2	14 (33%)	25 (58%)	**0.029**
Mortality	9 (21%)	10 (23%)	1

* Matching variables.

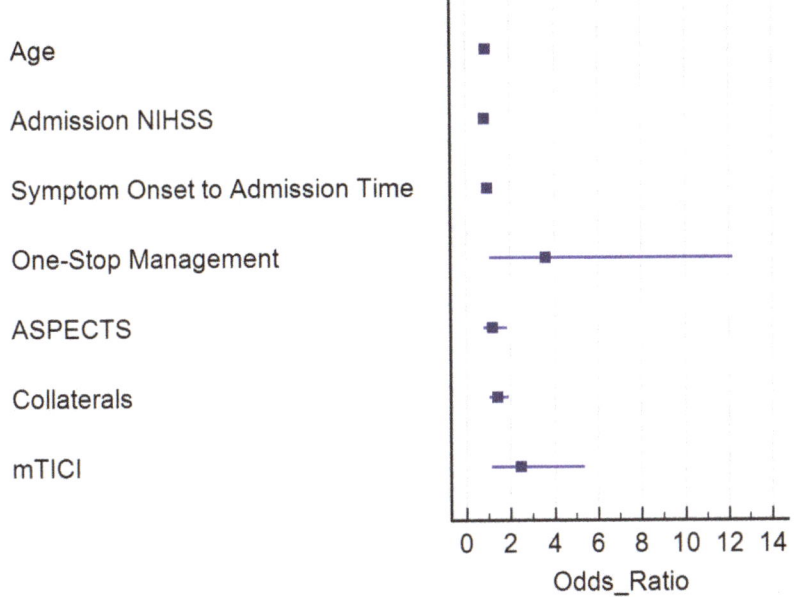

Figure 1. Logistic regression model comparing predictors of favorable clinical outcome in the matched population (one-stop management vs. normal management with MDCT).

4. Discussion

Our observational study establishes on a large scale the results from prior brief reports with median door-to-groin times under 30 min and median door-to-reperfusion times under 90 min for patients triaged with a one-stop management [8]. The proposed fast and commercially available protocol is safe for both direct admission and transfer patients. Intravenous rtPA was administered in 63% of our patients, with rates of any hemorrhage, symptomatic ICH and mortality comparable to larger trials. Regarding outcome results it should be noted that our observational study had no restrictions regarding pre-stroke mRS or initial ASPECTS. Compared to the thrombectomy trial from 2015 with focus on rapid endovascular treatment we observed markedly lower door-to-groin times with a 90th percentile of 50 min in our study vs. 147 min in the ESCAPE trial [6]. Door-to-reperfusion times were also markedly lower in our study with a 90th percentile of 117 min compared to 190 min in the ESCAPE trial [6]. Even in comparison to recent trials published in 2018 and performed in large-volume centers with daily training and standardized workflows, our median intrahospital times were more than 30 min lower with 29 min door-to-groin time (106 min in the 3D-Separator trial) and 59 min imaging-to-reperfusion time (97 min in the DEFUSE 3 trial) in our study [14,15].

In the period from 2014 to 2015 we were able to significantly reduce intrahospital times from a median door-to-groin time of 121 to 64 min by standardizing interdisciplinary operating procedures, conducting frequent team meetings, and providing mutual feedback [11]. However, despite the increased workload and training in the consecutive years we were not able to further reduce the intrahospital times through the MDCT-route [16]. The current case-matched analysis shows, indeed, that a one-stop management allows for and additional reduction of intrahospital times (Table 3). The decreased handling times together with the increased rates of successful reperfusion in the one-stop arm patient pool led to a significant increase in rates of favorable functional outcome at 90 days.

While the increased reperfusion rates are probably a result of increased use of sophisticated thrombectomy techniques [17], the earlier groin puncture times may also play a role in increased rates of complete reperfusion in one-stop patients. A recent study of the HERMES dataset has shown a decreased probability of successful reperfusion with prolonged intrahospital times in LVO patients [18]. Another interesting aspect of the one-stop management in stroke is the interaction of IV rtPA and remaining thrombi after incomplete thrombectomy. In the meta-analysis of the five positive thrombectomy trials in 2015, the median door-to-needle time was 35 min and the median door-to-reperfusion time 148 min [2]. As the thrombolytic effect of IV lysis is rapidly lost after termination of the 60 min infusion there is usually no effect of IV rtPA on distal emboli after incomplete mechanical reperfusion. In our setting, both the IV rtPA infusion and thrombectomy are initiated within a narrow time frame which frequently leads to substantial reperfusion prior to completion of the IV rtPA infusion. This fact could lead to resolution of emboli in new territories or distal emboli with a positive effect on functional outcome.

In order to establish a one-stop management of stroke patients with the proposed protocol there is obviously a need for angio-time capacity within the stroke center. Angiography suite capacity should not be a problem in off-hours. We did not encounter a relevant problem in our effort to establish a one-stop management as more than half of the interventions performed in our center are mechanical thrombectomies. For other centers with limited angiography availability, possible solutions include the installation of a dedicated stroke angiography or a pre-notification system. Even with a dedicated stroke angiography-suite there is always the possibility of another stroke patient arriving while performing mechanical thrombectomy on the 'stroke machine'. Regarding workload and safety, it should be noted that we decided to involve the senior physician in the exclusion of an ICH on FDCT images at all times, after a case of profound ICH which was missed by the resident on duty during off-hours (Figure 2). Discrepancies between residents and seniors in the interpretation of overnight head CTs and the detection of hemorrhages have been studied before for MDCT. The reported frequency of 1/230 cases in our study is comparable to the 141/22,590 cases in a study by Vagal et al. [19]. The workload of the stroke angiography can also be influenced by the NIHSS threshold chosen for the one-stop management. As of January 2017, we lowered our one-stop threshold to an admission NIHSS of ≥7 as a recent publication suggested that the best predictor for LVO is the NIHSS score with the aforementioned cut-off [20]. Other possibilities for a one-stop management include the combination of MDCT and C-arm in one room (so called MIYABI system) or the use of a mobile C-arm within the CT room [21]. Both systems have the disadvantages of a monoplanar angio system. The first solution has an additional drawback due to the increased costs for two machines, while with the second option the usually heavily utilized CT scanner is being blocked during thrombectomy. Our door-to-groin times were slightly higher (29 min) compared to the time metrics reported by Ribo et al. (17 min) and Jovin et al. (22 min). However, their door-to-reperfusion times (73 and 66 min respectively) were similar to ours (72 min) [22,23]. Furthermore, as we used non-invasive FDCT angiography for the delineation of LVOs, no unnecessary groin punctures were performed compared to a reported rate of 7% by Ribo et al. [24].

The main limitation of our study is the observational single-center design. All time metrics are prospectively documented in a stroke database, but the documentation is not performed in a blinded fashion. As this study was performed in a comprehensive stroke center, the number of LVO may be increased compared to regional stroke centers, which leads to an increased number of ischemic strokes compared to other centers. However, based on the observations including a significant reduction of door-to-groin times and secure triage of patients with hemorrhagic strokes, we have started a prospective, randomized trial in order to prove the effectiveness and safety of the proposed one-stop protocol.

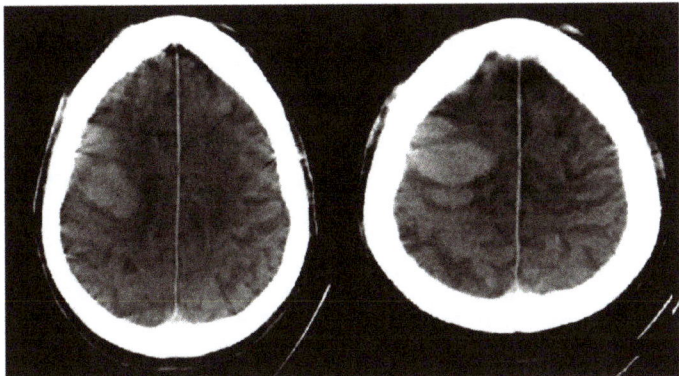

Figure 2. FDCT scan of intracranial hemorrhage which was missed by resident during off-hours.

5. Conclusions

One-stop management of stroke patients with a modern, FDCT-supporting angiography suite is feasible and allows for significantly shorter intrahospital times.

Author Contributions: Conception and Design of the work (M.-N.P., M.K., J.L., M.B.), Acquisition of the data (I.L.M., I.T., A.C.H., A.B., D.B., M.S., K.S.), Analysis and interpretation of the data (M.-N.P., I.P., D.S.L., M.G.), Drafting the work (M.-N.P.), Revising it critically for important intellectual property (All Authors), Final approval of the version to be published (All Authors), Accountable for all aspects of the work (M.-N.P., J.L.).

Funding: The Department of Neuroradiology, University Medical Center Goettingen, has a research agreement with Siemens Healthcare GmbH, Forchheim, Germany.

Conflicts of Interest: M.-N.P. and M.K. have received speaker's honoraria from Siemens Healthcare GmbH, Forchheim, Germany. The other authors have nothing to declare.

References

1. Goyal, M.; Menon, B.K.; van Zwam, W.H.; Dippel, D.W.J.; Mitchell, P.J.; Demchuk, A.M.; Dávalos, A.; Majoie, C.B.L.M.; van der Lugt, A.; de Miquel, M.A.; et al. Endovascular thrombectomy after large-vessel ischaemic stroke: A meta-analysis of individual patient data from five randomised trials. *Lancet* **2016**, *387*, 1723–1731. [CrossRef]
2. Saver, J.L.; Goyal, M.; van der Lugt, A.; Menon, B.K.; Majoie, C.B.; Dippel, D.W.; Campbell, B.C.; Nogueira, R.G.; Demchuk, A.M.; Tomasello, A.; et al. Time to Treatment With Endovascular Thrombectomy and Outcomes From Ischemic Stroke: A Meta-analysis. *JAMA* **2016**, *316*, 1279–1288. [CrossRef] [PubMed]
3. Berkhemer, O.A.; Fransen, P.S.; Beumer, D.; van den Berg, L.A.; Lingsma, H.F.; Yoo, A.J.; Schonewille, W.J.; Vos, J.A.; Nederkoorn, P.J.; Wermer, M.J.; et al. A randomized trial of intraarterial treatment for acute ischemic stroke. *N. Engl. J. Med.* **2015**, *372*, 11–20. [CrossRef]
4. Campbell, B.C.V.; Mitchell, P.J.; Kleinig, T.J.; Dewey, H.M.; Churilov, L.; Yassi, N.; Yan, B.; Dowling, R.J.; Parsons, M.W.; Oxley, T.J.; et al. Endovascular Therapy for Ischemic Stroke with Perfusion-Imaging Selection. *N. Engl. J. Med.* **2015**, *372*, 1009–1018. [CrossRef] [PubMed]
5. Saver, J.L.; Goyal, M.; Bonafe, A.; Diener, H.C.; Levy, E.I.; Pereira, V.M.; Albers, G.W.; Cognard, C.; Cohen, D.J.; Hacke, W.; et al. Stent-retriever thrombectomy after intravenous t-PA vs. t-PA alone in stroke. *N. Engl. J. Med.* **2015**, *372*, 2285–2295. [CrossRef] [PubMed]
6. Goyal, M.; Demchuk, A.M.; Menon, B.K.; Eesa, M.; Rempel, J.L.; Thornton, J.; Roy, D.; Jovin, T.G.; Willinsky, R.A.; Sapkota, B.L.; et al. Randomized Assessment of Rapid Endovascular Treatment of Ischemic Stroke. *N. Engl. J. Med.* **2015**, *372*, 1019–1030. [CrossRef]
7. Jovin, T.G.; Chamorro, A.; Cobo, E.; de Miquel, M.A.; Molina, C.A.; Rovira, A.; San Roman, L.; Serena, J.; Abilleira, S.; Ribo, M.; et al. Thrombectomy within 8 hours after symptom onset in ischemic stroke. *N. Engl. J. Med.* **2015**, *372*, 2296–2306. [CrossRef]

8. Psychogios, M.N.; Behme, D.; Schregel, K.; Tsogkas, I.; Maier, I.L.; Leyhe, J.R.; Zapf, A.; Tran, J.; Bahr, M.; Liman, J.; et al. One-Stop Management of Acute Stroke Patients: Minimizing Door-to-Reperfusion Times. *Stroke* **2017**, *48*, 3152–3155. [CrossRef]
9. Leyhe, J.R.; Tsogkas, I.; Hesse, A.C.; Behme, D.; Schregel, K.; Papageorgiou, I.; Liman, J.; Knauth, M.; Psychogios, M.-N. Latest generation of flat detector CT as a peri-interventional diagnostic tool: A comparative study with multidetector CT. *J. Neurointerv. Surg.* **2017**, *9*, 1253–1257. [CrossRef]
10. Maier, I.L.; Scalzo, F.; Leyhe, J.R.; Schregel, K.; Behme, D.; Tsogkas, I.; Psychogios, M.-N.; Liebeskind, D.S. Validation of collateral scoring on flat-detector multiphase CT angiography in patients with acute ischemic stroke. *PLoS ONE* **2018**, *13*, e0202592. [CrossRef]
11. Schregel, K.; Behme, D.; Tsogkas, I.; Knauth, M.; Maier, I.; Karch, A.; Mikolajczyk, R.; Hinz, J.; Liman, J.; Psychogios, M.N. Effects of Workflow Optimization in Endovascularly Treated Stroke Patients—A Pre-Post Effectiveness Study. *PLoS ONE* **2016**, *11*, e0169192. [CrossRef] [PubMed]
12. Psychogios, M.N.; Bahr, M.; Liman, J.; Knauth, M. One Stop Management in Acute Stroke: First Mothership Patient Transported Directly to the Angiography Suite. *Clin. Neuroradiol.* **2017**, *27*, 389–391. [CrossRef] [PubMed]
13. Holodinsky, J.K.; Kamal, N.; Wilson, A.T.; Hill, M.D.; Goyal, M. Workflow in Acute Stroke: What Is the 90th Percentile? *Stroke* **2017**, *48*, 808–812. [CrossRef] [PubMed]
14. Albers, G.W.; Marks, M.P.; Kemp, S.; Christensen, S.; Tsai, J.P.; Ortega-Gutierrez, S.; McTaggart, R.A.; Torbey, M.T.; Kim-Tenser, M.; Leslie-Mazwi, T.; et al. Thrombectomy for Stroke at 6 to 16 Hours with Selection by Perfusion Imaging. *N. Engl. J. Med.* **2018**, *379*, 708–718. [CrossRef] [PubMed]
15. Nogueira, R.G.; Frei, D.; Kirmani, J.F.; Zaidat, O.; Lopes, D.; Turk, A.S., 3rd; Heck, D.; Mason, B.; Haussen, D.C.; Levy, E.I.; et al. Safety and Efficacy of a 3-Dimensional Stent Retriever With Aspiration-Based Thrombectomy vs Aspiration-Based Thrombectomy Alone in Acute Ischemic Stroke Intervention: A Randomized Clinical Trial. *JAMA Neurol.* **2018**, *75*, 304–311. [CrossRef] [PubMed]
16. Schregel, K.; Behme, D.; Tsogkas, I.; Knauth, M.; Maier, I.; Karch, A.; Mikolajczyk, R.; Bähr, M.; Schäper, J.; Hinz, J.; et al. Optimized Management of Endovascular Treatment for Acute Ischemic Stroke. *J. Vis. Exp.* **2018**, *131*, e56397. [CrossRef]
17. Maus, V.; Behme, D.; Kabbasch, C.; Borggrefe, J.; Tsogkas, I.; Nikoubashman, O.; Wiesmann, M.; Knauth, M.; Mpotsaris, A.; Psychogios, M.N. Maximizing First-Pass Complete Reperfusion with SAVE. *Clin. Neuroradiol.* **2017**, *28*, 327–338. [CrossRef]
18. Bourcier, R.; Goyal, M.; Liebeskind, D.S.; Muir, K.W.; Desal, H.; Siddiqui, A.H.; Dippel, D.W.J.; Majoie, C.B.; van Zwam, W.H.; Jovin, T.G.; et al. Association of Time From Stroke Onset to Groin Puncture With Quality of Reperfusion After Mechanical Thrombectomy: A Meta-analysis of Individual Patient Data From 7 Randomized Clinical Trials. *JAMA Neurol.* **2019**, *76*, 405–411. [CrossRef]
19. Strub, W.M.; Leach, J.L.; Tomsick, T.; Vagal, A. Overnight preliminary head CT interpretations provided by residents: Locations of misidentified intracranial hemorrhage. *AJNR Am. J. Neuroradiol.* **2007**, *28*, 1679–1682. [CrossRef]
20. Heldner, M.R.; Hsieh, K.; Broeg-Morvay, A.; Mordasini, P.; Buhlmann, M.; Jung, S.; Arnold, M.; Mattle, H.P.; Gralla, J.; Fischer, U. Clinical prediction of large vessel occlusion in anterior circulation stroke: Mission impossible? *J. Neurol.* **2016**, *263*, 1633–1640. [CrossRef]
21. Pfaff, J.; Schonenberger, S.; Herweh, C.; Pham, M.; Nagel, S.; Ringleb, P.A.; Heiland, S.; Bendszus, M.; Mohlenbruch, M.A. Influence of a combined CT/C-arm system on periprocedural workflow and procedure times in mechanical thrombectomy. *Eur. Radiol.* **2017**, *27*, 3966–3972. [CrossRef] [PubMed]
22. Ribo, M.; Boned, S.; Rubiera, M.; Tomasello, A.; Coscojuela, P.; Hernández, D.; Pagola, J.; Juega, J.; Rodriguez, N.; Muchada, M.; et al. Direct transfer to angiosuite to reduce door-to-puncture time in thrombectomy for acute stroke. *J. Neurointerv. Surg.* **2018**, *10*, 221–224. [CrossRef] [PubMed]

23. Jadhav, A.P.; Kenmuir, C.L.; Aghaebrahim, A.; Limaye, K.; Wechsler, L.R.; Hammer, M.D.; Starr, M.T.; Molyneaux, B.J.; Rocha, M.; Guyette, F.X.; et al. Interfacility Transfer Directly to the Neuroangiography Suite in Acute Ischemic Stroke Patients Undergoing Thrombectomy. *Stroke* **2017**, *48*, 1884–1889. [CrossRef] [PubMed]
24. Mendez, B.; Requena, M.; Aires, A.; Martins, N.; Boned, S.; Rubiera, M.; Tomasello, A.; Coscojuela, P.; Muchada, M.; Rodríguez-Luna, D.; et al. Direct Transfer to Angio-Suite to Reduce Workflow Times and Increase Favorable Clinical Outcome. *Stroke* **2018**, *49*, 2723–2727. [CrossRef] [PubMed]

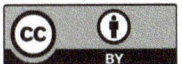

© 2019 by the authors. Licensee MDPI, Basel, Switzerland. This article is an open access article distributed under the terms and conditions of the Creative Commons Attribution (CC BY) license (http://creativecommons.org/licenses/by/4.0/).

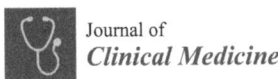

Article

Potential Utility of Neurosonology in Paroxysmal Atrial Fibrillation Detection in Patients with Cryptogenic Stroke

Chrissoula Liantinioti [1], Lina Palaiodimou [1], Konstantinos Tympas [2], John Parissis [2], Aikaterini Theodorou [1], Ignatios Ikonomidis [2], Maria Chondrogianni [1], Christina Zompola [1], Sokratis Triantafyllou [1], Andromachi Roussopoulou [1], Odysseas Kargiotis [3], Aspasia Serdari [4], Anastasios Bonakis [1], Konstantinos Vadikolias [4], Konstantinos Voumvourakis [1], Leonidas Stefanis [1,5], Gerasimos Filippatos [2] and Georgios Tsivgoulis [1,*]

[1] Second Department of Neurology, "Attikon" University Hospital, School of Medicine, National and Kapodistrian University of Athens, 12462 Athens, Greece; chrissa21@hotmail.com (C.L.); lina_palaiodimou@yahoo.gr (L.P.); katetheo24@gmail.com (A.T.); mariachondrogianni@hotmail.gr (M.C.); chriszompola@yahoo.gr (C.Z.); socrates_tr@hotmail.com (S.T.); an.rousso@yahoo.gr (A.R.); bonakistasos@yahoo.com (A.B.); cvoumvou@otenet.gr (K.V.); lstefanis@bioacademy.gr (L.S.)

[2] Second Department of Cardiology, "Attikon" University Hospital, Medical School, National and Kapodistrian University of Athens, 12462 Athens, Greece; kostas.tympas@yahoo.gr (K.T.); jparissis@yahoo.com (J.P.); ignoik@gmail.com (I.I.); geros@otenet.gr (G.F.)

[3] Stroke Unit, Metropolitan Hospital, 18547 Piraeus, Greece; kargiody@gmail.com

[4] Department of Neurology, University Hospital of Alexandroupolis, Democritus University of Thrace, School of Medicine, 68100 Alexandroupolis, Greece; aserdari@yahoo.com (A.S.); vadikosm@yahoo.com (K.V.)

[5] First Department of Neurology, Eginition Hospital, National and Kapodistrian University of Athens, School of Medicine, 11528 Athens, Greece

* Correspondence: tsivgoulisgiorg@yahoo.gr; Tel.: +30-693-717-8635; Fax: +30-210-583-2471

Received: 12 October 2019; Accepted: 14 November 2019; Published: 16 November 2019

Abstract: Background: Occult paroxysmal atrial fibrillation (PAF) is a common and potential treatable cause of cryptogenic stroke (CS). We sought to prospectively identify independent predictors of atrial fibrillation (AF) detection in patients with CS and sinus rhythm on baseline electrocardiogram (ECG), without prior AF history. We had hypothesized that cardiac arrhythmia detection during neurosonology examinations (Carotid Duplex (CDU) and Transcranial Doppler (TCD)) may be associated with higher likelihood of AF detection. Methods: Consecutive CS patients were prospectively evaluated over a six-year period. Demographics, clinical and imaging characteristics of cerebral ischemia were documented. The presence of arrhythmia during spectral waveform analysis of CDU/TCD was recorded. Left atrial enlargement was documented during echocardiography using standard definitions. The outcome event of interest included PAF detection on outpatient 24-h Holter ECG recordings. Statistical analyses were performed using univariate and multivariate logistic regression models. Results: A total of 373 patients with CS were evaluated (mean age 60 ± 11 years, 67% men, median NIHSS-score 4 points). The rate of PAF detection of any duration on Holter ECG recordings was 11% (95% CI 8%–14%). The following three variables were independently associated with the likelihood of AF detection on 24-h Holter-ECG recordings in both multivariate analyses adjusting for potential confounders: age (OR per 10-year increase: 1.68; 95% CI: 1.19–2.37; p = 0.003), moderate or severe left atrial enlargement (OR: 4.81; 95% CI: 1.77–13.03; p = 0.002) and arrhythmia detection during neurosonology evaluations (OR: 3.09; 95% CI: 1.47–6.48; p = 0.003). Conclusion: Our findings underline the potential utility of neurosonology in improving the detection rate of PAF in patients with CS.

Keywords: cryptogenic stroke; atrial fibrillation; neurosonology; Holter monitoring; transcranial Doppler; cervical duplex

1. Introduction

The etiology of acute cerebral ischemia (ACI) remains undetermined in more than one-third of all ischemic stroke (IS) patients upon discharge [1,2]. According to Trial of ORG 10172 in Acute Stroke Treatment (TOAST) classification, an IS is classified as cryptogenic stroke (CS) when no cause can be identified after the baseline diagnostic workup [3]. A well-defined etiopathogenic mechanism is cardioembolism, which actually accounts for 17% to 30% of all IS, with more than half of cardioembolic strokes being attributed to atrial fibrillation (AF) [4–6]. However, paroxysmal AF (PAF) is frequently undetected, due to episodic and asymptomatic nature and short duration [7]. It is therefore evident that a proportion of strokes labeled as CS are cardioembolic in origin because of occult PAF [8].

The detection of PAF is of utmost importance in order to provide the most suitable treatment for stroke secondary prevention. Antiplatelet treatment, advocated by current guideline recommendations for patients with CS [9], is known to provide inadequate protection from future cardioembolic events in patients with AF [10]. On the contrary, it has been estimated that the administration of anticoagulant therapy reduces the annual IS recurrence risk by 8.4% compared with antiplatelet therapy in IS patients with AF [11]. Both ESO/AHA guidelines recommend at least 24-h Holter monitoring in patients with CS to detect PAF [9,12].

Neurovascular imaging is also essential for accurate delineation of the stroke mechanism and the development of acute stroke therapies [13]. Carotid duplex ultrasound (CDU) and transcranial doppler ultrasound (TCD) are ancillary diagnostic tests in support of the etiological workup of IS and the evaluation of neurovascular status [14,15]. Both neurosonological modalities can be performed at the bedside in the very early stages of IS and are relatively inexpensive and noninvasive. Additionally, they allow monitoring and provide actual hemodynamic information. Thus, CDU and TCD may detect heart rhythm alterations in real-time during spectral waveform analysis [16,17] and provide complementary information to 24-h Holter-ECG recordings.

In view of former considerations, we sought to identify independent predictors of AF detection in patients with CS and sinus rhythm on baseline cardiac evaluation (electrocardiogram (ECG) and 24-h Holter-ECG recordings), without prior AF history. More specifically, we had hypothesized that cardiac arrhythmia detected during neurosonology evaluation (CDU and TCD) may be associated with higher likelihood of AF detection.

2. Methods

Consecutive patients with CS, no prior AF history and sinus rhythm on the baseline ECG and the 24-h Holter-ECG recordings were prospectively evaluated at a tertiary care stroke center ("Attikon" University Hospital, National and Kapodistrian University of Athens, Athens, Greece) over a six-year period. CS was defined according to TOAST criteria [3], following an extensive diagnostic workup of all patients presenting with symptoms of ischemic stroke (IS) or transient ischemic attack (TIA). More specifically, all patients underwent the following laboratory and imaging examinations: brain CT-scan or MRI-scan, full blood count, biochemical blood analysis (cholesterol and glucose values included), ECG, cardiac ultrasound, 24-h Holter heart-rhythm monitoring, CDU and TCD. Additional information regarding the diagnostic workup of CS patients in our center has been previously described [18,19].

Stroke severity at hospital admission was documented using National Institute of Health Stroke Scale (NIHSS) score [20] by certified vascular neurologists [18,19]. Baseline characteristics including demographics, vascular risk factors, admission NIHSS-scores, neuroimaging and neurosonology findings, echocardiographic measurements, and number of 24-h Holter monitoring evaluations were recorded. Radiologists blinded to the patients' clinical data analyzed neuroimaging examinations and cerebral infarctions were subsequently categorized according to their location as either cortical or non-cortical including subcortical, brainstem and cerebellar location [21].

CDU and TCD examinations were performed by a certified neurosonologist (GT) with a Refurbished Philips® CX50 portable ultrasound machine, using L12-3 and S5-1 ultrasound transducer probes respectively. Neurosonology examinations were performed in each patient within 48 h from hospital admission. Irregular duration of the intervals between consecutive peak-systolic velocities during spectral waveform analysis of extra- or intra-cranial arteries in at least three complexes indicated the presence of cardiac arrhythmia and this finding was prospectively documented. (Figure 1) [16,17]. Echocardiogram was performed by certified cardiologists and left atrial (LA) diameter was measured using standardized methodology as previously described [22]. LA enlargement was classified into mild, moderate or severe, according to the guidelines of the American Society of Echocardiography (ASE) [23].

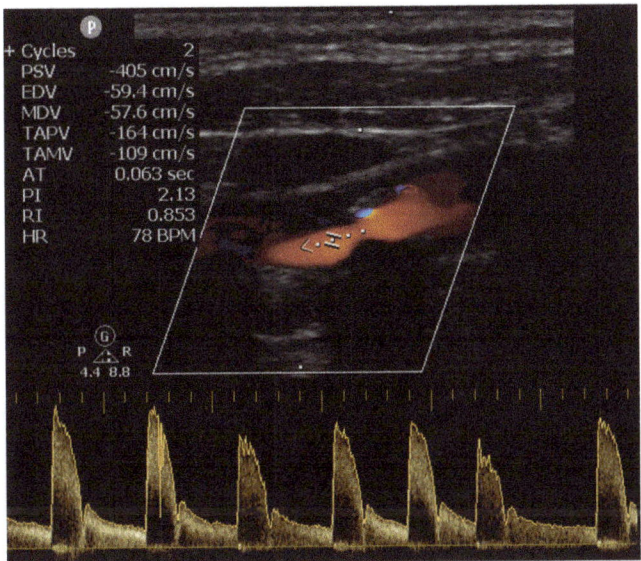

Figure 1. Detection of cardiac arrhythmia during spectral waveform analysis of external carotid artery in cervical duplex ultrasound.

Twenty-four-hour Holter ECG was performed using a 12-channel Holter monitoring Mortara H12+™ instrument. The inpatient recordings were completed within 96 h from hospital admission. It should be emphasized that sinus rhythm on baseline 24-h Holter ECG was a prerequisite for patients' inclusion in our study and for the diagnosis of CS [3]. During the follow-up period that varied between three to 60 months, CS patients underwent ≥1 outpatient 24-h Holter ECG recordings, based on the presence of premature atrial contractions on the baseline 24-h Holter ECG and that decision was not related to the neurosonology findings. The primary outcome event of interest included PAF detection of any duration as previously described [18]. Two blinded investigators using dedicated analysis software analyzed all ECG recordings [18]. Total time in AF was calculated as the sum of each individual AF episode for patients with multiple episodes during monitoring. The secondary outcome of interest included the current definition of PAF according to ACC/AHA/ESC guidelines, which applies to AF episodes without a reversible cause lasting >30 s [24].

The study protocol was approved by the ethics committee of our hospital and signed informed consent was obtained from the patient or legal representative before enrollment in all cases.

Statistical Analyses

Continuous variables are presented as mean ± SD (normal distribution) and as median with interquartile range (skewed distribution). Categorical variables are presented as percentages with their corresponding 95% Confidence Intervals (95% CI). Statistical comparisons between two groups were performed using χ^2 test, or in case of small expected frequencies, Fisher's exact test. Continuous variables were compared by the use of the unpaired t-test or Mann–Whitney U test, as indicated. Univariable and multivariable binary logistic regression models were used to evaluate associations between baseline characteristics (demographics, vascular risk factors, stroke severity, neuroimaging and neurosonology findings, echocardiographic measurements, and number of 24-h Holter monitoring evaluations) with the likelihood of detecting AF on Holter monitoring in patients with CS before and after adjusting for potential confounders. A cut-off of $p < 0.1$ was used to select variables for inclusion in multivariable analyses that were conducted using backward stepwise selection procedure. To confirm the robustness of multivariable models, we repeated all multivariable analyses using a forward selection procedure. Associations are presented as odds ratios (OR) with corresponding 95% confidence intervals (CI). Statistical significance was achieved if the p value was ≤0.05 in multivariable logistic regression analyses. The Statistical Package for Social Science (SPSS Inc., Armonk, NY, USA; version 23.0 for Windows) was used for statistical analyses.

3. Results

A total of 373 patients with CS (mean age 60 ± 11 years, 67% men, median NIHSS score on admission: four, IQR: 3–10) underwent 24-h Holter-ECG evaluations during the six-year study period. The baseline characteristics of the study population are presented in Table 1. The mean CHA2DS2-VASC score and the mean number of outpatient 24-h Holter-ECG recordings were 3.8 ± 1.3 and 1.5 ± 1.5 respectively. Moderate or severe left atrial enlargement were present in 6% of the study population, while in 20% we detected cardiac arrhythmia during neurosonology evaluations.

Table 1. Baseline characteristics of the study population ($n = 373$).

Variable	Overall
Age, years (mean ± SD)	60 ± 11
Female sex (%)	122 (33%)
NIHSS-Score, points (median, IQR)	4 (3–10)
Hypertension (%)	230 (62%)
Diabetes (%)	82 (22%)
Hyperlipidemia (%)	215 (58%)
Current Smoking (%)	158 (22.5%)
Coronary Artery Disease (%)	58 (16%)
Excessive Alcohol Intake (%)	37 (10%)
Previous History of TIA or Stroke (%)	74 (20%)
Heart Failure (%)	17 (5%)
Peripheral Arterial Disease (%)	15 (4%)
Vascular Disease (%)	70 (19%)
CHA2DS2-VASc Score, Points (mean ± SD)	3.8 ± 1.3
Left Atrial Enlargement (%)	155 (42%)
Mild	133 (36%)
Moderate	17 (5%)
Severe	5 (1%)
Cortical Location of Infarction (%)	76 (20%)
Cardiac Arrhythmia Detected during Neurosonology Evaluation (%)	66 (18%)
Number of 24-h Holter Recordings (mean ± SD)	1.5 ± 1.5
1	254 (68%)
2	85 (23%)
≥3	34 (9%)

IQR: interquartile range, TIA: transient ischemic attack.

AF of any duration was documented on outpatient 24-h Holter-ECG recordings in 40 patients with CS (11%, 95% CI: 8–14%). The mean duration of AF was 4940 ± 1043 s, while in 12 patients (30% of AF patients) AF duration was ≤30 s. The detection rate of AF ≥30 s was 8% (95% CI: 5–11%) in our cohort. AF detection rates differed significantly ($p < 0.001$) according to the degree of left atrial enlargement (Table 2). More specifically, the rates of AF detection were 7%, 12%, and 36% in patients with no, mild, moderate, or severe left atrial enlargement respectively (p for linear trend <0.001). AF detection rates also differed significantly ($p = 0.048$) according to the number of 24-h Holter-ECG recordings (Table 3). More specifically, the rates of AF detection were 8%, 14%, and 21% in patients with 1, 2, and ≥3 Holter recordings respectively (p for linear trend 0.014).

Table 2. Prevalence of atrial fibrillation detection on 24-h Holter monitoring stratified by degree of left atrial enlargement.

Left Atrial Enlargement	Atrial Fibrillation (−)	Atrial Fibrillation (+)	p-Value *	p-Value for Linear Trend **
None (%)	93%	7%		
Mild (%)	88%	12%	<0.001	<0.001
Moderate or Severe (%)	64%	36%		

* Pearson chi-square: 17.952 (df = 2); ** Linear by linear association: 12.887 (df = 1).

Table 3. Prevalence of atrial fibrillation detection on 24-h Holter monitoring stratified by the number of 24-h Holter-ECG recordings.

Number of 24-h Holter ECG Recordings	Atrial Fibrillation (−)	Atrial Fibrillation (+)	p Value *	p-Value for Linear Trend **
1 (%)	92%	8%		
2 (%)	86%	14%	0.048	0.014
≥3 (%)	79%	21%		

* Pearson chi-square: 6.079 (df = 2); ** Linear by linear association: 6.057 (df = 1).

Further evaluation regarding the cardiac structure was also conducted in a subset of our patients. Fifty-three percent of our patients (199/373) had undergone transesophageal echocardiogram (TEE). Cardiac CT and/or cardiac MRI were performed in three cases only, since these two investigations were not readily available in our hospital. All TEE, cardiac CT, and cardiac MRI investigations did not disclose any cardiogenic source of embolization in our cohort.

The univariable and multivariable associations of baseline characteristics with the likelihood of AF detection on 24-h Holter-ECG recordings are presented in Table 4. The following variables were associated with AF detection on initial univariable analyses using a p value of <0.1 as threshold for inclusion in multivariable models: age (OR per 10-year increase: 1.81; 95%CI: 1.31–2.50; $p < 0.001$), heart failure (OR: 2.74; 95% CI: 0.85–8.83; $p = 0.093$), CHA2DS2-VASC score (OR per 1-point increase: 1.53; 95% CI: 1.20–1.941; $p = 0.001$), ≥3 Holter recordings (OR: 2.40; 95% CI: 0.97–5.95; $p = 0.058$), moderate or severe left atrial enlargement (OR: 5.70; 95% CI: 2.22–14.61; $p < 0.001$), and cardiac arrhythmia detection during neurosonology evaluations (OR: 3.77; 95% CI: 1.87–7.60; $p < 0.001$). The following three variables were independently ($p < 0.05$) associated with the likelihood of AF detection on 24-h Holter-ECG recordings in multivariable logistic regression analyses conducted by backward selection procedure: age (OR per 10-year increase: 1.68; 95% CI: 1.19–2.37; $p = 0.003$), moderate or severe left atrial enlargement (OR: 4.81; 95% CI: 1.77–13.03; $p = 0.002$), and cardiac arrhythmia detection during neurosonology evaluations (OR: 3.09; 95%CI: 1.47–6.48; $p = 0.003$). We repeated the multivariable analyses using the forward selection procedure and obtained identical results. The independent associations of age (OR per 10-year increase: 1.68; 95% CI: 1.19–2.37; $p = 0.003$), moderate or severe left atrial enlargement (OR: 4.81; 95%CI: 1.77–13.03; $p = 0.002$) and cardiac arrhythmia detection during neurosonology evaluations (OR: 3.09; 95% CI: 1.47–6.48; $p = 0.003$) with the likelihood of AF detection persisted also on multivariable logistic regression analyses conducted by the forward selection procedure.

Table 4. Univariable and multivariable logistic regression analyses depicting the associations of baseline characteristics with the likelihood of atrial fibrillation detection during 24-h Holter monitoring.

Variable	Univariable Logistic Regression Analysis		Multivariable Logistic Regression Analysis	
	Odds Ratio (95%CI)	p *	Odds Ratio (95%CI)	p
Age (per 10-year increase)	1.81 (1.31–2.50)	<0.001	1.68 (1.19–2.37)	0.003
Female Sex	1.43 (0.73–2.80)	0.300		
NIHSS-Score at Admission (per 1-point increase)	0.97 (0.91–1.03)	0.295		
Hypertension	1.51 (0.74–3.08)	0.254		
Diabetes Mellitus	1.40 (0.67–2.94)	0.374		
Hyperlipidemia	1.60 (0.80–3.21)	0.185		
Previous History of TIA or Stroke	1.20 (0.54–2.64)	0.655		
Coronary Artery Disease	1.17 (0.49–2.80)	0.719		
Congestive Heart Failure	2.74 (0.85–8.83)	0.093	2.74 (0.85–8.83)	0.165
Current Smoking	1.22 (0.63–2.35)	0.558		
Excessive Alcohol Intake	1.34 (0.49–3.67)	0.565		
Peripheral Arterial Disease	1.30 (0.28–5.96)	0.739		
Vascular Disease	1.09 (0.48–2.49)	0.833		
CHA2DS2-VASc Score (per 1-point increase)	1.53 (1.20–1.94)	0.001	1.15 (0.80–1.66)	0.451
≥3 (24-h) Holter Evaluations	2.40 (0.97–5.95)	0.058	1.62 (0.58–4.52)	0.354
Cortical Location of Infarction	1.35 (0.63–2.90)	0.444		
Cardiac Arrhythmia Detected during Neurosonology Evaluation	3.77 (1.87–7.60)	<0.001	3.09 (1.47–6.48)	0.003
Moderate or Severe Left Atrial Enlargement	5.70 (2.22–14.61)	<0.001	4.81 (1.77–13.03)	0.002

* cutoff of $p < 0.1$ was used for selection of candidate variables for inclusion in multivariable logistic regression models.

4. Discussion

Our prospective single-center cohort study showed that detection of PAF in patients with CS is independently associated with increasing age, LA enlargement, and cardiac arrhythmia detection during neurosonology evaluations. In addition, the detection rates of AF of any duration and AF ≥ 30 s on outpatient 24-h Holter-ECG recordings were 11% and 8% respectively in our cohort.

There is mounting literature suggesting that newly diagnosed AF is identified in ≈5% of patients with stroke in the inpatient setting [25], while the rate of PAF detection in CS patients varies between 5–20%, according to different studies and prolonged Holter-ECG monitoring [26–28]. Repetition of 24-h Holter recording can detect AF at a higher rate, as it was also demonstrated in the present study, but it still carries lower diagnostic yield compared to continuous arrhythmia monitoring [29]. The detection of occult PAF has important therapeutic implications in CS patients, as anticoagulation is the optimal treatment for secondary stroke prevention in AF-associated stroke and can substantially reduce recurrent stroke and systemic embolism compared to antiplatelet therapy [30–34]. Furthermore, secondary prevention in CS includes oral anticoagulation when AF is detected, regardless of AF pattern (paroxysmal or chronic). Notably, the benefit of oral anticoagulation therapy in secondary stroke prevention in patients with AF has been established both for chronic and intermittent AF [35].

Another important finding is that AF duration was ≤30 s in 30% of the patients recognized with AF in outpatient Holter monitoring in our study, while the current American College of Cardiology/American Heart Association definition of PAF requires >30 s as a threshold for AF diagnosis [24]. However, AF of any duration should be considered clinically relevant in patients with CS, as recognized bursts of PAF may be markers of longer periods of AF that occur outside of the monitoring period. Interestingly, prior studies in CS patients have used a variety of time thresholds, ranging from 0 s to 5 minutes, reflecting the lack of consensus regarding AF duration yield [36–38].

Our study also disclosed an association between advancing age and detection of PAF in patients with CS, which persisted on multivariable analysis. This finding is consistent with other cohort studies, which demonstrated that older age was an independent predictor of occult PAF in CS patients [39,40].

AF detection on 24-h Holter monitoring is also associated with LA enlargement. According to our study, the rates of AF detection were 7%, 12% and 36% in patients with no, mild, moderate or severe left atrial enlargement respectively and that association was statistically significant. However, the metric used for indicating LA in our study was the LA diameter, whereas LA volume indexed to the subjects' body surface area, which represents a three-dimensional size of the LA is thought to be a superior metric of LA dimension in terms of predicting cardiovascular outcomes [41]. A recent study outlined the association of higher LA volume index with cardioembolic stroke and the rate of AF detection in patients with embolic stroke of undetermined source (ESUS), who completed four-week outpatient cardiac event monitoring [42]. ESUS is a subtype of CS and is used to describe non-lacunar CS in which embolism is a likely underlying mechanism [43]. However, ESUS constitutes a heterogenous group of patients, in whom other embolic mechanisms (patent foramen ovale, aortic plaque, non-stenosing unstable carotid plaque, cardiac valve disorders, coagulation disorders in patients with occult cancer) might be responsible for stroke, except for occult AF. Those underlying mechanisms mandate different management than oral anticoagulation, thus clinical utility of ESUS is debatable [44]. Consequently, our findings lend support to the recent concept that LA diameter measurement may help stratify ESUS patients with the greater benefit from anticoagulation due to underlying occult AF [44].

The potential diagnostic utility of neurosonology examinations (CDU and TCD) in the early detection of PAF in patients with CS is also supported by our results. Specifically, it was shown that cardiac arrhythmia detection during spectral waveform analysis in CDU/TCD evaluations was associated with the likelihood of AF detection on outpatient 24-h Holter-ECG recordings. A plausible explanation for this association may be related to the psychological stress induced by the TCD and CDU examinations to the patients that in turn may provoke episodes of arrhythmia, thus increasing the neurosonology rates of arrhythmia detection [45,46]. Being inexpensive, readily available, performed by-the-bed in the early stages of IS, even before the first 24-h Holter recording has been completed, CDU/TCD examination can be a useful tool for delineating stroke etiology in a multifactorial approach; both evaluating extracranial/intracranial vascular stenosis or occlusion and detecting cardiac arrhythmias in real-time [15–17]. One limiting factor is that, although neurosonology examinations can detect arrhythmias, it is not possible to differentiate them among the many different types and provide a certain diagnosis of AF. Abnormal neurosonology examination can represent AF as simple extra-systolic beats and consequently the specificity of this examination as a predictor of AF appears low. However, AF appears to account for a substantial proportion of rhythm abnormalities [47]. Even if the cardiac arrhythmia detected by neurosonology examinations is finally diagnosed as paroxysmal supraventricular tachycardia (PSVT) in ECG studies, this is also clinically relevant information, as PSVT patients have higher prevalence rate of AF [48]. Consequently, arrhythmia detection by CDU/TCD can be used as a potential marker that may assist in the identification of CS patients that should undergo prolonged cardiac monitoring using implantable cardiac monitors. If the present findings are externally validated, the echocardiographic and neurosonology findings may be included in current risk stratification scores (e.g., HAVOC) and other schemata for AF detection in CS [49,50].

Certain limitations of the present study need to be acknowledged. First, the sample size of the present single center study was moderate ($n = 373$). Second, there was no core laboratory analysis of CDU/TCD recordings for arrhythmia detection and no central adjudication of neuroimaging parameters. However, considering that investigators evaluating neuroimaging and neurosonology studies were blinded to the AF status of each patient, it is unlikely that this may have led to significant bias. Third, ECG detection of AF in CS patients was assessed by repetitive short-term (24-h) external monitoring devices in an outpatient setting and such an intermittent monitoring strategy has lower sensitivity and lower negative predictive value than continuous arrhythmia monitoring. Moreover, patients were not under continuous ECG monitoring during hospitalization, since the policy of our institution did not allow prolonged cardiac monitoring with repeated 24-h Holter-ECG recordings or cardiac telemetry or implantable cardiac monitoring during hospitalization. Fourth, the optimal duration of CDU/TCD recording for arrhythmia detection was not assessed in our study. It may be postulated that a more prolonged recording, for example continuous 1-h TCD monitoring using a headframe in search of arrhythmia and microembolic signals as well, could have identified more episodes of rhythm abnormalities, making the correlation with AF detection on ECG recordings even stronger. Finally, data about other possible confounders, such as secondary prevention therapies or patients' body mass index (BMI) were not collected.

5. Conclusions

In conclusion, to the best of our knowledge, this is the first study demonstrating an independent association between arrhythmia detection during neurosonology examinations in the early stages of IS and the detection of AF on outpatient 24-h Holter-ECG recordings in CS patients. Our findings appear to expand the utility of CDU/TCD studies in determining stroke etiology. However, our study was not designed to evaluate the diagnostic utility of neurosonology in comparison to outpatient prolonged cardiac monitoring. Further external validation of the present findings in larger cohorts of patients with more extensive duration of cardiac monitoring is required.

Author Contributions: Study concept and design: C.L., G.T.; Acquisition of Data: C.L., L.P., K.T., J.P., A.T., I.I., M.C., C.Z., S.T., A.R., G.T.; Analysis and interpretation: C.L., L.P., A.T., G.T.; Critical revision of the manuscript for important intellectual content: C.L., L.P., K.T., J.P., A.T., I.I., M.C., C.Z., S.T., A.R., O.K., A.S., A.B., K.V. (Konstantinos Vadikolias), K.V. (Konstantinos Voumvourakis), L.S., G.F., G.T.

Funding: This research received no external funding.

Conflicts of Interest: The authors declare no conflict of interest.

References

1. Schulz, U.G.; Rothwell, P.M. Differences in vascular risk factors between etiological subtypes of ischemic stroke: Importance of population based studies. *Stroke* **2003**, *34*, 2050–2059. [CrossRef] [PubMed]
2. Tsivgoulis, G.; Patousi, A.; Pikilidou, M.; Birbilis, T.; Katsanos, A.H.; Mantatzis, M.; Asimis, A.; Papanas, N.; Skendros, P.; Terzoudi, A.; et al. Stroke incidence and outcomes in Northeastern Greece: The Evros stroke registry. *Stroke* **2018**, *49*, 288–295. [CrossRef] [PubMed]
3. Adams, H.P., Jr.; Bendixen, B.H.; Kappelle, L.J.; Biller, J.; Love, B.B.; Gordon, D.L.; Marsh, E.E., 3rd. Classification of subtype of acute ischemic stroke. Definitions for use in a multicenter clinical trial. TOAST. Trial of Org 10172 in Acute Stroke Treatment. *Stroke* **1993**, *24*, 35–41. [CrossRef] [PubMed]
4. Murtagh, B.; Smalling, R.W. Cardioembolic stroke. *Curr. Atheroscler.* **2006**, *8*, 310–316. [CrossRef]
5. Khoo, C.W.; Lip, G.Y. Clinical outcomes of acute stroke patients with atrial fibrillation. *Expert. Rev. Cardiovasc. Ther.* **2009**, *7*, 371–374. [CrossRef]
6. Arboix, A.; Vericat, M.C.; Pujades, R.; Massons, J.; García-Eroles, L.; Oliveres, M. Cardioembolic infarction in the Sagrat Cor-Alianza Hospital of Barcelona Stroke Registry. *Acta Neurol. Scand.* **1997**, *96*, 407–412. [CrossRef]
7. Lip, G.Y.; Hee, F.L. Paroxysmal atrial fibrillation. *QJM* **2001**, *94*, 665–678. [CrossRef]

8. Kishore, A.; Vail, A.; Majid, A.; Dawson, J.; Lees, K.R.; Tyrrell, P.J.; Smith, C.J. Detection of atrial fibrillation after ischemic stroke or transient ischemic attack: A systematic review and meta-analysis. *Stroke* **2014**, *45*, 520–526. [CrossRef]
9. Kernan, W.N.; Ovbiagele, B.; Black, H.R.; Bravata, D.M.; Chimowitz, M.I.; Ezekowitz, M.D.; Fang, M.C.; Fisher, M.; Furie, K.L.; Heck, D.V. Guidelines for the prevention of stroke in patients with stroke and transient ischemic attack: A guideline for healthcare professionals from the American Heart Association/American Stroke Association. *Stroke* **2014**, *45*, 2160–2236. [CrossRef]
10. EAFT (European Atrial Fibrillation Trial) Study Group. Secondary prevention in non-rheumatic atrial fibrillation after transient ischaemic attack or minor stroke. *Lancet* **1993**, *342*, 1255–1262. [CrossRef]
11. Hart, R.G.; Benavente, O.; McBride, R.; Pearce, L.A. Antithrombotic therapy to prevent stroke in patients with atrial fibrillation: A meta-analysis. *Ann. Intern. Med.* **1999**, *131*, 492–501. [CrossRef] [PubMed]
12. European Stroke Organisation (ESO); Executive Committee; ESO Writing Committee. Guidelines for management of ischaemic stroke and transient ischaemic attack 2008. *Cerebrovasc Dis.* **2008**, *25*, 457–507. [CrossRef] [PubMed]
13. Masdeu, J.C.; Irimia, P.; Asenbaum, S.; Bogousslavsky, J.; Brainin, M.; Chabriat, H.; Herholz, K.; Markus, H.S.; Martínez-Vila, E.; Niederkorn, K.; et al. EFNS guideline on neuroimaging in acute stroke. Report of an EFNS task force. *Eur. J. Neurol.* **2006**, *13*, 1271–1283. [CrossRef] [PubMed]
14. Qureshi, A.I.; Alexandrov, A.V.; Tegeler, C.H.; Hobson, R.W.; Dennis Baker, J.; Hopkins, L.N.; American Society of Neuroimaging; Society of Vascular and Interventional Neurology. Guidelines for screening of extracranial carotid artery disease: A statement for healthcare professionals from the multidisciplinary practice guidelines committee of the American Society of Neuroimaging; cosponsored by the Society of Vascular and Interventional Neurology. *J. Neurol.* **2007**, *17*, 19–47.
15. Alexandrov, A.V.; Sloan, M.A.; Wong, L.K.; Douville, C.; Razumovsky, A.Y.; Koroshetz, W.J.; Kaps, M.; Tegeler, C.H.; American Society of Neuroimaging Practice Guidelines Committee. Practice standards for transcranial Doppler ultrasound: Part I–test performance. *J. Neurol.* **2007**, *17*, 11–18.
16. Tsivgoulis, G.; Alexandrov, A.V.; Sloan, M.A. Advances in transcranial doppler ultrasonography. *Curr. Neurol. Neurosci. Rep.* **2009**, *9*, 46–54. [CrossRef]
17. Alexandrov, A.V.; Sloan, M.A.; Tegeler, C.H.; Newell, D.N.; Lumsden, A.; Garami, Z.; Levy, C.R.; Wong, L.K.; Douville, C.; Kaps, M.; et al. Practice standards for transcranial Doppler (TCD) ultrasound. Part II. Clinical indications and expected outcomes. *J. Neurol.* **2012**, *22*, 215–224.
18. Liantinioti, C.; Tympas, K.; Katsanos, A.H.; Parissis, J.; Chondrogianni, M.; Zompola, C.; Papadimitropoulos, G.; Ioakeimidis, M.; Triantafyllou, S.; Roussopoulou, A.; et al. Duration of paroxysmal atrial fibrillation in cryptogenic stroke is not associated with stroke severity and early outcomes. *J. Neurol. Sci.* **2017**, *376*, 191–195. [CrossRef]
19. Katsanos, A.H.; Bhole, R.; Frogoudaki, A.; Giannopoulos, S.; Goyal, N.; Vrettou, A.R.; Ikonomidis, I.; Paraskevaidis, I.; Pappas, K.; Parissis, J.; et al. The value of transesophageal echocardiography for embolic strokes of undetermined source. *Neurology* **2016**, *87*, 988–995. [CrossRef]
20. National Institute of Health, National Institute of Neurological Disorders and Stroke. Stroke Scale. Available online: https://www.ninds.nih.gov/sites/default/files/NIH_Stroke_Scale_Booklet.pdf (accessed on 3 September 2019).
21. Tsivgoulis, G.; Kargiotis, O.; Katsanos, A.H.; Patousi, A.; Mavridis, D.; Tsokani, S.; Pikilidou, M.; Birbilis, T.; Mantatzis, M.; Zompola, C.; et al. Incidence, characteristics and outcomes in patients with embolic stroke of undetermined source: A population-based study. *J. Neurol. Sci.* **2019**, *401*, 5–11. [CrossRef]
22. Ikonomidis, I.; Frogoudaki, A.; Vrettou, A.R.; Andreou, I.; Palaiodimou, L.; Katogiannis, K.; Liantinioti, C.; Vlastos, D.; Zervas, P.; Varoudi, M.; et al. Impaired Arterial Elastic Properties and Endothelial Glycocalyx in Patients with Embolic Stroke of Undetermined Source. *Thromb. Haemost.* **2019**. [Epub ahead of print]. [CrossRef] [PubMed]
23. Lang, R.M.; Bierig, M.; Devereux, R.B.; Flachskampf, F.A.; Foster, E.; Pellikka, P.A.; Picard, M.H.; Roman, M.J.; Seward, J.; Shanewise, J.S.; et al. Recommendations for chamber quantification: A report from the American Society of Echocardiography's Guidelines and Standards Committee and the Chamber Quantification Writing Group, developed in conjunction with the European Association of Echocardiography, a branch of the European Society of Cardiology. *J. Am. Soc. Echocardiogr.* **2005**, *18*, 1440–1463. [PubMed]

24. Heart, R.S.; Zipes, D.P.; Camm, A.J.; Borggrefe, M.; Buxton, A.E.; Chaitman, B.; Fromer, M.; Gregoratos, G.; Klein, G.; Moss, A.J.; et al. ACC/AHA/ESC 2006 Guidelines for the Management of Patients with Atrial Fibrillation: A report of the American College of Cardiology/American Heart Association Task Force on Practice Guidelines and the European Society of Cardiology Committee for Practice Guidelines (Writing Committee to Revise the 2001 Guidelines for the Management of Patients With Atrial Fibrillation): Developed in collaboration with the European Heart Rhythm Association and the Heart Rhythm Society. *Circulation* **2006**, *114*, e257–e354.
25. Liao, J.; Khalid, Z.; Scallan, C.; Morillo, C.; O'Donnell, M. Noninvasive cardiac monitoring for detecting paroxysmal atrial fibrillation or flutter after acute ischemic stroke: A systematic review. *Stroke* **2007**, *38*, 2935–2940. [CrossRef]
26. Sanna, T.; Diener, H.C.; Passman, R.S.; Di Lazzaro, V.; Bernstein, R.A.; Morillo, C.A.; Rymer, M.M.; Thijs, V.; Rogers, T.; Beckers, F.; et al. Cryptogenic Stroke and underlying Atrial Fibrillation. *N. Engl. J. Med.* **2014**, *370*, 2478–2486. [CrossRef]
27. Flint, A.C.; Banki, N.M.; Ren, X.; Rao, V.A.; Go, A.S. Detection of paroxysmal atrial fibrillation by 30-day event monitoring in cryptogenic ischemic stroke: The Stroke and Monitoring for PAF in Real Time (SMART) Registry. *Stroke* **2012**, *43*, 2788–2790. [CrossRef]
28. Seet, R.C.; Friedman, P.A.; Rabinstein, A.A. Prolonged rhythm monitoring for the detection of occult paroxysmal atrial fibrillation in ischemic stroke of unknown cause. *Circulation* **2011**, *26*, 477–486. [CrossRef]
29. Choe, W.C.; Passman, R.S.; Brachmann, J.; Morillo, C.A.; Sanna, T.; Bernstein, R.A.; Di Lazzaro, V.; Diener, H.C.; Rymer, M.M.; Beckers, F.; et al. A Comparison of Atrial Fibrillation Monitoring Strategies After Cryptogenic Stroke (from the Cryptogenic Stroke and Underlying AF Trial). *Am. J. Cardiol.* **2015**, *116*, 889–893. [CrossRef]
30. Hylek, E.M.; Go, A.S.; Chang, Y.; Jensvold, N.G.; Henault, L.E.; Selby, J.V.; Singer, D.E. Effect of intensity of oral anticoagulation on stroke severity and mortality in atrial fibrillation. *N. Engl. J. Med.* **2003**, *349*, 1019–1026. [CrossRef]
31. Evans, A.; Perez, I.; Yu, G.; Kalra, L. Secondary stroke prevention in atrial fibrillation: Lessons from clinical practice. *Stroke* **2000**, *31*, 2106–2111. [CrossRef]
32. Nieuwlaat, R.; Prins, M.H.; Le Heuzey, J.Y.; Vardas, P.E.; Aliot, E.; Santini, M.; Cobbe, S.M.; Widdershoven, J.W.; Baur, L.H.; Lévy, S.; et al. Prognosis, disease progression, and treatment of atrial fibrillation patients during 1 year: Follow-up of the Euro Heart Survey on atrial fibrillation. *Eur. Heart J.* **2008**, *29*, 1181–1189. [CrossRef] [PubMed]
33. Puccio, D.; Novo, G.; Baiamonte, V.; Nuccio, A.; Fazio, G.; Corrado, E.; Coppola, G.; Muratori, I.; Vernuccio, L.; Novo, S. Atrial fibrillation and mild cognitive impairment: What correlation? *Minerva Cardioangiol.* **2009**, *57*, 143–150. [PubMed]
34. Coppola, G.; Manno, G.; Mignano, A.; Luparelli, M.; Zarcone, A.; Novo, G.; Corrado, E. Management of Direct Oral Anticoagulants in Patients with Atrial Fibrillation Undergoing Cardioversion. *Medicina* **2019**, *55*, 660. [CrossRef] [PubMed]
35. Van Walraven, C.; Hart, R.G.; Singer, D.E.; Laupacis, A.; Connolly, S.; Petersen, P.; Koudstaal, P.J.; Chang, Y.; Hellemons, B. Oral anticoagulants vs aspirin in nonvalvular atrial fibrillation: An individual patient meta-analysis. *JAM* **2002**, *288*, 2441–2448. [CrossRef]
36. Elijovich, L.; Josephson, S.A.; Fung, G.L.; Smith, W.S. Intermittent atrial fibrillation may account for a large proportion of otherwise cryptogenic stroke: A study of 30-day cardiac event monitors. *J. Stroke Cerebrovasc. Dis.* **2009**, *18*, 185–189. [CrossRef]
37. Ziegler, P.D.; Glotzer, T.V.; Daoud, E.G.; Wyse, D.G.; Singer, D.E.; Ezekowitz, M.D.; Koehler, J.L.; Hilker, C.E. Incidence of newly detected atrial arrhythmias via implant-able devices in patients with a history of thromboembolic events. *Stroke* **2010**, *41*, 256–260. [CrossRef]
38. Gaillard, N.; Deltour, S.; Vilotijevic, B.; Hornych, A.; Crozier, S.; Leger, A.; Frank, R.; Samson, Y. Detection of paroxysmal atrial fibrillation with transtelephonic EKG in TIA or stroke patients. *Neurology* **2010**, *74*, 1666–1670. [CrossRef]
39. Alhadramy, O.; Jeerakathil, T.J.; Majumdar, S.R.; Najjar, E.; Choy, J.; Saqqur, M. Prevalence and predictors of paroxysmal atrial fibrillation on Holter monitor in patients with stroke or transient ischemic attack. *Stroke* **2010**, *41*, 2596–2600. [CrossRef]

40. Favilla, C.G.; Ingala, E.; Jara, J.; Fessler, E.; Cucchiara, B.; Messé, S.R.; Mullen, M.T.; Prasad, A.; Siegler, J.; Hutchinson, M.D.; et al. Predictors of finding occult atrial fibrillation after cryptogenic stroke. *Stroke* **2015**, *46*, 1210–1215. [CrossRef]
41. Tsang, T.S.; Abhayaratna, W.P.; Barnes, M.E.; Miyasaka, Y.; Gersh, B.J.; Bailey, K.R.; Cha, S.S.; Seward, J.B. Prediction of cardiovascular outcomes with left atrial size: Is volume superior to area or diameter? *J. Am. Coll. Cardiol.* **2006**, *47*, 1018–1023. [CrossRef]
42. Jordan, K.; Yaghi, S.; Poppas, A.; Chang, A.D.; Mac Grory, B.; Cutting, S.; Burton, T.; Jayaraman, M.; Tsivgoulis, G.; Sabeh, M.K.; et al. Left Atrial Volume Index Is Associated With Cardioembolic Stroke and Atrial Fibrillation Detection After Embolic Stroke of Undetermined Source. *Stroke* **2019**, *50*, 1997–2001. [CrossRef] [PubMed]
43. Hart, R.G.; Diener, H.C.; Coutts, S.B.; Easton, J.D.; Granger, C.B.; O'Donnell, M.J.; Sacco, R.L.; Connolly, S.J.; Cryptogenic Stroke/ESUS International Working Group. Embolic strokes of undetermined source: The case for a new clinical construct. *Lancet Neurol.* **2014**, *13*, 429–438. [CrossRef]
44. Tsivgoulis, G.; Katsanos, A.H.; Köhrmann, M.; Caso, V.; Lemmens, R.; Tsioufis, K.; Paraskevas, G.P.; Bornstein, N.M.; Schellinger, P.D.; Alexandrov, A.V.; et al. Embolic strokes of undetermined source: Theoretical construct or useful clinical tool? *Ther. Adv. Neurol. Disord.* **2019**, *12*, 1756286419851381. [CrossRef] [PubMed]
45. Hansson, A.; Madsen-Härdig, B.; Olsson, S.B. Arrhythmia-provoking factors and symptoms at the onset of paroxysmal atrial fibrillation: A study based on interviews with 100 patients seeking hospital assistance. *BMC Cardiovasc. Disord.* **2004**, *4*, 13. [CrossRef] [PubMed]
46. Severino, P.; Mariani, M.V.; Maraone, A.; Piro, A.; Ceccacci, A.; Tarsitani, L.; Maestrini, V.; Mancone, M.; Lavalle, C.; Pasquini, M.; et al. Triggers for Atrial Fibrillation: The Role of Anxiety. *Cardiol. Res. Pract.* **2019**, *2019*, 1208505. [CrossRef] [PubMed]
47. Khurshid, S.; Choi, S.H.; Weng, L.C.; Wang, E.Y.; Trinquart, L.; Benjamin, E.J.; Ellinor, P.T.; Lubitz, S. Frequency of Cardiac Rhythm Abnormalities in a Half Million Adults. *Circ. Arrhythm. Electrophysiol.* **2018**, *11*, e006273. [CrossRef]
48. Hamer, M.E.; Wilkinson, W.E.; Clair, W.K.; Page, R.L.; McCarthy, E.A.; Pritchett, E.L. Incidence of symptomatic atrial fibrillation in patients with paroxysmal supraventricular tachycardia. *J. Am. Coll. Cardiol.* **1995**, *25*, 984–988. [CrossRef]
49. Kwong, C.; Ling, A.Y.; Crawford, M.H.; Zhao, S.X.; Shah, N.H. A Clinical Score for Predicting Atrial Fibrillation in Patients with Cryptogenic Stroke or Transient Ischemic Attack. *Cardiology* **2017**, *138*, 133–140. [CrossRef]
50. Lip, G.Y.; Nieuwlaat, R.; Pisters, R.; Lane, D.A.; Crijns, H.J. Refining clinical risk stratification for predicting stroke and thromboembolism in atrial fibrillation using a novel risk factor-based approach: The euro heart survey on atrial fibrillation. *Chest* **2010**, *137*, 263–272. [CrossRef]

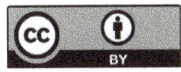

© 2019 by the authors. Licensee MDPI, Basel, Switzerland. This article is an open access article distributed under the terms and conditions of the Creative Commons Attribution (CC BY) license (http://creativecommons.org/licenses/by/4.0/).

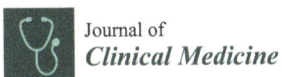 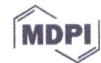

Article

Impact of the Total Number of Carotid Plaques on the Outcome of Ischemic Stroke Patients with Atrial Fibrillation

Hyungjong Park [1,2], Minho Han [1], Young Dae Kim [1], Joonsang Yoo [2], Hye Sun Lee [3], Jin Kyo Choi [1], Ji Hoe Heo [1] and Hyo Suk Nam [1,*]

[1] Department of Neurology, Yonsei University College of Medicine, Seoul 03722, Korea; hjpark209042@gmail.com (H.P.); UMSTHOL18@yuhs.ac (M.H.); neuro05@yuhs.ac (Y.D.K.); JKSNAIL85@yuhs.ac (J.K.C.); jhheo@yuhs.ac (J.H.H.)
[2] Department of Neurology, Keimyung University School of Medicine, Daegu 42601, Korea; quarksea@gmail.com
[3] Biostatistics Collaboration Unit, Yonsei University College of Medicine, university, Seoul 03722, Korea; HSLEE1@yuhs.ac
* Correspondence: hsnam@yuhs.ac; Tel.: +82-2-2228-1617; Fax: +82-2-393-0705

Received: 10 September 2019; Accepted: 31 October 2019; Published: 7 November 2019

Abstract: Background: Atrial fibrillation (AF) shares several risk factors with atherosclerosis. We investigated the association between total carotid plaque number (TPN) and long-term prognosis in ischemic stroke patients with AF. Methods: A total of 392 ischemic stroke patients with AF who underwent carotid ultrasonography were enrolled. TPN was assessed using B-mode ultrasound. The patients were categorized into two groups according to best cutoff values for TPN (TPN ≤ 4 vs. TPN ≥ 5). The long-term risk of major adverse cardiovascular events (MACE) and mortality according to TPN was investigated using a Cox hazard model. Results: After a mean follow-up of 2.42 years, 113 patients (28.8%) had developed MACE and 88 patients (22.4%) had died. MACE occurred more frequently in the TPN ≥ 5 group than in the TPN ≤ 4 group (adjusted hazard ratio [HR], 1.50; 95% confidence interval [CI], 1.01–2.21; $p < 0.05$). Moreover, the TPN ≥ 5 group showed an increased risk of all-cause mortality (adjusted HR, 2.69; 95% CI, 1.40–5.17; $p < 0.05$). TPN along with maximal plaque thickness and intima media thickness showed improved prognostic utility when added to the variables of the $CHAD_2DS_2$-VASc score. Conclusion: TPN can predict the long-term outcome of ischemic stroke patients with AF. Adding TPN to the $CHAD_2DS_2$-VASc score increases the predictability of outcome after stroke.

Keywords: atrial fibrillation; cerebral infarction; carotid stenosis; ultrasonography; outcomes

1. Introduction

Atrial fibrillation (AF) is the most common cause of cardioembolic stroke and is associated with poor prognosis in survivors after ischemic stroke. AF was reported to increase the annual risk of cardiovascular events by 5-fold [1,2]. In efforts to prevent cardiovascular events due to AF, researchers have focused on the identification of patients at high risk of developing cardiovascular events [3]. Several studies have suggested that atherosclerosis is associated with both the development and the outcome of AF [4]. For example, among the components of the $CHAD_2DS_2$-VASc score, age, hypertension, diabetes, history of stroke/transient ischemic attack, and vascular disease are known to be the important risk factors for atherosclerosis [5,6].

Carotid atherosclerosis ≥ 50% in patients with AF is well known to be an independent risk factor for future ischemic stroke and vascular events [7–9]. However, the prognostic implication of carotid atherosclerosis < 50% is not well known. Carotid ultrasonography can easily detect mild carotid atherosclerosis through measurements of the carotid intima media thickness (IMT) and carotid plaque thickness [8–10]. However, little is known about the prognostic impact of the number of carotid plaques on the outcome of patients with AF. In this regard, we evaluated the association between the total carotid plaque number (TPN) and long-term prognosis in ischemic stroke patients with AF.

2. Materials and Methods

2.1. Study Population

This is a hospital-based observational study in ischemic stroke patients who were prospectively registered to a stroke registry from January 2007 to December 2013 in Severance Hospital, Seoul, South Korea. [11]. The registry enrolled consecutive patients with acute ischemic stroke within 7 days of onset. During admission, all patients were evaluated with brain magnetic resonance imaging and/or computed tomography, as well as cerebral angiography (magnetic resonance angiography, computed tomography angiography, or digital subtraction angiography). Systemic evaluation included 12-lead electrocardiography (ECG), chest radiography, standard blood tests, lipid profile, and continuous ECG monitoring during stay in the stroke unit. Specific evaluation for finding the cardioembolic source, such as transthoracic echocardiography, transesophageal echocardiography, and 24-h Holter monitoring was done.

The stroke subtypes according to the Trial of ORG 10172 in Acute Stroke Treatment (TOAST) classification [12] and the presence of angiographic abnormalities were prospectively determined using neuroradiologist reports and the consensus of stroke specialists in weekly stroke conferences, and prospectively entered into a computerized database.

This study was approved by the institutional review board of Severance Hospital, Yonsei University Health System, which waived the requirement for informed consent from patients owing to the retrospective nature of the analysis.

2.2. Clinical Variables

We collected data on demographics and risk factors of stroke including hypertension, diabetes, hyperlipidemia, coronary artery disease, peripheral artery disease, history of stroke, transient ischemic accident or thromboembolism, and smoking habit. Hypertension was defined as a systolic blood pressure of ≥ 140 mmHg or a diastolic blood pressure of ≥ 90 mmHg, or any history of anti-hypertensive agent use. Diabetes was defined as fasting glucose level ≥ 7.0 mmol/L, random blood glucose level ≥ 11.0 mmol/L, glycated hemoglobin ≥ 6.5%, or a history of oral hypoglycemic agent or insulin use. Hyperlipidemia was defined as serum total cholesterol ≥ 6.21 mmol/L, low-density lipoprotein cholesterol ≥ 4.14 mmol/L, or any history of use of lipid-lowering agents after a diagnosis of hyperlipidemia. AF was diagnosed on the basis of the findings of routine ECG, Holter monitoring, or continuous ECG monitoring on the current admission or before admission. Paroxysmal AF was also considered the presence of AF. Congestive heart failure was determined from the history of heart failure diagnosis, treatment with loop diuretics, and ejection fraction ≤35% on echocardiography. Coronary artery occlusive disease (CAOD) was defined as any history of unstable angina, myocardial infarction, and CAOD. Peripheral artery occlusive disease was defined as any history of a diagnosis of peripheral artery disease at any hospital regardless of the presence or absence of intervention or medication for peripheral artery disease. Patients were considered current smokers if they had smoked any cigarettes within 1 year before admission. Medication history including anti-coagulant, anti-platelet, anti-hypertensive, and lipid-lowering agent use was collected. Laboratory data were also obtained for complete blood count, lipid profile, blood urea nitrogen level, and creatinine level. The severity of stroke was determined using the National Institute Health Stroke Scale (NIHSS) score at admission.

2.3. Carotid Artery Assessment

Carotid artery plaques were assessed using B-mode ultrasound (iU22 ultrasound system; Philips, Bothell, WA, USA) with a 3-9-MHz multifrequency linear array transducer. All measurements were done in a semi-dark room by two trained ultrasonographers. Bilateral longitudinal and transverse images of the common carotid arteries (CCAs) and internal carotid arteries (ICAs) were always obtained and the presence of plaque was decided after comparison of longitudinal and transverse images. The IMT in the CCAs was defined as the distance of the interface between the lumen-intima and the media-adventitia. The far wall of the carotid artery was visualized bilaterally in the CCAs (20–50 mm proximal to the bifurcation of blood flow), carotid bulb (0–20 mm proximal to the bifurcation of blood flow), and internal and external carotid arteries (0–20 mm distal to the bifurcation of blood flow). At 20, 25, and 30 mm proximal to the bifurcation of blood flow, IMT was bilaterally measured at the far wall of the CCAs during end-diastole, and calculated as the mean value for each patient. According to the Mannheim criteria [13], carotid plaque was defined as a focal structure encroaching into the arterial lumen by at least 0.5 mm, > 50% of surrounding IMT values, or thickness ≥ 1.5 mm above the distance of the interface between the lumen-intima and the media-adventitia.

The thickness of each plaque in the carotid arteries in the whole scanned area was also bilaterally measured. The TPN was determined by simply counting (bilaterally) the number of plaques in proximal ICAs and CCAs. The best cutoff values for TPN were determined using the Contal and O'Quigley method, which calculates the maximum hazard ratio (HR) based on log-rank statistics [14].

2.4. Follow-Up and Outcomes

After discharge, each patient was followed up with regularly at 3 months, 1 year, and yearly thereafter. At each follow-up visit, medical information including occurrence of any cardiovascular events, newly detected vascular risk factors, lifestyle modification after stroke, and re-admission to another hospital was obtained via face-to-face interviews with neurologists or through clinical research associates in the outpatient clinic. When the patients missed a scheduled visit, we obtained the information from the patients or their proxy through a telephone interview with a structured questionnaire [15]. In addition, we also obtained mortality data based on death certificates from the Korean National Statistical Office (http://www.kostat.go.kr).

The primary end point was major adverse cardiovascular events (MACE; cardiovascular mortality, non-cardiovascular mortality, and occurrence of non-fatal stroke or myocardial infarction). Cardiovascular mortality was defined as any mortality due to stroke, myocardial infarction, other cardiac disease, or unobserved sudden death. The secondary outcome was all-cause mortality. The censoring date was December 31, 2013.

2.5. Statistical Analysis

The data were presented as mean ± standard deviation or medians (interquartile range [IQR]), as appropriate. Differences between the two groups were compared with the chi-square test, Fisher's exact test, Student's *t*-test, and the Mann–Whitney U-test, as appropriate. Survival analysis was conducted, and survival curves were plotted using Kaplan–Meier analysis. The difference of survival time between groups was analyzed using a log-rank test. To determine the independent predictor of MACE and all-cause mortality, Cox proportional hazard regression analysis was used, and HR and 95% confidence interval (CI) values were summarized. Cox proportional hazard regression analysis was conducted with adjustments for age, sex, initial NIHSS score, and variables with $p < 0.1$ in the univariate analysis.

To evaluate the added value of carotid plaque burden for the prognosis of ischemic stroke caused by AF, we constructed the model incorporating variables in the CHA_2DS_2-VAS_c score and other variables associated with carotid plaque burden such as IMT, maximal carotid plaque thickness, and TPN. We compared the following five models: (1) CHA_2DS_2-VAS_c score variables alone; (2) addition of IMT; (3) addition of maximal carotid plaque thickness; (4) addition of TPN; and (5) addition of IMT, maximal carotid plaque thickness, and TPN. For internal validation of the newly developed model, time-dependent receiver-operating characteristic curves and areas under the curve (AUCs) were determined based on Heagerty's incident / dynamic AUCs during the median follow-up time [16]. A boot strapping method with 1000 re-samplings for calculating the 95% CI and the difference between the c-indices of each model was applied [17]. All tests were two-sided, and $p < 0.05$ was considered statistically significant. Statistical analysis was performed using R software, version 3.1.3 (R Foundation of Statistical Computing, Vienna, Austria).

3. Results

3.1. Patients' Characteristics

A total of 3727 consecutive ischemic stroke/transient ischemic attack patients were enrolled during the study period. After the exclusion of 2896 patients without AF, a total of 831 patients with AF remained. Among them, 150 patients without carotid ultrasonography and 76 patients with valvular heart disease were excluded. Patients who had > 50% stenosis in the intracranial or extracranial arteries ($n = 143$), complex aortic atheroma (≥ 4 mm or mobile atheroma) ($n = 6$), lacunar infarction ($n = 50$), and other rare etiologies ($n = 14$) according to the TOAST classification were also excluded. Finally, a total of 392 patients were analyzed (Figure 1).

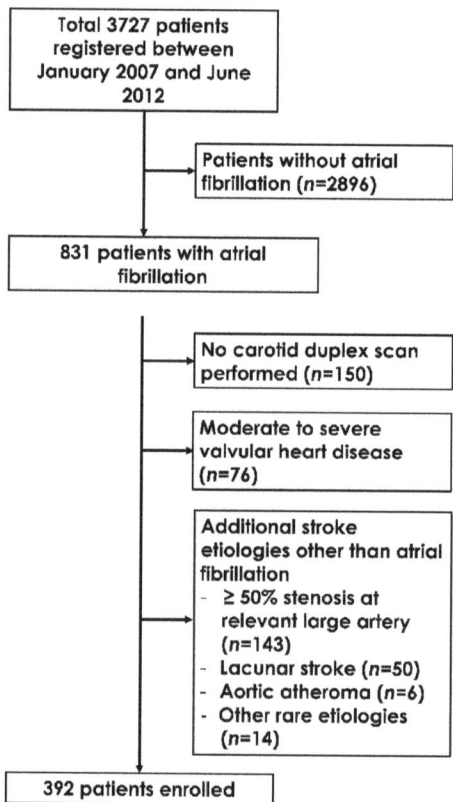

Figure 1. Flow sheet for study patients' selection.

The baseline characteristics of the enrolled patients are summarized in Table 1. The mean age of the total enrolled patients was 69.2 ± 10.3 years, and 225 (57.5%) patients were men. The median NIHSS score at admission was 5.5 (IQR 2–13). Before admission, 88 (22.4%) patients were taking oral anticoagulants. Carotid plaques were found in 343 (87.5%) patients. The median TPN was 3 (IQR 2–6). The median IMT and plaque thickness was 0.8 (IQR 0.7–0.9) and 2.1 (IQR 1.7–2.9), respectively. The inter-rater reliability based on the intraclass correlation coefficient (ICC) between ultrasonographers for carotid duplex sonography parameters was excellent, as follows: TPN (ICC: 0.983, $p < 0.001$), IMT (ICC: 0.966, $p < 0.001$), and maximal plaque thickness (ICC: 0.892, $p = 0.001$). In case of disagreement between ultrasonographers regarding parameters of the carotid duplex sonography, any disagreement was resolved by consensus. Following the Contal and O'Quigley method, the patients were categorized into two groups according to the best cutoff values for TPN (TPN ≤ 4 vs. TPN ≥ 5). The TPN ≤ 4 group consisted of 239 (71.0%) patients, and the TPN ≥ 5 group comprised 153 (39.0%) patients. Patients in the TPN ≥ 5 group were older and more likely to have hypertension, CAOD, statin use, or anti-hypertensive drug use. In addition, the TPN ≥ 5 group had higher IMT (0.9 ± 0.2 vs. 0.8 ± 0.2, $p < 0.001$) and larger maximal plaque thickness (3.0 ± 0.9 vs. 1.7 ± 1.1, $p < 0.001$) than the TPN ≤ 4 group.

Table 1. Clinical characteristics of study patients according to the total carotid plaque number (TPN).

	TPN ≤ 4 (N = 239)	TPN ≥ 5 (N = 153)	P Value
Demographics			
Age, years	66.4 ± 10.5	73.5 ± 8.4	< 0.001
Sex, men	134 (56.1)	91 (59.5)	0.575
Initial NIHSS score	5 (2–13)	6 (2–13)	0.639
Risk factors			
Hypertension	155 (64.9)	126 (82.4)	< 0.001
Diabetes mellitus	53 (22.2)	46 (30.1)	0.102
Smoking	38 (15.9)	23 (15.0)	0.930
Hyperlipidemia	38 (15.9)	37 (24.2)	0.057
PAOD	5 (2.1)	7 (4.6)	0.275
CAOD	47 (19.7)	50 (32.7)	0.005
CHF	33 (13.8)	21 (13.7)	1.000
Laboratory findings			
Hemoglobin, g/dL	14.1 ± 2.1	13.5 ± 1.5	0.001
White blood cell, × 10^9/L	8202.7 ± 2827.0	7830.1 ± 2939.5	0.211
Platelet, × 10^9/L	225.6 ± 69.9	224.6 ± 70.0	0.885
Blood urea nitrogen, mmol/L	17.4 ± 6.3	18.8 ± 9.6	0.190
Creatinine, μmol/L	1.0 ± 0.8	1.3 ± 1.6	0.128
Total cholesterol, mmol/L	170.8 ± 35.8	167.2 ± 39.4	0.361
Triglyceride, mmol/L	96.2 ± 50.2	89.5 ± 45.3	0.184
HDL-cholesterol, mmol/L	45.0 ± 11.5	44.8 ± 11.9	0.865
LDL-cholesterol, mmol/L	106.5 ± 32.3	103.6 ± 35.7	0.399
Premorbid medication			
Antiplatelet agent	98 (41.0)	76 (49.7)	0.114
Anticoagulants	60 (25.1)	28 (18.3)	0.147
Statin	36 (15.1)	44 (28.8)	0.002
Antihypertensive agent	93 (38.9)	81 (52.9)	0.009
Carotid duplex measurement			
IMT, mm	0.8 ± 0.2	0.9 ± 0.2	< 0.001
Maximal plaque thickness, mm	1.7 ± 1.1	3.0 ± 0.9	< 0.001
Total plaque number, n	2 (1–3)	7 (5–10.5)	< 0.001

Data are shown as n (%), mean ± SD, or median (IQR). SD, standard deviation; IQR, interquartile range; NIHSS, National Institute of Health Stroke Scale; PAOD, peripheral artery occlusive disease; CAOD, coronary artery occlusive disease; CHF, congestive heart failure;; HDL, high density lipoprotein; LDL, low density lipoprotein; IMT, intimal medial thickness.

3.2. Outcome

The mean follow-up period was 2.42 ± 1.83 years. During the follow-up, a total of 113 (28.8%) MACE occurred in 60 (25.1%) patients of the TPN ≤ 4 group and in 53 (34.6%) patients of the TPN ≥ 5 group. In Kaplan–Meier analysis, the TPN ≥ 5 group showed a higher MACE rate than the TPN ≤ 4 group (log-rank test, $p < 0.001$) (Figure 2A). Multivariate Cox proportional regression analysis showed that the TPN ≥ 5 group had a significantly higher MACE rate than the TPN ≤ 4 group after adjusting for age, sex, and variables with $p < 0.1$ in univariate analysis (adjusted hazard ratio [HR], 1.50; 95% CI, 1.01–2.21; $p < 0.05$) (Table 2).

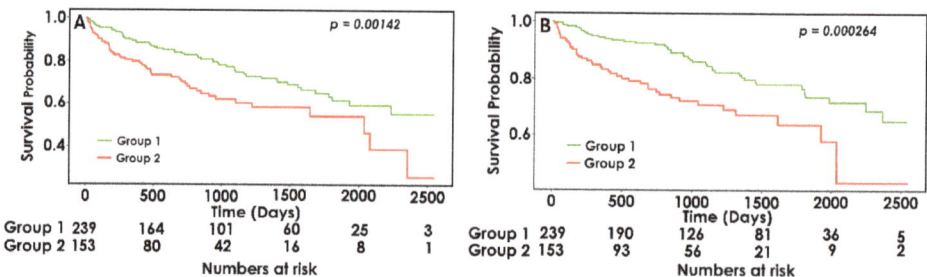

Figure 2. Kaplan–Meier analysis for (**A**) major adverse cardiovascular event (MACE); (**B**) all-cause mortality according to the total carotid plaque number (TPN).

In terms of all-cause mortality, 88 (22.4%) patients had died during the follow up period. In Kaplan–Meier curve analysis, the TPN ≥ 5 group showed a higher mortality rate than the TPN ≤ 4 group (log-rank test, $p < 0.001$) (Figure 2B). In multivariate Cox proportional regression analysis after adjusting for age, sex, and variables with $p < 0.10$ in univariate analysis, patients in the TPN ≥ 5 group showed an increased risk of all-cause mortality (adjusted HR, 2.69; 95% CI, 1.40–5.17; $p < 0.05$) compared with patients in the TPN ≤ 4 group (Table 2).

Table 2. Unadjusted and adjusted hazard ratio for MACE and all-cause mortality according to the total carotid number of plaque.

	MACE				All-Cause Mortality			
	Univariate Analysis		Multivariate Analysis		Univariate Analysis		Multivariate Analysis	
	HR (95% CI)	P Value	HR (95% CI)	P Value	HR (95% CI)	P Value	HR (95% CI)	P Value
Demographics								
Age	1.05 (1.03–1.07)	0.000	1.04 (1.01–1.06)	0.002	1.07 (1.05–1.10)	0.000	1.05 (1.02–1.08)	0.003
Sex	0.66 (0.45–0.95)	0.027	1.03 (0.67–1.59)	0.887	0.66 (0.43–1.00)	0.051	0.95 (0.49–1.84)	0.874
Initial NIHSS score	1.06 (1.03–1.08)	0.000	1.05 (1.02–1.08)	0.001	1.07 (1.04–1.00)	0.446	1.07 (1.03–1.11)	0.000
Risk factors								
Hypertension	1.32 (0.86–2.04)	0.208			1.21 (0.74–1.96)	0.446		
Diabetes mellitus	1.02 (0.66–1.56)	0.933			1.10 (0.68–1.78)	0.106		
Smoking	1.18 (0.72–1.93)	0.512			1.16 (0.66–2.02)	0.603		
PAOD	1.70 (0.69–4.18)	0.247			2.68 (1.08–6.65)	0.033	1.25 (0.36–4.41)	0.727
CAOD	1.51 (1.01–2.26)	0.046	1.14 (0.75–1.75)	0.532	1.74 (1.11–2.73)	0.016	1.18 (0.64–2.16)	0.588
CHF	1.66 (1.05–2.61)	0.029	1.22 (0.76–1.97)	0.411	2.31 (1.43–3.72)	0.001	1.72 (0.83–3.57)	0.148
Laboratory findings								
Hemoglobin	0.88 (0.80–0.95)	0.002	0.91 (0.82–1.01)	0.909	0.86 (0.79–0.94)	0.001	0.94 (0.79–1.11)	0.466
White blood cell	1.00 (1.00–1.00)	0.831			1.00 (1.00–1.00)	0.836		
Platelet	1.00 (1.00–1.00)	0.361			1.00 (0.99–1.00)	0.040	1.00 (0.99–1.00)	0.998
BUN	1.02 (0.99–1.05)	0.157			1.03 (1.01–1.06)	0.018	1.01 (0.98–1.05)	0.590
Creatinine	1.05 (0.88–1.24)	0.600			1.08 (0.91–1.28)	0.371		
Total cholesterol	1.00 (0.99–1.00)	0.089			0.99 (0.99–1.00)	0.067		
Triglyceride	1.00 (1.00–1.00)	0.929	1.00 (0.99–1.01)	0.184	1.00 (1.00–1.00)	0.974		
HDL–cholesterol	1.00 (0.98–1.01)	0.844			1.00 (0.98–1.02)	0.987		
LDL–cholesterol	0.99 (0.99–1.00)	0.071	1.00 (0.99–1.00)	0.234	0.99 (0.99–1.00)	0.051		
Premorbid medication								
Antiplatelet agent	1.03 (0.71–1.49)	0.867			1.02 (0.67–1.56)	0.916		
Anticoagulants	0.78 (0.49–1.23)	0.288			0.83 (0.50–1.40)	0.494		
Statin	1.41 (0.92–2.16)	0.117			1.28 (0.78–2.11)	0.330		
Antihypertensive agent	1.45 (0.99–2.13)	0.056			1.75 (1.13–2.70)	0.011	1.73 (0.89–3.38)	0.106
Total plaque number								
TPN ≤ 4 (reference)	1		1		1		1	
TPN ≥ 5	1.82 (1.25–2.64)	0.002	1.50 (1.01–2.21)	0.044	2.16 (1.41–3.29)	<0.001	2.69 (1.40–5.17)	0.003

MACE, major adverse cardiovascular events; HR, hazard ratio; CI, confidential interval; National Institute of Health Stroke Scale; PAOD, peripheral artery occlusive disease; CAOD, coronary artery occlusive disease; CHF, congestive heart failure; BUN, blood urea nitrogen; HDL, high density lipoprotein; LDL, low density lipoprotein; IMT, intimal medial thickness.

3.3. Prognostic Utility of Carotid Plaque Burden on Ischemic Stroke Caused by AF

During the median follow-up period, the c-indices of Heagerty's incident/dynamic AUC of each model were calculated (Table 3 and Supplementary Figure S1). The baseline model consisted of age, sex, congestive heart failure, diabetes mellitus, CAOD, and peripheral artery occlusive disease, which are the same variables of the $CHAD_2DS_2$-VASc score. The c-index for the baseline model was 0.651 (95% CI, 0.605–0.705) in MACE and 0.712 (95% CI, 0.658–0.766) in all-cause mortality. In model 5, including of all parameters of carotid plaque burden including TPN, maximal plaque thickness, and IMT improved prognostic utility that with the $CHAD_2DS_2$-VASc score alone in MACE (c-index, 0.686, 95% CI, 0.638–0.737, $p = 0.045$) and all-cause mortality (c-index, 0.734, 95% CI (0.686–0.786, $p = 0.025$).

Table 3. C-indices of Heagerty's incident/dynamic AUC for predicting MACE and all-cause mortality

	MACE			All–Cause Mortality		
	c–Index (95% CI)	Difference	P-Value	c–Index	Difference	P-Value
Model 1 *	0.651 (0.605–0.705)	Reference		0.696 (0.647–0.753)	Reference	
Model 2 †	0.661 (0.613–0.714)	0.010 (−0.005–0.033)	0.267	0.712 (0.658–0.766)	0.016 (−0.005–0.046)	0.218
Model 3 ‡	0.672 (0.626–0.726)	0.020 (0.001–0.049)	0.214	0.716 (0.670–0.769)	0.019 (0.001–0.045)	0.113
Model 4 §	0.657 (0.609–0.710)	0.006 (0–0.022)	0.317	0.701 (0.651–0.756)	0.005 (−0.001–0.021)	0.405
Model 5 ‖	0.686 (0.638–0.737)	0.034 (0.006–0.071)	0.045	0.734 (0.686–0.786)	0.038 (0.006–0.075)	0.025

AUC, area under the curve; MACE, major adverse cardiovascular events; CI, confidence interval. * Model 1: CHA_2DS_2-VASc variables (age, sex, hypertension, diabetes mellitus, congestive heart failure, coronary artery occlusive disease, peripheral artery occlusive disease) † Model 2: Model 1 plus carotid intima medial thickness; ‡ Model 3: Model 1 plus total number of plaque; § Model 4: Model 1 plus maximal thickness of plaque; ‖ Model 5: Model 1 plus carotid intima medial thickness plus maximal plaque thickness plus total number of plaque.

4. Discussion

The present study revealed that carotid plaque burden of < 50% carotid stenosis was a strong prognostic marker in patients with AF. Among the parameters of carotid plaque burden, TPN is easily counted during carotid ultrasonography examination. It showed an impact on the outcome of ischemic stroke patients with AF. Moreover, the carotid plaque burden improved the predictive value of the $CHAD_2DS_2$-VASc score in predicting cardiovascular events and mortality in ischemic stroke patients with AF.

AF is the most common cause of cardioembolic stroke. Patients with AF had markedly reduced survival compared with those without AF. In the Framingham Heart Study, the risk factor-adjusted odds ratio for death was 1.5 and 1.9 in men and women, respectively [18]. Patients with AF frequently have concomitant cerebral atherosclerosis (20–50% of cases) [19,20]. It is well known that atherosclerosis is a systemic disorder that plays an important role in the prognosis of patients with AF [4]. It can be assumed that patients with AF are more likely to have additional atherosclerotic burden and may have poor prognosis. We previously reported that patients who have both large artery atherosclerosis (>50% atherosclerotic stenosis in the relevant artery) and cardioembolism showed higher cardiovascular mortality than patients with a single cause of either large artery atherosclerosis or cardioembolism [21]. Thus, it can be inferred that concomitant carotid atherosclerosis with AF is associated with the development of cardiovascular events despite the presence of < 50% stenosis.

To date, little is known about the impact of < 50% atherosclerotic stenosis of the carotid artery on the outcome of ischemic stroke patients with AF. The presence of large artery atherosclerosis can be screened using luminography including computed tomography angiography, magnetic resonance angiography, or digital subtraction angiography. However, arterial wall changes including small plaques or increased IMT in the carotid artery cannot be detected using luminography. Carotid ultrasonography is a noninvasive imaging examination that can easily and accurately evaluate carotid plaques and IMT in the arterial lumen.

We found that the TPN ≥ 5 group had a 1.5-fold higher MACE rate than the TPN ≤ 4 group after adjustments. Moreover, considering all parameters of carotid plaque burden, including TPN, maximal plaque thickness, and IMT, contributed to the improvement of the risk stratification of ischemic stroke patients with AF over that with the $CHAD_2DS_2$-VASc risk score alone. The components of the $CHAD_2DS_2$-VASc score are clinical variables including old age, hypertension, diabetes, and vascular disease. These variables are also well-known risk factors for atherosclerosis [6]. Therefore, adding the carotid plaque burden to the model improves the risk prediction.

In line with our findings, cohort studies including non-stroke patients also reported similar results. In ARAPACIS (Atrial Fibrillation Registry for Ankle-brachial Index Prevalence Assessment: Collaborative Italian Study), a prospective nationwide observational cohort study in patients with non-valvular AF, the investigators reported that carotid plaque detection improves the predictive value of the $CHAD_2DS_2$-VASc score in patients with AF [22]. The ARIC (Atherosclerosis Risk in Communities) study investigators also reported that carotid IMT and the presence of carotid plaque are associated with an increased risk of ischemic stroke in patients with AF. The addition of carotid IMT and carotid plaque to the model provided an incremental predictive value for the risk of stroke over the $CHAD_2DS_2$-VASc score alone in adults with AF who had no prior ischemic stroke. Although we reached similar findings, a difference of the present study from the two cohort studies is that we enrolled only ischemic stroke patients with AF. Another difference is that we adopted TPN because this variable can be easily and acutely measured on routine carotid ultrasonography [10].

Currently, the method for the secondary prevention of ischemic stroke caused by AF is anticoagulation with a vitamin K antagonist or a direct oral anticoagulant (DOAC) [23]. However, vitamin K antagonists can prevent only 67% of future ischemic stroke events and DOAC did not show superiority over vitamin K antagonists [24,25]. Identification of high-risk patients for future events despite anticoagulation treatment is important. Carotid atherosclerosis and atherosclerotic burden can be easily detected using carotid duplex ultrasonography. Although TPN is less accurate and operator-dependent method than quantification measurement of carotid plaque such as total plaque area [26,27], TPN can be easily counted and may be helpful in identifying high risk patients in daily clinical practice. Our study has several limitations. First, unstable plaque morphology and hypoechoic plaque are associated with an increased risk of ischemic stroke; however, we did not analyze the characteristics of individual plaques. Nevertheless, unstable carotid plaque is known to be prevalent in advanced carotid atherosclerosis, and our study did not include patients with >50% stenosis in an intracranial or extracranial artery. Thus, the influence of the morphologic feature of carotid plaques may be little. Second, carotid duplex ultrasonography was conducted by two ultrasonographers; however, the measurement agreement between them was high. Third, potential selection bias may exist. To minimize selection bias, we recruited consecutive ischemic stroke patients with AF.

5. Conclusions

In conclusion, TPN is an important risk predictor in ischemic stroke patients with AF. In addition, considering all parameters of carotid plaque burden including TPN, maximal plaque thickness, and IMT may contribute to improving the risk prediction in ischemic stroke patients with AF, compared with the prediction with the clinical variables of $CHAD_2DS_2$-VASc score alone. These findings suggest that carotid ultrasonography may be useful in reclassifying these patients.

Supplementary Materials: The following are available online at http://www.mdpi.com/2077-0383/8/11/1897/s1, Figure S1. The c-indices of Heagerty's incident/dynamic AUC of each model (**A**) major adverse cardiovascular event (MACE); (**B**) all-cause mortality.

Author Contributions: Conceptualization, H.P. and H.S.N.; Methodology, Y.D.K., and J.Y.; Formal analysis, M.H., H.S.L., and J.K.C.; Investigation, H.P., Y.D.K., and J.Y.; Writing—original draft preparation, H.P and H.S.N.; Writing—review and editing, H.P., J.H.H., and H.S.N.; Supervision, H.P., M.H., Y.D.K., J.Y., H.S.L., J.K.C., J.H.H., and H.S.N. Read and approved the final manuscript, all authors.

Funding: This work was supported by a grant from the National Research Foundation of Korea (NRF) funded by the Korean government (MSIT) (2019R1H1A1079907); the Korea Health Technology R&D project through the Korea Health Industry Development Institute (KHIDI) funded by the Ministry of Health & Welfare, Republic of Korea (grant no. HC15C1056); and the Basic Science Research Program through the NRF funded by the Ministry of Education (NRF-2018R1A2A3074996).

Acknowledgments: We thank Junghye Choi, BS, for her efforts in data collection.

Conflicts of Interest: The authors declare no conflict of interest.

Disclosures: None.

Co-investigators: None.

References

1. Schnabel, R.B.; Yin, X.; Gona, P.; Larson, M.G.; Beiser, A.S.; McManus, D.D.; Newton-Chen, C.; Lubitz, S.A.; Magnani, J.W.; Ellinor, P.T.; et al. 50 year trends in atrial fibrillation prevalence, incidence, risk factors, and mortality in the framingham heart study: A cohort study. *Lancet* **2015**, *386*, 154–162. [CrossRef]
2. Wolf, P.A.; Mitchell, J.B.; Baker, C.S.; Kannel, W.B.; D'Agostino, R.B. Impact of atrial fibrillation on mortality, stroke, and medical costs. *Arch. Intern. Med.* **1998**, *158*, 229–234. [CrossRef]
3. Lau, D.H.; Nattel, S.; Kalman, J.M.; Sanders, P. Modifiable risk factors and atrial fibrillation. *Circulation* **2017**, *136*, 583–596. [CrossRef]
4. Bekwelem, W.; Jensen, P.N.; Norby, F.L.; Soliman, E.Z.; Agarwal, S.K.; Lip, G.Y.; Pan, W.; Folsom, A.R.; Longstreth, W.T., Jr.; Alonso, A.; et al. Carotid atherosclerosis and stroke in atrial fibrillation: The atherosclerosis risk in communities study. *Stroke* **2016**, *47*, 1643–1646. [CrossRef] [PubMed]
5. European Heart Rhythm Association; European Association for Cardio-Thoracic Surgery; Camm, A.J.; Kirchhof, P.; Lip, G.Y.; Schotten, U.; Savelieva, I.; Ernst, S.; van Gelder, I.C.; Al-Attar, N.; et al. Guidelines for the management of atrial fibrillation: The task force for the management of atrial fibrillation of the European Society of Cardiology (ESC). *Eur. Heart J.* **2010**, *31*, 2369–2429. [PubMed]
6. Cha, M.J.; Kim, Y.D.; Nam, H.S.; Kim, J.; Lee, D.H.; Heo, J.H. Stroke mechanism in patients with non-valvular atrial fibrillation according to the $CHADS_2$ and $CHAD_2DS_2$-VASc score. *Eur. J. Neurol.* **2012**, *19*, 473–479. [CrossRef]
7. Nagai, Y.; Kitagawa, K.; Sakaguchi, M.; Shimizu, Y.; Hashimoto, H.; Yamagami, H.; Narita, M.; Ohtsuki, T.; Hori, M.; Matsumoto, M. Significance of earlier carotid atherosclerosis for stroke subtypes. *Stroke* **2001**, *32*, 1780–1785. [CrossRef]
8. Steinvil, A.; Sadeh, B.; Bornstein, N.M.; Havakuk, O.; Greenberg, S.; Arbel, Y.; Konigstein, M.; Finkelstein, A.; Banai, S.; Halkin, A. Impact of carotid atherosclerosis on the risk of adverse cardiac events in patients with and without coronary disease. *Stroke* **2014**, *45*, 2311–2317. [CrossRef] [PubMed]
9. Störk, S.; van den Beld, A.W.; von Schacky, C.; Angermann, C.E.; Lamberts, S.W.; Grobbee, D.E.; Bots, M.L. Carotid artery plaque burden, stiffness, and mortality risk in elderly men: A prospective, population-based cohort study. *Circulation* **2004**, *110*, 344–348. [CrossRef] [PubMed]
10. Maeda, S.; Sawayama, Y.; Furusyo, N.; Shigematsu, M.; Hayashi, J. The association between fatal vascular events and risk factors for carotid atherosclerosis in patients on maintenance hemodialysis: Plaque number of dialytic atherosclerosis study. *Atherosclerosis* **2009**, *204*, 549–555. [CrossRef] [PubMed]
11. Lee, B.I.; Nam, H.S.; Heo, J.H.; Kim, D.I. Yonsei stroke registry. Analysis of 1,000 patients with acute cerebral infarctions. *Cerebrovasc. Dis.* **2001**, *12*, 145–151. [CrossRef] [PubMed]
12. Adams, H.P., Jr.; Bendixen, B.H.; Kappelle, L.J.; Biller, J.; Love, B.B.; Gordon, D.L.; Marsh, E.E. Classification of subtype of acute ischemic stroke. Definitions for use in a multicenter clinical trial. Toast. Trial of org 10172 in acute stroke treatment. *Stroke* **1993**, *24*, 35–41. [CrossRef] [PubMed]

13. Touboul, P.J.; Hennerici, M.G.; Meairs, S.; Adams, H.; Amarenco, P.; Bornstein, N.; Csiba, L.; Desvarieux, M.; Ebrahim, S.; Hernadez, R.H.; et al. Mannheim carotid intima-media thickness and plaque consensus (2004–2006–2011). An update on behalf of the advisory board of the 3rd, 4th and 5th watching the risk symposia, at the 13th, 15th and 20th european stroke conferences, Mannheim, Germany, 2004, Brussels, Belgium, 2006, and Hamburg, Germany, 2011. *Cerebrovasc. Dis.* **2012**, *34*, 290–296. [PubMed]
14. Contal, C.; O'Quigley, J. An application of changepoint methods in studying the effect of age on survival in breast cancer. *Comput. Stat. Data Anal.* **1999**, *30*, 253–270. [CrossRef]
15. Yoo, J.; Song, D.; Baek, J.H.; Kim, K.; Kim, J.; Song, T.J.; Lee, H.S.; Choi, D.; Kim, Y.D.; Nam, H.S.; et al. Poor long-term outcomes in stroke patients with asymptomatic coronary artery disease in heart CT. *Atherosclerosi* **2017**, *265*, 7–13. [CrossRef]
16. Heagerty, P.J.; Zheng, Y. Survival model predictive accuracy and ROC curves. *Biometrics* **2005**, *61*, 92–105. [CrossRef]
17. Uno, H.; Cai, T.; Pencina, M.J.; D'Agostino, R.B.; Wei, L. On the C-statistics for evaluating overall adequacy of risk prediction procedures with censored survival data. *Stat. Med.* **2011**, *30*, 1105–1117. [CrossRef] [PubMed]
18. Benjamin, E.J.; Wolf, P.A.; D'Agostino, R.B.; Silbershatz, H.; Kannel, W.B.; Levy, D. Impact of atrial fibrillation on the risk of death: The framingham heart study. *Circulation* **1998**, *98*, 946–952. [CrossRef] [PubMed]
19. Chang, Y.J.; Ryu, S.J.; Lin, S.K. Carotid artery stenosis in ischemic stroke patients with nonvalvular atrial fibrillation. *Cerebrovasc. Dis.* **2002**, *13*, 16–20. [CrossRef]
20. Kanter, M.C.; Tegeler, C.H.; Pearce, L.A.; Weinberger, J.; Feinberg, W.M.; Anderson, D.C.; Gomez, C.R.; Rothrock, J.F.; Helgason, C.M.; Hart, R.G.; et al. Carotid stenosis in patients with atrial fibrillation. Prevalence, risk factors, and relationship to stroke in the Stroke Prevention in Atrial Fibrillation Study. *Arch. Intern. Med.* **1994**, *154*, 1372–1377. [CrossRef] [PubMed]
21. Kim, Y.D.; Cha, M.J.; Kim, J.; Lee, D.H.; Lee, H.S.; Nam, C.M.; Nam, H.S.; Heo, J.H. Long-term mortality in patients with coexisting potential causes of ischemic stroke. *Int. J. Stroke* **2015**, *10*, 541–546. [CrossRef] [PubMed]
22. Basili, S.; Loffredo, L.; Pastori, D.; Proietti, M.; Farcomeni, A.; Vestri, A.R.; Pignatelli, P.; Daví, G.; Hiatt, W.R.; Lip, G.Y.H.; et al. Carotid plaque detection improves the predictive value of cha2ds2-vasc score in patients with non-valvular atrial fibrillation: The ARAPACIS study. *Int. J. Cardiol.* **2017**, *231*, 143–149. [CrossRef] [PubMed]
23. Kirchhof, P.; Benussi, S.; Kotecha, D.; Ahlsson, A.; Atar, D.; Casadei, B.; Castella, M.; Diener, H.-C.; Heidbuchel, H.; Hendriks, J.; et al. 2016 ESC guidelines for the management of atrial fibrillation developed in collaboration with EACTS. *Eur. Heart J.* **2016**, *37*, 2893–2962. [CrossRef] [PubMed]
24. Hart, R.G.; Pearce, L.A.; Aguilar, M.I. Meta-analysis: Antithrombotic therapy to prevent stroke in patients who have nonvalvular atrial fibrillation. *Ann. Intern. Med.* **2007**, *146*, 857–867. [CrossRef] [PubMed]
25. Lip, G.Y.; Lane, D.A. Stroke prevention in atrial fibrillation: A systematic review. *JAMA* **2015**, *313*, 1950–1962. [CrossRef]
26. Mitchel, C.; Korcarz, C.E.; Genper, A.D.; Kaufman, J.D.; Post, W.; Tracy, R.; Gassett, A.J.; Ma, N.; McClelland, R.L.; Stein, J.H. Ultrasound carotid plaque features, cardiovascular disease risk factors and events: The Multi-Ethnic Study of Atherosclerosis. *Atheroslcerosis* **2018**, *276*, 195–202. [CrossRef]
27. López-Melgar, B.; Fernández-Friera, L.; Sánchez-González, J.; Vilchez, J.P.; Cecconi, A.; Mateo, J.; Peñalvo, J.L.; Oliva, B.; García-Ruiz, J.M.; Kauffman, S.; et al. Accurate quantification of atherosclerotic plaque volume by 3D vascular ultrasound using the volumetric linear array method. *Atherosclerosis* **2016**, *248*, 230–237. [CrossRef]

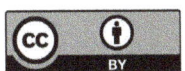

© 2019 by the authors. Licensee MDPI, Basel, Switzerland. This article is an open access article distributed under the terms and conditions of the Creative Commons Attribution (CC BY) license (http://creativecommons.org/licenses/by/4.0/).

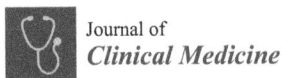

Review

Twenty Years of Cerebral Ultrasound Perfusion Imaging—Is the Best yet to Come?

Jens Eyding [1,2,*], Christian Fung [3], Wolf-Dirk Niesen [4] and Christos Krogias [5]

1. Department of Neurology, Klinikum Dortmund gGmbH, Beurhausstr 40, 44137 Dortmund, Germany
2. Department of Neurology, University Hospital Knappschaftskrankenhaus, Ruhr University Bochum, 44892 Bochum, Germany
3. Department of Neurosurgery, Universityhospital, University of Freiburg, 79106 Freiburg, Germany; christian.fung@uniklinik-freiburg.de
4. Department of Neurology, Universityhospital, University of Freiburg, 79106 Freiburg, Germany; wolf-dirk.niesen@uniklinik-freiburg.de
5. Department of Neurology, St. Josef-Hospital, Ruhr University Bochum, 44791 Bochum, Germany; christos.krogias@rub.de
* Correspondence: jens.eyding@rub.de

Received: 10 February 2020; Accepted: 10 March 2020; Published: 17 March 2020

Abstract: Over the past 20 years, ultrasonic cerebral perfusion imaging (UPI) has been introduced and validated applying different data acquisition and processing approaches. Clinical data were collected mainly in acute stroke patients. Some efforts were undertaken in order to compare different technical settings and validate results to gold standard perfusion imaging. This review illustrates the evolution of the method, explicating different technical aspects and milestones achieved over time. Up to date, advancements of ultrasound technology as well as data processing approaches enable semi-quantitative, gold standard proven identification of critically hypo-perfused tissue in acute stroke patients. The rapid distribution of CT perfusion over the past 10 years has limited the clinical need for UPI. However, the unexcelled advantage of mobile application raises reasonable expectations for future applications. Since the identification of intracerebral hematoma and large vessel occlusion can also be revealed by ultrasound exams, UPI is a supplementary multi-modal imaging technique with the potential of pre-hospital application. Some further applications are outlined to highlight the future potential of this underrated bedside method of microcirculatory perfusion assessment.

Keywords: ultrasound; acute ischemic stroke; perfusion imaging; contrast agent; intracerebral hematoma; subarachnoid hemorrhage

---

1. Introduction: Cerebral Ultrasound Perfusion Imaging (UPI), First Clinical Applications

Ultrasound imaging is a key diagnostic tool in clinical medicine. Even if an expert examiner is needed to obtain and interpret the images, it is advantageous to other diagnostic entities for various reasons, two of them being the mobile bedside character of the examination and the absence of radiation exposure. Besides gray-scale B-mode imaging for tissue characterization, vessel imaging by Doppler-based duplex-sonography is the basis in most diagnostic work-up settings. After application of specific contrast enhancing substances, improved vessel imaging and contrast-enhanced tissue imaging (CEUS) can provide sophisticated information like vascular occlusion or tissue perfusion imaging in various indications. In neurosonology, ischemic stroke and its diagnostic work up is the leading indication for ultrasound imaging questioning the vessel status of extra- and intracranial arteries. With the invention of contrast-enhanced perfusion imaging, the question of transferability to cerebral imaging quickly emerged. In 1998, the first report on the ability of tracing contrast enhancer in the cerebral microcirculation of healthy volunteers by transient harmonic imaging was published [1], followed by a case report on two acute stroke patients displaying impaired contrast increase in later infarcted areas in 1999 [2]. The technical approach was adapted from echocardiography, where size of myocardial infarct had been visualized before [3]. Various case series could reproduce the initial results by demonstrating missing signal increase in affected ischemic brain areas [4–6]. In the cerebral application, the temporal bone hampers ultrasound transmission resulting in relatively poor imaging quality. Therefore, different variations of harmonic imaging techniques and data acquisition and processing approaches have been introduced since to improve imaging quality [7–10]. Hereby, a novel approach displaying both hemispheres in one examination for isochronal comparison of normal and ischemic brain areas (bilateral or mirror approach) was introduced in 2003 [11] (compare "Data Acquisition and Processing" below for comparison of unilateral and bilateral approach). Using a bolus kinetic approach, time-based parameters such as TPI (time-to-peak intensity) could distinguish between areas of normal, impaired, and nullified parenchymal perfusion [12,13]. Figure 1 illustrates the conventional transversal insonation plane using the transtemporal bone window. Figure 2 illustrates an early unilateral examination of an acute stroke patient displaying missing contrast enhancement in later infarction, and Figure 3 an up-to-date bilateral examination of a normal person and an acute stroke patient displaying different areas of impaired perfusion. A systematical review of the literature on the method has recently summarized an overview until early 2017 [14].

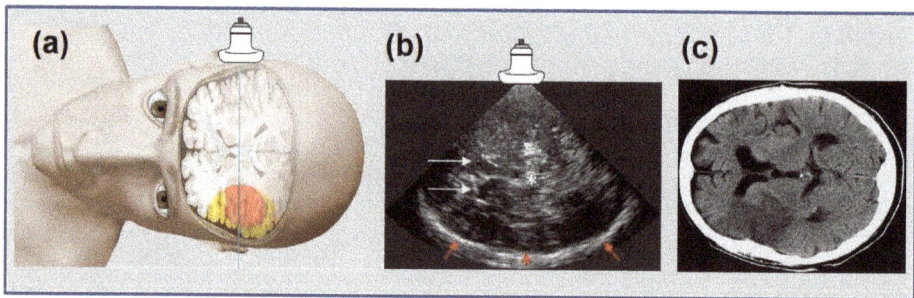

Figure 1. Schematic representation of insonation plane in transtemporal ultrasound imaging (**a**), adapted from [13] (with permission of copyright owner) with a corresponding "bilateral" B-mode image (**b**) with explanatory anatomical landmarks: white arrows = frontal horns of side ventricles; * = midline, third ventricle; red arrows = contralateral skull. Infarcted areas cannot be displayed in B-mode ultrasound. For orientation, comparison to conventional cerebral computed tomography scan, CCT, (**c**) with plane shifted by 90° accordingly, with an infarction in the hemisphere "contralateral" to the probe.

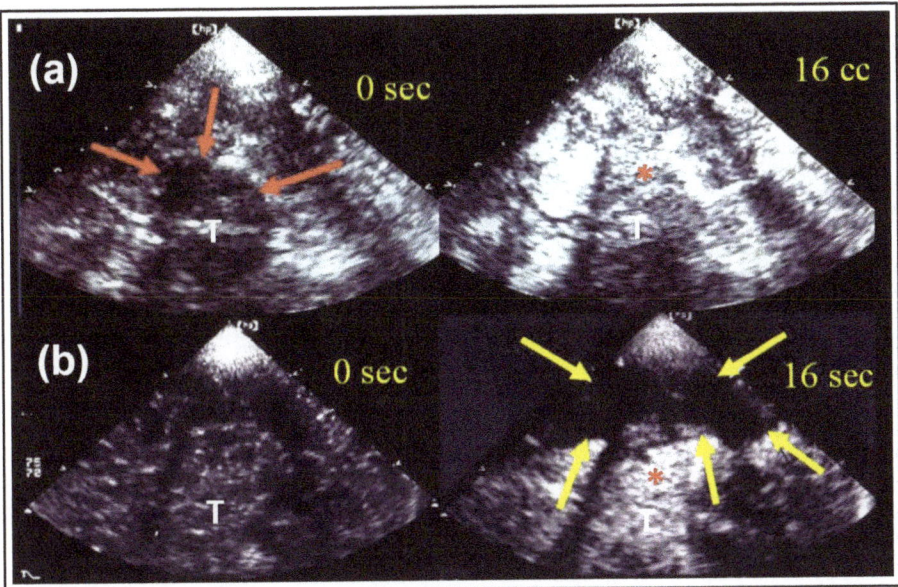

Figure 2. Ultrasound perfusion imaging in the course of time. Early "unilateral" gray-scale imaging in a healthy volunteer (**a**) and an acute stroke patient (**b**) corresponding to Figure 1: at baseline (0 s) and after contrast enhancer application at the time of maximal contrast enhancement (16 s). The thalamic region (red arrows) is marked with increase of brightness in both examples (*), whereas the regions of the lentiform nucleus and temporoparietal lobe are spared (yellow arrows), where later infarction was demonstrated in CCT follow-up. (T) indicates the third ventricle, adapted from [15] with permission from Elsevier.

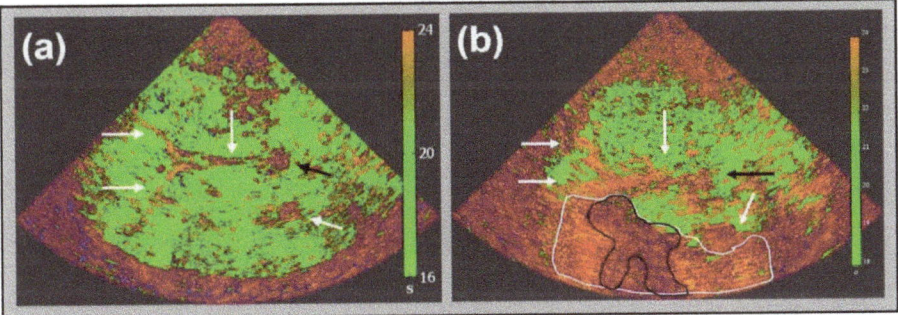

Figure 3. Up to date "bilateral" perfusion imaging corresponding to Figure 1: parametric image of time-to-peak intensity (TPI) in a healthy volunteer (**a**) with homogeneously distributed greenish parts of parenchymal structures (TPI 16 to 20 s) and the depiction of frontal and posterior horns of side ventricles as well as third ventricle (white arrows), and pineal gland (black arrow), adapted from [12]. Note the near field artifact. TPI parameter image of an acute stroke patient 2.5 h after symptom onset (**b**) of a severe stroke caused by occlusion of the M1 segment of the middle cerebral artery. Note the core of infarction (pink area, surrounded by black line) and hypo-perfused nature, and potentially salvageable area (orange area, surrounded by white line) due to collateral flow; adapted from [12] with the publisher's permission.

2. Technical Aspects

2.1. Microbubbles and Harmonic Imaging

The use of ultrasound contrast enhancers (US-CE) is a prerequisite in the application of ultrasound perfusion imaging (UPI). US-CEs consist of gaseous microbubbles (diameter ranging between 1 and 10 µm), which are stabilized by various types of shells, aiming to provide high microbubble stability with improved signal-to-noise ratio and a sufficient examination time [16]. These microbubbles show strong backscattering of beamed ultrasound pulses, not only with linear scattering, but mainly with non-linear scattering, which usually is not relevantly present in most tissues. The different composition of the US-CEs that have been used so far in UPI are displayed in Table 1.

Table 1. Ultrasound contrast enhancers having been used in brain perfusion studies (adapted from [16]).

Name	First Approved	Gas	Shell Material	Producer/Distributor
Levovist®	1993, withdrawn	Air	Galactose microparticles	Schering AG, Berlin, DE
Optison®	1998	Octafluoropropane, C_3F_8	Cross-linked serum albumin	GE healthcare, Buckinghamshire, UK
SonoVue®	2001	Sulphurhexafluoride, SF_6	Phospholipid	Bracco diagnostics, Milano, Italy

With increasing acoustic power, the microbubbles can be set into resonance vibrations, a process that results in the additional emission of harmonic frequencies—multiples of the fundamental frequency. This attribute enables various contrast harmonic imaging modes to detect the US-CE with high sensitivity and to differentiate it from the surrounding tissue. This goal is usually achieved by a band pass filter, which suppresses the fundamental frequencies.

Depending on the applied acoustic power, various interactions between the ultrasound beam and the US-CEs occur. By further increasing the ultrasound energy, the microbubbles can burst. This effect is referred to as "stimulated acoustic emission", since bursting microbubbles emit their own ultrasound, which in turn can be used for ultrasound imaging. The mechanical index (MI), originally defined to predict the onset of cavitation in fluids, gives an on-screen indication of the likelihood of microbubble destruction during examination. MI is defined as maximum value of the peak negative pressure divided by the square root of the acoustic center frequency. The threshold between a low MI and high MI is not clearly defined in cerebral imaging; however, an MI > 1.0 is needed for the destruction of the microbubbles to compensate for the ultrasound absorption of the skull [10]. Therefore, actual acoustic intensity in brain parenchyma is far less than in other organs as expected by mere MI values because of the strong absorption of the skull. Overall, data acquisition modes can be divided in "non-destructive" and "destructive" imaging modes:

2.1.1. "Non-Destructive Imaging Modes":

Conventional Harmonic Imaging

Conventional harmonic imaging is a single pulse modality based on the described stronger non-linear oscillation of US-CEs compared to the surrounding tissue. The non-linear oscillation results in harmonic frequencies (multiples of the fundamental frequency), enabling the differentiation between the signals of tissue and microbubbles by the use of band pass filters (Figure 4).

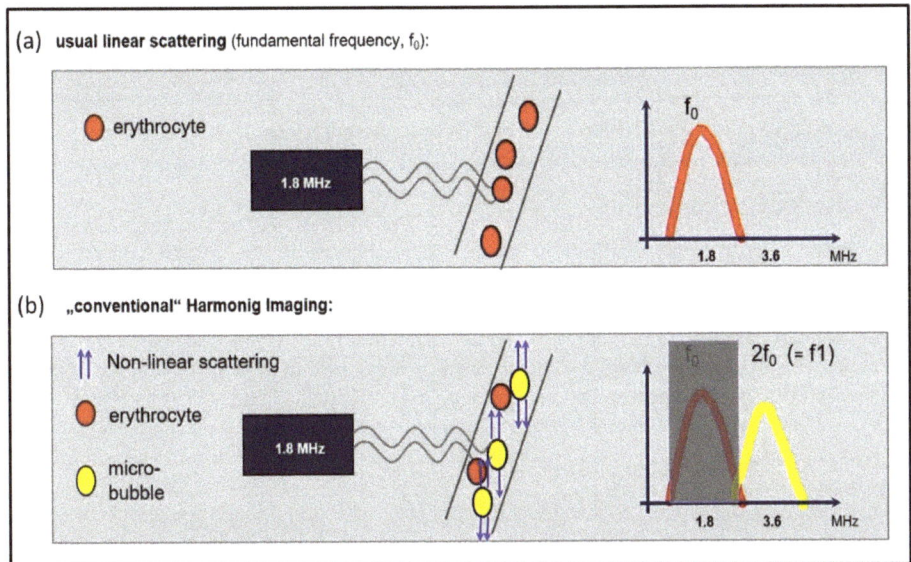

Figure 4. The basic principle of harmonic imaging. (**a**) When an ultrasound wave passes through tissue, the predominantly linear scattering of the erythrocytes results in a frequency, which is reflected back to the probe, which is equal to the transmitted frequency (here: fundamental frequency of 1.8 MHz). (**b**) "Harmonic imaging" due to non-linear scattering of the microbubbles: the resonance frequency of the microbubbles is typically a multiple of the transmitted (or fundamental) frequency. The harmonic frequencies are sent back to the probe, where they are used to create the image. Specifically, the second harmonic frequency (2f0) is used. The fundamental component is filtered out, so that that the received frequency of 3.6 MHz is two-fold higher than the transmitted frequency of 1.8 MHz.

Phase Inversion Harmonic Imaging

In phase (or pulse-) inversion harmonic imaging (PIHI), two echoes are acquired per line, resulting from a pair of mirror-inverted transmit pulses. An acoustic wave in a medium (i.e., the first transmit pulse) shows sinus-wave characteristics, so that a zone of overpressure is followed by a symmetric zone of negative pressure. In case of a linear scatterer, the summation of the two scattered and acquired echoes results in a reciprocative elimination, so that the fundamental is cancelled out. With the use of US-CEs, the non-linear oscillation changes according to the absolute pressure, so that the summation of the two echoes results in a mismatch, as the overpressure in the first echo will not be equal to the negative pressure in the second echo. This mismatch is the same for both half cycles, so that the result of the summation, in principle, is the second harmonic. Only this mismatch is visualized, so that PIHI performs the separation of the second harmonic from the fundamental [8].

Power Modulation Harmonic Imaging

Like in PIHI, power modulation harmonic imaging (PMHI) represents a further multi-pulse technique. Using multiple pulses with differences in amplitude, PMHI aims to detect the harmonic response by sending several pulses and subtracting the responses, as the linear response reduces with multi-pulsing and the harmonic response remains.

2.1.2. "Destructive Imaging modes":

Contrast Burst Imaging and Time Variance Imaging

Contrast burst imaging (CBI) and time variance imaging (TVI) are derived from Power Doppler in which pulses are broadband with high acoustic power. Power Doppler uses the Doppler shift in frequency induced by the movement of the scattering objects, displaying the amplitude of the Doppler signal, instead of displaying this frequency shift. This technique can also be combined with a harmonic bandpass filter. In this context, CBI detects the changes in the acoustic properties of microbubbles that are caused by ultrasound-induced destruction, while suppressing tissue and clutter signals by multiple echo measurements. TVI also depicts the time variant acoustic properties of microbubbles by analyzing multiple pulse echo measurements, but TVI uses a contrast-agent-specific analysis strategy to improve the suppression of noise and artifacts [9,17].

2.2. Data Acquisition and Processing

In order to detect the distribution of contrast enhancer in the micro vascular space, various approaches of data acquisition as well as data processing have been applied [14]. Data acquisition, in this context, means the kind of ultrasound application, i.e., the specific harmonic imaging technique used (see above). This can be done either with a constant setting during the examination as well as with varying, e.g., the mechanical index (MI) in the course of the examination in order to achieve specific effects on the course of received ("reflected") noise. Data processing, on the other hand, means the kind of analysis of the expected course of received noise alterations followed by specific US-CE application (either as a bolus application or as a constant infusion) according to the applied harmonic imaging regimen.

First reports were based on second harmonic imaging following a single application of US-CE (bolus kinetics) [1,2,4–7]. Depth of insonation was initially restricted to 10 cm due to technical constraints, i.e., only one hemisphere of the brain could be analyzed by the time (later called the "unilateral" approach). Received time intensity curves (TIC) were analyzed by dedicated algorithms, which derive specific parameters of wash-in and wash-out (such as time-to-peak intensity, TPI) by fitting the actual information (TIC) to the expected course defined by pre-described mathematical model functions [15] (compare Figure 5). Subsequent studies initially analyzed different harmonic imaging modes like phase inversion harmonic imaging (PIHI) [8] and also adapted "destructive" modes (applying higher MI) with the aim to increase signal-to-noise ratio (CBI and TVI) [10,17]. Due to the unilateral character of the examination, only qualitative information was extracted, i.e., perfusion could be classified as either normal or constricted. Another technical constraint of the unilateral approach is the fact that tissue close to the probe cannot be analyzed due to nearfield artifacts. Therefore, cortical areas of the brain cannot be evaluated.

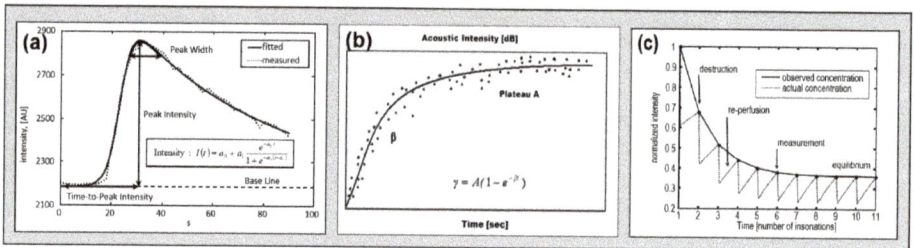

Figure 5. Theoretical course-of-time intensity curves in three different kinetic models as measured in models. Dotted lines represent measured concentration and straight lines represent course of fitted model function. (**a**) Bolus kinetic [8], (**b**) refill kinetic [18], and (**c**) depletion kinetic [15] with permission of the original publishers.

Further technical approaches intended to extract qualitative information (i.e., the degree of perfusion restriction) by applying different acquisition and processing approaches. The refill kinetics approach applied a combination of low MI and high MI imaging during a constant infusion of contrast enhancer [18]. The hypothesis was to destroy the US-CE by an ultra-quick series of high MI pulses and then to display the "refilling" of tissue perfusion by low MI imaging, which should be dependent on the state of perfusion. A given algorithm extracts specific parameters, which have been proven to represent semi-quantitative parameters in myocardial perfusion imaging. A different approach was to apply a longer series of relatively slow frequent and high MI pulses during a constant infusion of US-CE and thereby to evaluate the "depletion" of tissue perfusion, which should also be dependent on the state of perfusion (CODIM) [9]. Figure 5 displays considerations on the mathematical function describing three theoretical courses of time intensity curves of different kinetic models.

Another attempt to extract (semi-) quantitative data was introduced as the so-called bilateral approach [8]. Here, imaging depth was set to 15 cm, visualizing not only one but both hemispheres in one examination (compare Figures 2 and 3). This became possible due to improved ultrasound machines and the introduction of second generation US-CEs (Optison®, SonoVue®), improving signal-to-noise ratio. Two potential advantages were claimed. First, utilizing the so-called mirror approach, intra-individual comparison of perfusion parameters in both affected and unaffected hemispheres could facilitate semi-quantitative analyses. A prerequisite would be the depth-independence of at least one relevant parameter, which could especially be proven for the time dependent parameter, time-to-peak intensity (TPI) [11]. Second, once the affected hemisphere was on the far side of the probe, cortical areas of the affected hemisphere could also be evaluated for perfusion impairments. Since cortical areas are frequently involved in territorial infarction, this was seen as a relevant improvement.

Irrespective of data acquisition and processing modality, the evaluation of specific parameters can be performed two-fold, either by the analysis of pre-defined regions of interest (ROI) or by the presentation of parametric images, where data analysis is carried out by pixel-wise presentation according to one specific parameter (e.g., time-to-peak intensity) [8]. Both processing modalities are offered by industrial providers by now and have been tested against dedicated solutions recently [13]. Figure 6 displays both ROI-wise analysis and a parametric image in an acute stroke patient.

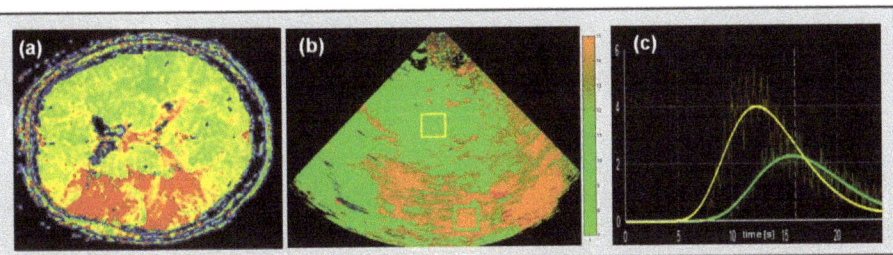

Figure 6. Perfusion MRI time-to-peak (TTP) map of an acute stroke patient with expanded penumbral perfusion delay in the territory of the middle cerebral artery (MCA) omitting basal ganglia (**a**). Ultrasonic cerebral perfusion imaging UPI parametric image with a corresponding depiction of time-to-peak intensity (TPI) delay in the MCA territory omitting basal ganglia (**b**). Exemplary depiction of ROI-wise course-of-time intensity curve in normal perfused brain tissue (yellow curve corresponding yellow box in (**c**) in basal ganglia of the unaffected hemisphere) and penumbral tissue (green curve and box) in an acute stroke patient with MCA occlusion and apparent collateral compensation.

3. Validation to Standard Imaging

Validating different UPI approaches to standard imaging has been crucial from the beginning. In the early studies, patients presenting with ischemic strokes were evaluated in a sub-acute time window up to 24–48 h after symptom onset [1,2,4–7]. Therefore, the actual target was the identification of already infarcted tissue, which was tested mainly against follow-up, non-contrast CCT. Since the focus of interest shifted toward the differentiation between ischemic and penumbral tissue, validation tools needed to become more sophisticated. However, CT (or MRI) perfusion imaging has not always been as well accessible as it is today. Hence, one approach was to define parenchymal tissue as normal, delayed-, or not-perfused in the acute UPI examination and correlate this classification to infarcted and non-infarcted tissue in follow-up CCT according to early clinical course [12]. The hypothesis was that both delayed- and not-perfused tissue of initial UPI should be infarcted in follow-up CCT once there had not been clinical improvement in the meantime. Once there had been distinctive clinical improvement, only not-perfused tissue of the initial UPI exam should be infarcted in the follow-up CCT.

As a matter of fact, especially CT perfusion imaging gained a lot of interest at that time and started its impressive road of success not just in clinical stroke medicine. Nowadays, CT perfusion imaging is widely accessible, probably being the most important factor why the significance of UPI has not further evolved. However, later UPI studies employed timely, correlated CT or MRI perfusion imaging and recently proved that the bilateral approach of high MI bolus imaging, in particular, could distinguish between unimpaired, delayed, and nullified perfusion [19]. Pre specified ROIs in both hemispheres were determined; TPI values of the unaffected hemisphere served as an intra-individual normal value. Values of the affected hemisphere yielded the perfusion status, either for specified ROIs or displayed as parameter image for the whole imaging plane. Once TPI was within ±4 s as compared with the intra-individual normal value, perfusion was unimpaired; a delay of more than 4 s indicated critically hypo-perfused tissue, and nullified rise of TIC indicated infarction. Hereby, the ability of the method to detect penumbral tissue in acute stroke was claimed.

4. Clinical Applications up to Date and Future Indications

Most of the UPI studies have been so far performed in acute stroke patients as described above. Besides contrast-enhanced imaging of cerebral vessels, UPI has already been mentioned in the EFSUMB guidelines and recommendations on the clinical practice of contrast-enhanced ultrasound (CEUS) in 2012 [20]. Studies have mainly been performed in territorial infarction due to main vessel occlusion. One study proved that infarctions as small as 2 cm in diameter can be reliably detected [21]. Case series have demonstrated detectable perfusion impairments in non-occlusive diseases as well [22,23]. In these applications, the bilateral approach utilizing a high MI setting following a bolus application of contrast enhancer seems to deliver the most robust information on the clinical questioning, focusing on vessel occlusion and penumbral imaging. Future challenges of UPI in acute stroke should focus on multicenter validation of up-to-date study results as well as the potential of mobile application. First attempts of mobile cerebral ultrasound imaging in acute stroke have focused on vessel imaging [24], but also basic perfusion imaging is challenged in one industrial project [25]. In addition to being a bedside method, UPI may also be used for serial studies in order to follow-up on brain perfusion. One indication may be early detection of successful recanalization. Serial assessment of UPI may also be used for the guidance of hemodynamic therapy to optimize cerebral perfusion with UPI as a surrogate marker. In a small study in stroke patients, improvement of cerebral perfusion detected by UPI was achieved due to systemic hemodynamic optimization [26].

However, different indications may require different technical settings. Whilst ischemic stroke remains the domain of UPI, it also has been used for identifying different acute or subacute cerebral lesions other than ischemic. There are a few studies on patients with intracranial hemorrhage (ICH) where UPI was used either to improve sonographic detectability of ICH or to describe perihemorrhagic penumbral perfusion (compare Figure 7). ICH can be detected as a hyperechogenic mass lesion within the brain parenchyma with a high sensitivity and specificity [27]. Detection and especially clear distinction of ICH from the adjacent tissue may be difficult in severe cerebral microangiopathy, in lobar hemorrhage, or in only small lesions. Comparable to CT-perfusion studies with a recess or severe hypo-perfusion of contrast media within the hemorrhagic lesion [28], UPI shows a recess of ultrasound contrast media especially within the ICH core and massive reduction of contrast media within the hemorrhagic lesion. Consecutively, ICH appears hypo-echogenic compared to the adjacent tissue, which is perfused normally as shown by the contrast agent with a clear delineation of the border of ICH from the surrounding tissue. Thus, detection of ICH volume may be improved significantly, especially in serial measurements [29]. Despite perihemorrhagic edema, the area of hypo-perfusion or non-perfusion in ICH is fairly restricted to the hemorrhagic lesion itself with no or a very narrow area of hypo-perfused tissue, e.g., perifocal penumbral perfusion. Conversely, parenchymal hemorrhagic transformation of ischemic stroke due to early spontaneous recanalization is difficult to distinguish from primary ICH on native scan but is characterized by a significantly larger perifocal penumbral zone of hypo-perfused tissue exceeding the hemorrhagic lesion by far [30]. Thus, UPI not only helps delineating the border of ICH for more valid volume measurement but also allows distinction of primary ICH from PHI.

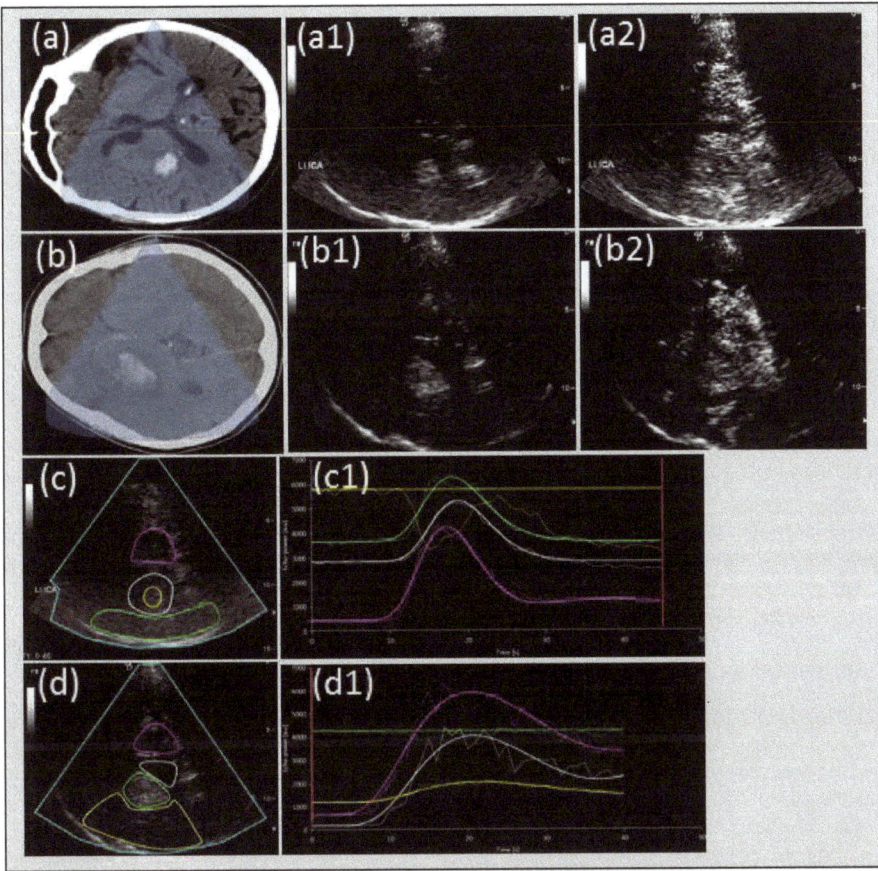

Figure 7. Perfusion imaging in intracerebral hemorrhage and hemorrhagic transformation of cerebral infarction. Cerebral CT of intracerebral hemorrhage (ICH) of the right basal ganglia, (**a**) native transcranial gray-scale sonography with hyperechogenic depiction of ICH (**a1**) and UPI with relative hypo-echogenicity of ICH compared to contrast perfusion of cerebral tissue (**a2**) due to non-perfusion constricted to the hemorrhagic lesion (**c,c1**). Cerebral CT of ICH due to hemorrhagic transformation (**b**), native transcranial gray-scale sonography with hyperechogenic depiction of hemorrhagic transformation (**b1**) and UPI with persistent hyperechogenicity of the hemorrhagic lesion due to omitted perfusion of the surrounding tissue due to acute stroke (**b2**) with slowed or missing tissue perfusion (**b2,d,d1**).

Even though bedside monitoring of cerebral perfusion in brain trauma and acute or chronic subdural hematoma is extremely interesting and theoretically may help in guiding therapy—for instance by defining a surgical need in chronic SDH by detection of cortical hypo-perfusion due to venous compromise—studies on UPI are lacking and data on brain perfusion in these patients generally are scarce. Another application of UPI currently under scientific evaluation is the setting of aneurysmal subarachnoid hemorrhage (NCT02907879). UPI is evaluated with respect to its potential to diagnose cerebral hypo-perfusion in the course of cerebral vasospasm.

Various authors have evaluated cerebral tumors and their ultrasound perfusion patterns [31–35]. UPI is not only able to increase the differentiation of normal brain tissue from brain tumors but it is also helpful to differentiate different tumor types according to their perfusion pattern [32]. Tumor tissue shows a dramatic rise of contrast enhancement and high peak intensities compared to normal brain parenchyma [32]. When comparing benign and malignant tumors, there were no significant differences in peak intensities of the time–intensity curves, yet malignant tumors showed shorter times-to-peak intensities [32]. In the eyes of the authors, UPI is a rapid, practical and cost-effective technique, especially in critically ill patients or if multiple consecutive examinations are necessary. During intraoperative application, ultrasound allows the surgeon to localize a lesion in real-time even before the opening of the dura. This facilitates the surgical access and is a useful add-on to neuronavigation [36,37]. In addition, UPI enables the surgeon to assess tumor enhancement, vascularity, and perfusion, and to control for completeness of resection [38–40]. UPI has been applied in a variety of different brain tumors, e.g., gliomas and metastases [40,41]. In a recent study, Prada et al. characterized intraoperative contrast-enhanced ultrasound images of various brain tumors [40]. They also found a high accuracy between US-based real-time neuronavigation and preoperative MRI findings. The authors concluded that contrast application is useful for the localization, definition of borders, and depiction of the vascularization and perfusion pattern of brain tumors [40]. In another study, UPI was specifically evaluated in brain space-occupying lesions and could identify specific patterns of brain perfusion [42]. It could be shown that meningeomas and glioblastomas, if no large areas of necrosis were present, showed an increased perfusion, while in tumors with necrosis the perfusion was reduced as compared to normal tissue, although in total only 15 brain tumors were evaluated. In another study, it was shown that the differentiation between tumor and normal brain tissue was superior after administration of US-CE [41]. US-CE also enabled the control of completeness of resection, yet this was dependent on technical aspects like the position of the resection cavity. UPI has the potential to become a helpful tool for the surgeon during intraoperative application, yet larger studies are needed.

5. Restrictions of the Method and Safety Considerations

Despite the proven evidence of reproducibility and robustness, especially of time-based parameters of the bolus kinetic, no widespread application of UPI modalities has yet been achieved. Partly, this may be due to some well-known limitations of the method. First, a sonolucent transtemporal bone window is needed. Up to 15%–20% of the elderly patients present with an insufficient bone window, so that UPI is not applicable. Second, patients need to be compliant, so that the transducer can be held in position for the 45–60 s of data acquisition. Especially, severely affected patients may be agitated and therefore unsuitable for the method, bearing in mind that the procedure is hand-held. Third, using the bolus kinetic approach only one two-dimensional imaging plane can be evaluated per bolus application. Therefore, quantification is restricted to an investigation plane that has to be chosen beforehand. However, future development of three-dimensional insonation systems may overcome these limitations. Fourth, quantification is yet only semi-quantitative, i.e., no absolute values can be determined. However, quantification (in acute stroke) as described above utilizes the mirror approach, which is also common in CT and MRI perfusion imaging. In addition, quantification has only been proven for one parameter (TPI). Other parameters have to be challenged in future studies. Regarding safety of UPI, there have been apprehensions of side effects of both US-CE and administration of ultrasound pulses on brain integrity. These have mainly been triggered by results of studies applying long-lasting, whole brain, low-frequency insonation in the setting of ultrasound-enhanced thrombolysis, resulting in massive hemorrhage and blood–brain barrier disruption [43,44]. However, applying standard settings of transcranial insonation, UPI is regarded safe with no evidence of blood–brain barrier affection [45,46].

6. Conclusions

Cerebral ultrasound perfusion imaging has the potential to serve as a supplementary tool to conventional diagnostics in various clinical questionings. As long as temporal bone window is present, a multi-modal approach of vascular imaging for the detection of vessel occlusion, microvascular perfusion impairment or intracerebral hemorrhage is covered by the method. In addition, conventional contrast-enhanced imaging omitting the quantification of perfusion may serve as an extension of diagnostic properties. The unique feature of mobility facilitates application at the bedside. This could enable pre-hospital diagnostics, but also easy-to-apply follow-up diagnostics in the intensive care unit or stroke unit as well as in the operating room. Future developments should focus on multi-center studies to validate the findings described in this manuscript and the development of automated algorithms for examiner independence.

Author Contributions: Conceptualization, J.E., C.F., W.-D.N., and C.K.; methodology, J.E., C.F., W.-D.N., and C.K.; writing—original draft preparation, J.E., C.F., W.-D.N., and C.K.; writing—review and editing, J.E., C.F., W.-D.N., and C.K. All authors have read and agree to the published version of the manuscript.

Funding: This research received no external funding. The APC was funded by the DFG Open Access Publication Funds of the Ruhr-University Bochum.

Conflicts of Interest: The authors declare no conflict of interest.

References

1. Postert, T.; Muhs, A.; Meves, S.; Federlein, J.; Przuntek, H.; Büttner, T. Transient response harmonic imaging: An ultrasound technique related to brain perfusion. *Stroke* **1998**, *29*, 1901–1907. [CrossRef] [PubMed]
2. Postert, T.; Federlein, J.; Weber, S.; Przuntek, H.; Büttner, T. Second harmonic imaging in acute middle cerebral artery infarction: Preliminary results. *Stroke* **1999**, *30*, 1702–1706. [CrossRef]
3. Firschke, C.; Lindner, J.R.; Wie, K.; Goodman, N.C.; Skyba, D.M.; Kaul, S. Myocardial perfusion imaging in the setting of coronary artery stenosis and acute myocardial infarction using venous injection of a second generation echocardiographic contrast agent. *Circulation* **1997**, *96*, 959–967. [PubMed]
4. Federlein, J.; Postert, T.; Meves, S.; Weber, S.; Przuntek, H.; Büttner, T. Ultrasonic evaluation of pathological brain perfusion in acute stroke using second harmonic imaging. *J. Neurol. Neurosurg. Psychiatry* **2000**, *69*, 616–622. [CrossRef]
5. Wiesmann, M.; Meyer, K.; Albers, T.; Seidel, G. Parametric imaging with contrast-enhanced ultrasound in acute ischemic stroke. *Stroke* **2004**, *35*, 508–513. [CrossRef] [PubMed]
6. Seidel, G.; Meyer-Wiethe, K.; Berdien, G.; Hollstein, D.; Toth, D.; Aach, T. Ultrasound perfusion imaging in acute middle cerebral artery infarction predicts outcome. *Stroke* **2004**, *35*, 1107–1111. [CrossRef]
7. Postert, T.; Hoppe, P.; Federlein, J.; Helbeck, S.; Ermert, H.; Przuntek, H.; Büttner, T.; Wilkening, W. Contrast agent specific imaging modes for the ultrasonic assessment of parenchymal cerebral echo contrast enhancement. *J. Cereb. Blood Flow. Metab.* **2000**, *20*, 1709–1716. [CrossRef]
8. Eyding, J.; Krogias, C.; Wilkening, W.; Meves, S.; Ermert, H.; Postert, T. Parameters of cerebral perfusion in phase inversion harmonic imaging (PIHI) ultrasound examinations. *Ultrasound. Med. Biol.* **2003**, *29*, 1379–1385. [CrossRef]
9. Eyding, J.; Wilkening, W.; Reckhardt, M.; Schmid, G.; Meves, S.; Ermert, H.; Przuntek, H.; Postert, T. Contrast Burst Depletion Imaging (CODIM): A new imaging procedure and analysis method for semi-quantitative ultrasonic perfusion imaging. *Stroke* **2003**, *34*, 77–83. [CrossRef]
10. Kern, R.; Perren, F.; Schoeneberger, K.; Gass, A.; Hennerici, M.; Meairs, S. Ultrasound microbubble destruction imaging in acute middle cerebral artey stroke. *Stroke* **2004**, *35*, 1665–1670. [CrossRef]
11. Krogias, C.; Postert, T.; Wilkening, W.; Meves, S.; Przuntek, H.; Eyding, J. Semiquantitative analysis of ultrasonic cerebral perfusion imaging. *Ultrasound Med. Biol.* **2005**, *31*, 1007–1012. [CrossRef] [PubMed]
12. Eyding, J.; Schöllhammer, M.; Eyding, D.; Wilkening, W.; Meves, S.; Schröder, A.; Przuntek, H.; Krogias, C.; Postert, T. Contrast-enhanced ultrasonic parametric perfusion imaging detects tissue at risk in acute stroke. *J. Cereb. Blood Flow. Metab.* **2006**, *26*, 576–582. [CrossRef] [PubMed]

13. Reitmeir, R.; Eyding, J.; Oertel, M.F.; Wiest, R.; Gralla, J.; Fischer, U.; Giquel, P.Y.; Weber, S.; Raabe, A.; Mattle, H.P.; et al. Is ultrasound perfusion imaging capable of detecting mismatch? A proof of-concept study in acute stroke patients. *J. Cereb. Blood Flow. Metab.* **2017**, *37*, 1517–1526. [CrossRef] [PubMed]
14. Vinke, E.J.; Kortenbout, J.; Eyding, J.; Slump, C.H.; van der Hoeven, J.G.; de Korte, C.L.; Hoedemaekers, C.W.E. Potential of contrast enhanced ultrasound as a bedside monitoring technique of cerebral perfusion: A systematic review. *Ultrasound Med. Biol.* **2017**, *43*, 2751–2757. [CrossRef]
15. Eyding, J.; Wilkening, W.; Postert, T. Brain perfusion and ultrasonic imaging techniques. *Eur. J. Ultrasound.* **2002**, *16*, 91–104. [CrossRef]
16. Paefgen, V.; Doleschel, D.; Kiessling, F. Evolution of contrast agents for ultrasound imaging and ultrasound-mediated drug delivery. *Front. Pharmacol.* **2015**, *6*, 197. [CrossRef]
17. Meves, S.H.; Wilkening, W.; Thies, T.; Eyding, J.; Holscher, T.; Finger, M.; Schmid, G.; Ermert, H.; Postert, T. Ruhr Center of Competence for Medical Engineering. Comparison between echo contrast agent specific imaging modes and perfusion-weighted magnetic resonance imaging for the assessment of brain perfusion. *Stroke* **2002**, *33*, 2433–2437. [CrossRef]
18. Kern, R.; Diels, A.; Pettenpohl, J.; Kablau, M.; Brade, J.; Hennerici, M.G.; Meairs, S. Real-time ultrasound brain perfusion imaging with analysis of microbubble replenishment in acute MCAstroke. *J. Cereb. Blood Flow. Metab.* **2011**, *31*, 1716–1724. [CrossRef]
19. Eyding, J.; Reitmair, R.; Oertel, M.; Fischer, U.; Wiest, R.; Gralla, J.; Raabe, A.; Zubak, I.; Z'Graggen, W.; Beck, J. Ultrasonic quantification of cerebral perfusion in acute arterial occlusive stroke-a comparative challenge of the refill- and the bolus-kinetics approach. *PLoS ONE* **2019**, *14*, e0220171. [CrossRef]
20. Piscaglia, F.; Nolsøe, C.; Dietrich, C.F.; Cosgrove, D.O.; Gilja, O.H.; Bachmann Nielsen, M.; Albrecht, T.; Barozzi, L.; Bertolotto, M.; Catalano, O.; et al. The EFSUMB Guidelines and Recommendations on the Clinical Practice of Contrast Enhanced Ultrasound (CEUS). Update 2011 on non-hepatic applications. *Ultraschall Med.* **2012**, *33*, 33–59. [CrossRef]
21. Nolte, C.H.; Gruss, J.; Steinbrink, J.; Jungehulsing, G.J.; Brunecker, P.; Hopt, A.M.; Schreiber, S.J. Ultrasound Perfusion Imaging of Small Stroke Involving the Thalamus. *Ultraschall Med.* **2008**, *29*, 1–5. [CrossRef] [PubMed]
22. Krogias, C.; Henneböhl, C.; Geier, B.; Hansen, C.; Hummel, T.; Meves, S.H.; Lukas, C.; Eyding, J. Transcranial ultrasound perfusion imaging and perfusion-MRI–a pilot study on the evaluation of cerebral perfusion in severe carotid artery stenosis. *Ultrasound Med. Biol.* **2010**, *36*, 1973–1980. [CrossRef] [PubMed]
23. Krogias, C.; Meves, S.H.; Hansen, C.; Mönnings, P.; Eyding, J. Ultrasound Perfusion Imaging of the brain–Routine and novel applications. Uncommon cases and review of the literature. *J. Neuroimaging* **2011**, *21*, 255–258. [CrossRef]
24. Herzberg, M.; Boy, S.; Hölscher, T.; Ertl, M.; Zimmermann, M.; Ittner, K.P.; Pemmerl, J.; Pels, H.; Bogdahn, U.; Schlachetzki, F. Prehospital stroke diagnostics based on neurological examination and transcranial ultrasound. *Crit. Ultrasound. J.* **2014**, *6*, 3. [CrossRef]
25. Lima, F.O.; Mont'Alverne, F.J.A.; Bandeira, D.; Nogueira, R.G. Pre-hospital assessment of large vessel occlusion strokes: Implications for modeling and planning stroke systems of care. *Front. Neurol.* **2019**, *10*, 955. [CrossRef] [PubMed]
26. Fuhrer, H.; Reinhard, M.; Niesen, W.D. Paradigm change? Cardiac output better associates with cerebral perfusion than blood pressure in ischemic stroke. *Front. Neurol.* **2017**, *8*, 706. [CrossRef]
27. Seidel, G.; Kaps, M.; Dorndorf, W. Transcranial color-coded duplex sonography of intracerebral hematomas in adults. *Stroke* **1993**, *24*, 1519–1527. [CrossRef]
28. Fainardi, E.; Borrelli, M.; Saletti, A.; Schivalocchi, R.; Azzini, C.; Cavallo, M.; Ceruti, S.; Tamarozzi, R.; Chieregato, A. CT perfusion mapping of hemodynamic disturbances associated to acute spontaneous intracerebral hemorrhage. *Neuroradiology* **2008**, *50*, 729–740. [CrossRef]
29. Kern, R.; Kablau, M.; Sallustio, F.; Fatar, M.; Stroick, M.; Hennerici, M.G.; Meairs, S. Improved detection of intracerebral hemorrhage with transcranial ultrasound perfusion imaging. *Cerebrovasc. Dis.* **2008**, *26*, 277–283. [CrossRef]
30. Niesen, W.; Schläger, A.; Reinhard, M.; Fuhrer, H. Transcranial sonography to differentiate primary intracerebral hemorrhage from cerebral infarction with hemorrhagic transformation. *J. Neuroimaging* **2018**, *28*, 370–373. [CrossRef]

31. Harrer, J.U.; Hornen, S.; Oertel, M.F.; Stracke, C.P.; Klötzsch, C. Comparison of perfusion harmonic imaging and perfusion mr imaging for the assessment of microvascular characteristics in brain tumors. *Ultraschall. Med.* **2008**, *29*, 45–52. [CrossRef] [PubMed]
32. Harrer, J.U.; Mayfrank, L.; Mull, M.; Klötzsch, C. Second harmonic imaging: A new ultrasound technique to assess human brain tumour perfusion. *J. Neurol. Neurosurg. Psychiatry* **2003**, *74*, 333–338. [CrossRef]
33. Harrer, J.U.; Möller-Hartmann, W.; Oertel, M.F.; Klötzsch, C. Perfusion imaging of high-grade gliomas: A comparison between contrast harmonic and magnetic resonance imaging. Technical note. *J. Neurosurg.* **2004**, *101*, 700–703. [CrossRef] [PubMed]
34. Wu, D.F.; He, W.; Lin, S.; Han, B.; Zee, C.S. Using Real-Time Fusion Imaging Constructed from Contrast-Enhanced Ultrasonography and Magnetic Resonance Imaging for High-Grade Glioma in Neurosurgery. *World Neurosurg.* **2019**, *125*, e98–e109. [CrossRef] [PubMed]
35. Della Pepa, G.M.; Ius, T.; Menna, G.; La Rocca, G.; Battistella, C.; Rapisarda, A.; Mazzucchi, E.; Pignotti, F.; Alexandre, A.; Marchese, E.; et al. "Dark corridors" in 5-ALA resection of high-grade gliomas: Combining fluorescence-guided surgery and contrast-enhanced ultrasonography to better explore the surgical field. *J. Neurosurg. Sci.* **2019**, *63*, 688–696. [CrossRef]
36. Nagelhus Hernes, T.A.; Lindseth, F.; Selbekk, T.; Wollf, A.; Solberg, O.V.; Harg, E.; Rygh, O.M.; Tangen, G.A.; Rasmussen, I.; Augdal, S.; et al. Computer-assisted 3D ultrasound-guided neurosurgery: Technological contributions, including multimodal registration and advanced display, demonstrating future perspectives. *Int. J. Med. Robot* **2006**, *2*, 45–59. [CrossRef] [PubMed]
37. Rasmussen, I.A., Jr.; Lindseth, F.; Rygh, O.M.; Berntsen, E.M.; Selbekk, T.; Xu, J.; Nagelhus Hernes, T.A.; Harg, E.; Håberg, A.; Unsgaard, G. Functional neuronavigation combined with intra-operative 3D ultrasound: Initial experiences during surgical resections close to eloquent brain areas and future directions in automatic brain shift compensation of preoperative data. *Acta Neurochir. (Wien)* **2007**, *149*, 365–378. [CrossRef]
38. Lassau, N.; Chami, L.; Chebil, M.; Benatsou, B.; Bidault, S.; Girard, E.; Abboud, G.; Roche, A. Dynamic contrast-enhanced ultrasonography (DCE-US) and anti-angiogenic treatments. *Discov. Med.* **2011**, *11*, 18–24.
39. Solbiati, L.; Ierace, T.; Tonolini, M.; Cova, L. Guidance and monitoring of radiofrequency liver tumor ablation with contrast-enhanced ultrasound. *Eur. J. Radiol.* **2004**, *51*, S19–S23. [CrossRef]
40. Prada, F.; Perin, A.; Martegani, A.; Aiani, L.; Solbiati, L.; Lamperti, M.; Casali, C.; Legnani, F.; Mattei, L.; Saladino, A.; et al. Intraoperative contrast-enhanced ultrasound for brain tumor surgery. *Neurosurgery* **2014**, *74*, 542–552. [CrossRef]
41. Engelhardt, M.; Hansen, C.; Eyding, J.; Wilkening, W.; Brenke, C.; Krogias, C.; Scholz, M.; Harders, A.; Ermert, H.; Schmieder, K. Feasibility of contrast-enhanced sonography during resection of cerebral tumours: Initial results of a prospective study. *Ultrasound. Med. Biol.* **2007**, *33*, 571–575. [CrossRef] [PubMed]
42. Vicenzini, E.; Delfini, R.; Magri, F.; Puccinelli, F.; Altieri, M.; Santoro, A.; Giannoni, M.F.; Bozzao, L.; Di Piero, V.; Lenzi, G.L. Semiquantitative human cerebral perfusion assessment with ultrasound in brain space-occupying lesions: Preliminary data. *J. Ultrasound. Med.* **2008**, *27*, 685–692. [CrossRef] [PubMed]
43. Daffertshofer, M.; Gass, A.; Ringleb, P.; Sitzer, M.; Sliwka, U.; Els, T.; Sedlaczek, O.; Koroshetz, W.J.; Hennerici, M.G. Transcranial lowfrequency ultrasound-mediated thrombolysis in brain ischemia: Increased risk of hemorrhage with combined ultrasound and tissue plasminogen activator: Results of a phase II clinical trial. *Stroke* **2005**, *36*, 1441–1446. [CrossRef] [PubMed]
44. Reinhard, M.; Hetzel, A.; Kruger, S.; Kretzer, S.; Talazko, J.; Ziyeh, S.; Weber, J.; Els, T. Blood-brain barrier disruption by low-frequency ultrasound. *Stroke* **2006**, *37*, 1546–1548. [CrossRef]
45. Jungehulsing, G.J.; Brunecker, P.; Nolte, C.H.; Fiebach, J.B.; Kunze, C.; Doepp, F.; Villringer, A.; Schreiber, S.J. Diagnostic transcranial ultrasound perfusion-imaging at 2.5 MHz does not affect the blood–brain barrier. *Ultrasound Med. Biol.* **2008**, *34*, 147–150. [CrossRef]
46. Harrer, J.U.; Eyding, J.; Ritter, M.; Schminke, U.; Schulte-Altedorneburg, G.; Köhrmann, M.; Nedelmann, M.; Schlachetzki, F. The potential of neurosonography in neurological emergency and intensive care medicine: Basic principles, vascular stroke diagnostics, and monitoring of stroke-specific therapy-part 1. *Ultraschall. Med.* **2012**, *33*, 218–235.

© 2020 by the authors. Licensee MDPI, Basel, Switzerland. This article is an open access article distributed under the terms and conditions of the Creative Commons Attribution (CC BY) license (http://creativecommons.org/licenses/by/4.0/).

MDPI
St. Alban-Anlage 66
4052 Basel
Switzerland
Tel. +41 61 683 77 34
Fax +41 61 302 89 18
www.mdpi.com

Journal of Clinical Medicine Editorial Office
E-mail: jcm@mdpi.com
www.mdpi.com/journal/jcm

www.ingramcontent.com/pod-product-compliance
Lightning Source LLC
LaVergne TN
LVHW070654100526
838202LV00013B/965